Microscopic and Endoscopic Surgery with the CO_2 Laser

Albert H. Andrews, Jr.
Editor

Thomas G. Polanyi
Associate Editor

John Wright • PSG Inc
Boston Bristol London
1982

Library of Congress Cataloging in Publication Data

Main entry under title:

Microscopic and endoscopic surgery with the CO_2 laser.

Bibliography: p.
Includes index.
1. Microsurgery. 2. Lasers in surgery.
3. Endoscope and endoscopy. I. Andrews, Albert Henry, 1907–
II. Polanyi, Thomas G.
[DNLM: 1. Lasers—Therapeutic use. 2. Microsurgery—Methods.
WO 512 M6245]
RD33.6.M46 617′.05 81-15989
ISBN 0-7236-7009-9 AACR2

Published by:
John Wright • PSG Inc, 545 Great Road, Littleton,
Massachusetts 01460, U.S.A.
John Wright & Sons Ltd, 42-44 Triangle West,
Bristol BS8 1EX, England

Printed in Great Britain by
John Wright & Sons (Printing) Ltd. at The Stonebridge Press, Bristol.

International Standard Book Number: 0-7236-7009-9

Library of Congress Catalog Card Number: 81-15989

This book is dedicated to the physicists, engineers, technicians, administrators, nurses, and physicians whose interest and cooperation have made possible the development and application of the CO_2 laser for microsurgery and endoscopic surgery.

PREFACE

The CO_2 laser, a relatively new addition to surgical instrumentation, has been used in clinical surgery for almost ten years. Up to this time, its most widespread use has been with microsurgery and endoscopic surgery, therefore this book will confine itself principally to these two topics.

The introduction presents the information on which the clinical uses are based. Otolaryngology was the first specialty to accept this new modality and gynecology was next, and the sections on these two specialties are the most extensive and have the most contributors.

Out intent in this book is to present the use of the CO_2 laser in clinical and experimental surgery. In so doing, an understanding of the generation of the laser beam, and its properties, hazards, safety procedures, and of tissue responses to electromagnetic radiation are essential. The specific uses in the different surgical fields are presented following a discussion of these topics and of other technical details related to the application of lasers in surgery. We hope we have supplied a manual of value to the newcomer and a reference for the experienced surgeon.

The principal objective of this book, however, is to present information to assist the clinician in determining the appropriateness of the CO_2 laser for an individual patient or for clinic or hospital use. The advantages and disadvantages of surgery with CO_2 lasers provide a basis for such a decision. The advantages are summarized as follows:

- The beam may be used to incise or to destroy tissue, and precise control of the area and the depth of destruction is assured by visualization—most frequently with an operating microscope.
- Bleeding is reduced or absent, which improves visualization, reduces trauma from blood control procedures, and minimizes bleeding in blood coagulopathies.
- Blood vessels are sealed when the blood flow is stopped.
- Spot size is generally 2 mm or less in diameter depending on the laser, the focus, and the delivery device.
- The area of destruction is sharply limited and the zone of devitalized and affected tissue is narrow.
- Application to regions of difficult access is benefited.
- The method is usable in neoplastic disease.
- Postoperative complications are fewer than after conventional surgery.
- Postoperative pain is low.
- Healing is rapid.
- Scar formation is minimal.
- Hospitalization time is reduced.

The disadvantages to the CO_2 laser are summarized as follows:

- Fire hazards must be understood and the safety procedures rigidly followed, especially in procedures about head, neck, and airways, and in cooperation with the anesthesiologists.
- Training, experience, and surgical skill are prerequisites to successful use.
- The CO_2 laser should be used only when there are clear cut advantages over conventional procedures.
- Healing of skin is generally slower than after scalpel incision.
- Blood flowing from a vessel larger than about 0.5 mm prevents sealing.
- Oxidized solids, ie, char, impedes beam absorption by underlying tissue and increases tissue reaction.
- The cost of the equipment is appreciable; however, if the cost is amortized over several years, the cost is reduced. The total cost is further lessened by decreased length of hospital stay and increased speed of recovery.

The term *laser* is the acronym of "light amplification by stimulated emission of radiation." Different grammatical forms based on the term laser have come into use. In this book the word laser is used as both a noun and adjective, *to lase* is used as the infinitive (instead of *to laser*), *lased* is used for the past tense, past participle, and passive voice (instead of *lasered*), and *lasing* is used as the participle (instead of *lasering*). It is hoped that purists in language will forgive these shortcuts and recognize the affectation associated with the use of laser as the stem word.

The senior contributors were invited by the editors and the associate contributors by the senior contributors. Doctors Goldman and McBurney were invited to collaborate on dermatology. The selection of the contributors was based on their knowledge, experience, authorship of publications, and contributions to surgery with the CO_2 laser.

We express our appreciation to the contributors for their cooperation and excellence of their contributions and, above all else, their willingness to share their expertise.

ACKNOWLEDGMENTS

We gratefully acknowledge the valuable assistance and support of Edward L. Applebaum, MD, Professor and Head of the Department of Otolaryngology, Abraham Lincoln School of Medicine, University of Illinois, and for making available the facilities of the Department; the editorial assistance of Jane Lantz; and the secretarial services of Frances Dimas, Ramona Sandoval and Julius Union and especially Angelina Rodriguez who did much of the typing for the Editor.

CONTRIBUTORS

Albert H. Andrews, Jr., MS, MD
Professor of Bronchoesophagology Emeritus
The Abraham Lincoln School of Medicine
University of Illinois
Consultant in Surgery (Otolaryngology)
Ravenswood Hospital
Professor of Otolaryngology and Bronchoesophagology
Rush Medical College
Rush-Presbyterian-St. Luke's Hospital Medical Center
President, Midwest Biolaser Institute
Chicago, Illinois

Peter W. Ascher, MD
Neurochirurgische Universitätsaklinik
Graz
Austria

Michael S. Baggish, MD
Chairman, Department Obstetrics and Gynecology
Mt. Sinai Hospital
Professor of Obstetrics and Gynecology and Professor of Pathology
University of Connecticut School of Medicine
Hartford, Connecticut

Howard M. Baim, MD
Instructor in Otolaryngology
Abraham Lincoln School of Medicine
University of Illinois
Courtesy Staff, Ravenswood Hospital
Chicago, Illinois

Hugh Beckman, MD
Chairman, Department of Ophthalmology
Sinai Hospital of Detroit
Detroit, Michigan

Joseph H. Bellina, MD, PhD, FACOG
Clinical Professor
Louisiana State University
Department of Obstetrics and Gynecology
Director, Laser Research Foundation
New Orleans, Louisiana

James H. Dorsey, MD, FACOG
Head, Division of Gynecologic Oncology
Greater Baltimore Medical Center
Assistant Professor
Gynecology and Obstetrics
The Johns Hopkins School of Medicine
Baltimore, Maryland

I. Farine, MD
Chaim Sheba Medical Center
Tel Hashomer Hospital
Part of Tel Aviv University
Sackler Medical School
Tel Hashomer
Israel

Ronald J. French, MD
Assistant Clinical Professor of Otolaryngology
Tulane University School of Medicine
Active Staff, Touro Infirmary
Active Staff, Eye, Ear, Nose and Throat Infirmary
Chief of Otolaryngology
East Jefferson General Hospital
New Orleans, Louisiana

Terry A. Fuller, PhD
Chief, Laser Surgery Laboratories
Sinai Hospital of Detroit
Detroit, Michigan

Leon Goldman, MD
Professor Emeritus
Department of Dermatology
Director of Laser Laboratory
University of Cincinnati
Medical Center
Director, Laser Treatment Center
Jewish Hospital
Cincinnati, Ohio

R.R. Hall, MS, FRCS
Senior Lecturer in Urological Surgery
University of Newcastle Upon Tyne
Consultant Urologist
Freeman Hospital
Newcastle Upon Tyne
England

Gerald B. Healy, MD
Associate Professor of Otolaryngology
Boston University School of Medicine
and Harvard Medical School
Otolaryngologist-in-Chief
The Children's Hospital
Medical Center
Boston, Massachusetts

M. Heim, MD
Chaim Sheba Medical Center
Tel Hashomer Medical Hospital
Part of Tel Aviv University
Sackler Medical School
Tel Hashomer
Israel

H. Horoszowski, MD
Chaim Sheba Medical Center
Tel Hashomer Hospital
Part of Tel Aviv University
Sackler Medical School
Tel Hashomer
Israel

Geza J. Jako, MD
Professor of Otolaryngology
Boston University School of
Medicine
Boston, Massachusetts

Rocco V. Lobraico, MD, FACS,
FACOG
Clinical Professor
Obstetrics and Gynecology
The Abraham Lincoln School of
Medicine
University of Illinois
Chairman, Department of Obstetrics
and Gynecology
Chief, Laser Section of Surgery
Ravenswood Hospital Medical Center
Chicago, Illinois

Elizabeth I. McBurney, MD
Clinical Assistant Professor
of Dermatology
Tulane University School of Medicine
Clinical Associate Professor
of Dermatology
Louisiana State University
Head, Department of Dermatology
Howard Clinic
Slidell, Louisiana

Martin L. Norton, MD, JD
Director of Anesthesia
St. Luke's Hospital
Lecturer in Law
(Health Law Institute)
Cleveland-Marshall College of Law
Cleveland State University
(Formerly Professor of
Anesthesiology, Boston University
School of Medicine)
Cleveland, Ohio

J. Oldhoff, MD
Division of Oncology
Department of Surgery
University Hospital
Groningen
The Netherlands

J. Wolter Oosterhuis, MD
Assistant Professor of Surgical
Pathology
Department of Pathology
University of Groningen
Groningen
The Netherlands

Thomas G. Polanyi, PhD
Director of Research and Development
Merrimack Laboratories, Inc.
Hudson, Massachusetts

Stanley M. Shapshay, MD
Assistant Professor of Otolaryngology
Boston University School of Medicine
Assistant Surgeon
Boston University Medical Center
Assistant Visiting Surgeon
Boston City Hospital
Assistant Otolaryngologist
Children's Hospital Medical Center
Boston, Massachusetts

George T. Simpson, MD
Director of Otolaryngology and
Visiting Surgeon
Boston City Hospital
Assistant Professor and Surgeon
Boston University Medical Center
Assistant Otolaryngologist
Veterans Administration Hospital
Chief Otolaryngologist
Massachusetts Institute of Technology
Cambridge, Massachusetts
Assistant Otolaryngologist
Children's Hospital Medical Center
Boston, Massachusetts

Steven F. Soltes, MD
Instructor in Otolaryngology
The Abraham Lincoln School of
Medicine
University of Illinois
Chicago, Illinois

M. Stuart Strong, MD
Chief of Otolaryngology
University Hospital
Professor of Otolaryngology
Boston University School of Medicine
Boston, Massachusetts

William M. Strouse, MS (Physics)
Consultant
Great Pasture Road
West Redding, Connecticut

Charles W. Vaughan, MD
Chief of Otolaryngology
Veterans Administration
Medical Center
Associate Professor of
Otolaryngology
Boston University School of Medicine
Boston, Massachusetts

R.C.J. Verschueren, MD
Division of Oncology
Department of Surgery
University Hospital
Groningen
The Netherlands

CONTENTS

PART IV Other Applications of the CO_2 Laser in Surgery

PART I
Introduction

1 History of the CO_2 Laser in Surgery

Thomas G. Polanyi, PhD

The use of lasers in medicine, in particular for surgery, is still in its infancy, but in ophthalmological surgery as well as in several areas of microsurgery, the role of lasers has been firmly established. In the aerodigestive tract, for example, the number of surgeons using CO_2 lasers as the modality of choice is continuously increasing and so are the applications in this field. In the endoscopic treatment of selected bronchial lesions, lasers fulfill a unique role. Treatment of lesions of the female genital tract with CO_2 lasers is becoming another major area of application of these lasers to microsurgery. Additional endoscopic and microsurgical applications of CO_2 and argon ion lasers can be anticipated in such areas as neuromicrosurgery, otology, orthopedic surgery, and pelvic surgery. In the near future, the endoscopic treatment of gastric hemorrhages and of disorders of the urinary tract by means of neodymium or argon ion lasers could likely emerge as new, important applications of lasers in medicine.[1]

In this chapter, the development of surgery with lasers will be sketched, including some technical, experimental, and clinical aspects. The earliest period of surgery with lasers started in 1961 and ended in 1967. It coincides approximately with the period of time during which only pulsed lasers were available. In 1965, exploration into the possibility of using CO_2 lasers in surgery began. The findings that stimulated this search and the initial results on laboratory animals, will be summarized in this chapter. Significant results of further research and the endeavors to use CO_2 lasers as *light scalpels,* or direct substitutes for the cold knife or the electrosurgical knife, will also be reviewed. Despite initial high hopes that CO_2 lasers would lead to a major breakthrough in bloodless surgery, these endeavors have not led to definitive applications. The use of CO_2 lasers in combination with the operating microscope for the treatment of lesions in the aerodigestive tract will be reviewed in more detail, because this work has opened the way to the major applications of CO_2 lasers in microsurgery and endoscopic surgery.

THE EARLY PERIOD OF SURGERY WITH LASERS (1961-1967)

In 1960, the first laser discovered by Maiman[2] emitted light at a wavelength of 0.69 microns (μ) in short pulses lasting one millisecond or less. Soon afterwards, the output power of these ruby lasers had been so increased that they could pierce a stack of steel razor blades. The neodymium (Nd)-in-glass laser, operating in the pulsed mode at a wavelength of 1.06 μ, was discovered soon afterwards in 1961 by Snitzer,[3] and the output power of this laser exceeded by far that of the ruby laser. These new, extraordinarily intense sources of light excited the interest of researchers in many fields, including medical researchers whose workers hoped that lasers would become new weapons in the fight against cancer.

Surgical experiments soon began with both ruby and Nd-in-glass lasers, in which various organs and tumors implanted in the experimental animals were exposed to laser light and the biological effects studied. Unfortunately, difficulties in controlling the level of output power of these early lasers led to many conflicting results and early reports, such as that of irradiating even part of a tumor would cause a regression of the entire mass, which could not be confirmed in other laboratories. Soon afterwards, it was found that to obtain a *cure*, the entire mass of the tumor had to be destroyed.

It became apparent, as well, that the major obstacle to achieving complete destruction was the small absorption by nonpigmented biological tissues of the 0.69 and 1.06 μ wavelengths of the lasers used in this work, since the low absorption of tissues required the delivery of large amounts of energy whose thermal effect could not be localized to the diseased tissue volume. In the course of experiments on such tissues, researchers were led to use more and more energy and higher and higher power densities. At the higher power densities mechanical tissue disruption effects occurred, in addition to tissue heating, and this caused viable cancer cells to be propelled into the laboratory environment.[4] This important finding, in conjunction with the less than promising results obtained up until that time in the treatment of experimental tumors, effectively brought to an end this line of research with ruby and Nd-in-glass lasers and exercised, as well, a strongly negative effect on any surgical research with any laser.

Notwithstanding the discouraging results, these early investigations were valuable. Medical researchers were alerted to possible applications of lasers—the idea of differential absorption of electromagnetic radiation by tissues, such as tattoos and melanomas, which could be destroyed by light energy while healthy tissues were preserved. Possible future developments in staining techniques and laser engineering might lead some day to cancer treatment methods involving optimized differential therapeutic absorption of light.

Highly successful, on the other hand, was the application of ruby lasers to ophthalmology to produce small, precisely located, therapeutic lesions on the retina. The small energy needed for this work and the high absorption of the retina for visible radiation made this application possible. Clinical instruments using ruby lasers for photocoagulation were developed in the mid-1960s. The argon ion laser (A^+), discovered in the mid-1960s, essentially replaced the ruby laser in applications to ophthalmic surgery by the early 1970s, because the wavelength of operations of the A^+ laser, 0.48 μ, is absorbed not only by the retina but also by hemoglobin. In addition, the A+ laser operates in the continuous (CW) mode—a definite advantage, since dosage is easier to control with CW lasers.

RECOGNITION OF THE SURGICAL POTENTIAL OF THE CO_2 LASER (1965)

In 1965, about the same time that disillusionment with ruby and Nd-in-glass lasers for cancer therapy was deepening, the potential utility in surgery of the newly developed carbon dioxide laser operating in the infrared at 10.6 μ[5] was first explored.

Yahr and Strully,[6] in the author's laboratory at the American Optical Corporation, found that a focused 20 watt (W) CO_2 laser beam, when moved along a line, would separate skin similarly to a steel scalpel. Encouraged by this finding, Yahr carried out a laparotomy on a dog, exposed the liver and performed a partial liver resection. Blood loss during the laparotomy was negligible and minimal during the liver operation. These first experiments were made with a typical physics laboratory laser installed on an optical bench; the laser was stationary and horizontal. The beam was made vertical and focused on the experimental animal; the anesthetized dog was secured onto a wheeled typewriter table. To perform the operation, the table was moved under the beam and the focused CO_2 laser beam acted as a noncontacting light scalpel with a high degree of hemostasis.

DEVELOPMENT OF THE FIRST CO_2 LASER SYSTEM FOR SURGERY

The findings and the enthusiasm of Yahr and Strully stimulated the development in the laboratories of the American Optical Corporation of a CO_2 laser system for surgery, which would permit systematic exploration of the potential of this new source of energy. The system consisted of a carbon dioxide laser whose output beam was directed into an articulated

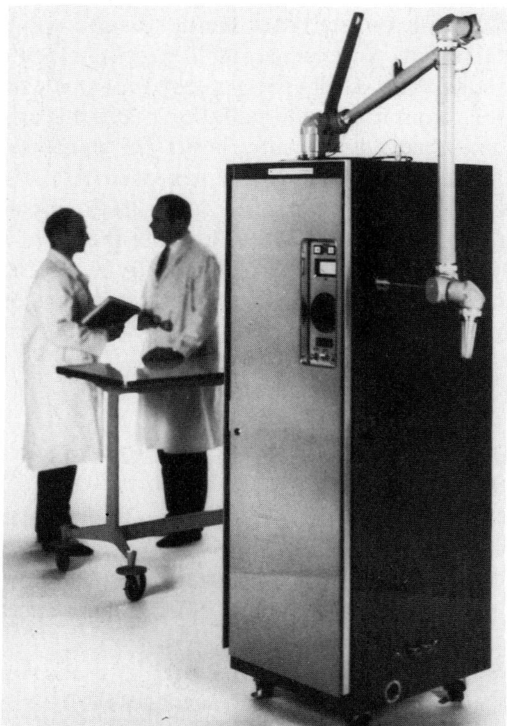

Figure 1-1 Instrument for surgery with carbon dioxide lasers developed in the research laboratory of the American Optical Corporation, 1967, called AO-100. The beam from the vertically positioned laser in the cabinet is directed into the articulated beam manipulating arm, and is focused by lenses at the distal end of the arm. These lenses are contained in the handpieces described in Figure 1-2.

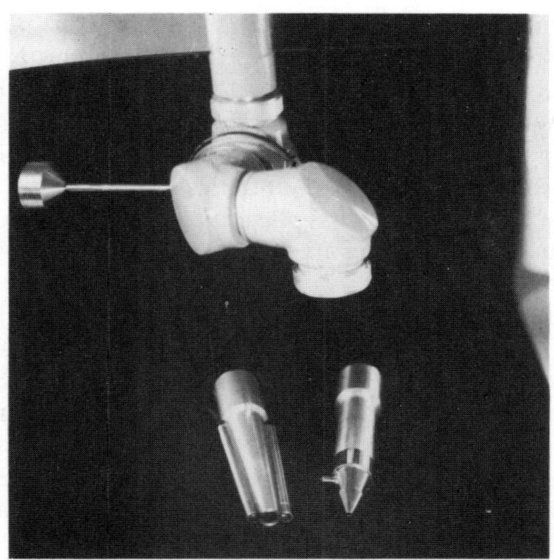

Figure 1-2 Handpiece attachments to the laser beam manipulating arm (1967). The handpiece on the left has a long focal length and the focal point is well beyond the end of the handpiece. Each of the two barrels located on this handpiece contains a light source and an optical system, which projects a luminous line on the work piece. The focal spot of the laser beam is where the two lines bisect and form a symmetrical cross. This preserves the no-touch feature of the light scalpel. The handpiece on the right contains a short focal length lens; the focal spot is at the tip of the sharp truncated cone, which can be located by visually terminating the cone. (Reproduced by permission from Polanyi TG, Bredemeier HC, Davis TW Jr: A CO_2 laser for surgical research. *Med Biol Eng Comput* 8:541–548, 1970.)

beam manipulating arm, carrying at its distal end a handpiece containing a focusing lens. The arm enabled the surgeon to apply the focused or unfocused beam, from any direction, freely to tissues in as wide a volume as is required by surgical practice. Laser, power source, and electrical controls for dosage of the energy applied to tissues were all contained in a movable cabinet, which also supported the manipulating arm. The system is shown in Figure 1-1 and the handpieces in Figure 1-2. The maximum power delivered to tissues from this system was 50 W.[7,8]

FIRST INVESTIGATIONS WITH THE CO_2 LASER (1967-1972)

In the years between 1967 and 1972, numerous concurrent investigations were undertaken with systems similar to the one shown in Figure 1-1, later supplemented with endoscopic and microscopic attachments. Toward the end of this period, the instrumentation was used increasingly for clinical work as well.

The initial investigations, which stimulated the development of surgery with CO_2 lasers, will be reviewed briefly. Interestingly, already at this early stage several, distinct broad areas of application started to emerge: 1) tissue devitalization[9] and coagulation of hemorrhages with low power density unfocused beams, 2) excisional surgery as is practiced in freehand general surgery, and 3) endoscopic surgery and microsurgery. In some of these areas, definitive applications have been found, notably in endoscopic surgery and microsurgery; in others, applications are still in a stage of definition.

The first systematic surgical research following the initial experiments of Yahr and Strully was undertaken in 1967 by R.F. Edlich in the laboratory of Prof O. Wangensteen at the Medical School of the University of Minnesota. Edlich used the broad, unfocused CO_2 laser beam to devitalize the mucosa of the stomachs of dogs. He demonstrated this could be done without damage to the muscularis mucosae and that healing would take place normally.[10] In the same laboratory between 1968 and 1970, Gonzalez and Edlich investigated control of superficial hepatic hemorrhages,[11] and Goodale et al[12] investigated control of gastric hemorrhages in the exposed canine stomach. Goodale later also used a rigid gastroscope developed by Bredemeier[13] for this canine work. Madden et al[14] compared healing of laser skin incisions in rats with other modalities. With exception of the latter, all other investigations in this laboratory were made with unfocused beams of about 4 cm^2 area and a power density of about 12 W/cm^2 or less.

In the same year, 1967, G.J. Jako brought to the author's laboratory a cadaver larynx. In a quick experiment, it was found possible to produce discrete localized lesions of controllable size using the focusing handpieces. Continuation of the experiment in vivo on canine larynges required the development of an endoscopic delivery system, and later of an attachment permitting use of the focused CO_2 laser beam in conjunction with an operating microscope. The successful development of these delivery systems by H.C. Bredemeier[13,15] during the following years, 1968 to 1970, was stimulated by the continued excellent surgical results obtained by Jako. This work, which has opened the major applications of CO_2 lasers to surgery, is reviewed in more detail in the section on microsurgery and endoscopic surgery.

Fidler in the following year, 1968, started surgical research with an AO-100 system in the Laser Laboratory of Dr. L. Goldman at the University of Cincinnati. He studied hemostatic properties of incisions made with a sharply focused CO_2 laser beam and the healing of the surgical wounds thus produced (Fidler JP, personal communication, 1968). His first work was on burn debridement in rats, and later in pigs. Experimental surgery with the CO_2 laser continued at the University of Cincinnati for many years: A. Naprstek, in 1969, experimented with cardiovascular surgery[16] and partial liver and kidney resections in dogs. This work was continued by Goldman et al[17] and taken up again by Fidler et al.[18]

Mullins et al, in 1968, investigated liver resections in rhesus monkeys with a laboratory-type set up similar to that used by Yahr and Strully in 1965.[19]

Stanley S. Stellar, joined the ranks of the early pioneers of surgery with CO_2 lasers in 1969, stimulated by Fidler's 1969 report to the Gordon Research Conference on Lasers in Medicine and Biology. Stellar had prior experience with pulsed ruby lasers, and he used the CO_2 laser system extensively for surgical research. He investigated the cutting of skin, subcutaneous fat, fascia, muscles, periosteum and spinal cord in cats and rats. He produced minimal lesions in the brain and spinal cord of cats under the operating microscope (Figure 1-3) using the beam-focusing handpieces.[20] He also studied resection and vaporization of malignant tumors implanted in rats.[21] Later, 1970 to 1972, with Ger, Levine and Stellar,[22,23] he investigated burn debridement in pigs following Ger's suggestions for an animal model for decubitus ulcers.

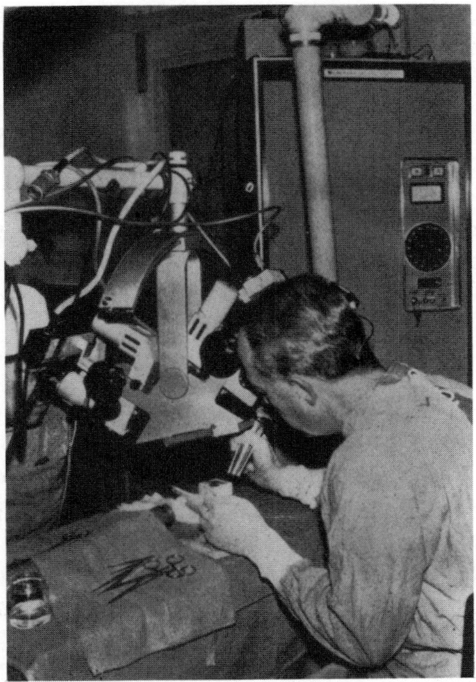

Figure 1-3 Freehand surgery with CO_2 lasers using handpieces and an operating microscope (1969). (Reproduced by permission from Stellar S, Polanyi TG, Bredemeier HC: Lasers in surgery, in Wolbarsht ML [ed]: *Laser Applications in Medicine and Biology,* vol 2. New York, Plenum Publishing Co, 1974.)

R. R. Hall, also in 1968, independently from the work reported thus far, initiated a project to explore the advantages of CO_2 lasers in surgery at the Royal College of Surgeons in London, England. Hall and his colleagues investigated skin incisions in rats,[24] liver resection in dogs,[25] wound healing,[26] and the mechanism of interaction of CO_2 laser energy with biological tissues.[27] Hall used instrumentation developed in the Applied Physics Division of the Atomic Weapons Research Establishment, Aldermaston, England, in cooperation with the Research Department of Anesthetics of The Royal College of Surgeons.

Stellar[29] stressed the extraordinary capacity of the CO_2 laser beam to gently reduce tissue masses to vapor from a distance with a sterilizing effect, and with precision and high localization of the area of destruction. He emphasized the potential of this surgical modality in neurosurgery. In general, precision of tissue removal seemed limited only by instrument design factors and the surgeon's skill.

Hemostasis was investigated extensively. Capillary bleeding was absent in all cases. Vessels up to about 1 mm or less in diameter could be transected with no or minimal bleeding; however, bleeding from larger vessels could be controlled only with difficulty. The original finding—and enthusiasm—regarding the hemostatic nature of the light scalpel had slowly to be qualified.

FURTHER DEVELOPMENT OF SURGERY WITH CO_2 LASERS

Following the initial investigations, the number of workers in the field multiplied; earlier findings were reexamined, and research progressed parallel to experimental surgery and clinical applications. This, in essence, continues to be the state-of-the-field today.

Research

In connection with burn debridement, studies were continued on tissue damage and wound healing in pigs by Levine et al.[30,31] It was found that the take of split skin grafts was as good as that with conventional surgery.

Liver surgery in dogs was studied extensively by Fidler et al.[32] He concluded that in clinical hepatic surgery, the CO_2 laser might be used as an ancillary tool only.

R. Verschueren reached similar negative conclusions regarding liver surgery. He investigated osteotomies in dogs and found that bone healing is delayed when compared to conventional methods, but he suggested the CO_2 laser might be used with advantage for bone biopsies.[33] Morein et al[34] investigated laser induced epiphysiodesis in rabbits, and thought that the CO_2 laser also might be useful for the shortening of extremities. Ben-Bassat et al[35] studied the healing process in bowel surgery on cats and found a slight delay in healing compared with cold knife surgery. Ben-Basset et al[36] investigated by light and electron microscopy the cut edges of human skin and mucous membranes. They found: "The ultrasections, cut after a distance of 250 μ from the border, showed well preserved tissue. The control blocks (excision by surgical knife) revealed preserved tissue already from the beginning of the cut edge, and no necrosis was found."

Extensive studies were made of the interaction of CO_2 laser energy with nervous tissues by Ascher,[37] using light microscopy and high magnification scanning electron microscopy. At a magnification of 2200x, Ascher found dramatic differences in the appearance of brain tissue cut with the CO_2 laser or the cold knife: "The appearance of a surface cut with the CO_2 laser is as smooth as a 'golf course,' while that cut with a scalpel is replete with cleavages and covered with blood cells.[37p61] At a magnification of 5000x, sciatic nerve fibers cut with the CO_2 laser appear rounded, smooth and encapsulated while electric knife cuts present a frazzled and honeycombed appearance."[37p66] Ascher also found that nerves severed with the CO_2 laser will not anastomose.[38] His findings may explain, at least in part, recurrent reports by patients that after surgery with CO_2 lasers, postoperative pain is reduced.

Verschueren addressed the important problem of tissue damage using rabbit livers.[33] He found that the thermal damage at the margins of a CO_2 laser wound increased with exposure time and was independent of laser beam power. Mihasi et al[39] also studied tissue damage on dog tongues and found results similar to Verschueren.

Oosterhuis et al in 1975[40] and Mihasi et al in 1976[39] investigated the *allowability* of using the CO_2 laser in cancer surgery and found no contraindications. Oosterhuis in 1977[41] sought to answer the question of whether or not the CO_2 laser has *advantages* in cancer surgery. He found indications that surgery with the CO_2 laser decreased lymphatic spread of tumor cells when compared with other modalities. He concluded, however, that it would be prudent for the time being to recommend surgery with CO_2 lasers only in those cases where it offered clear-cut technical advantages over other methods; eg, in selected cases of endoscopic surgery, orthopedic surgery, or where reduction in blood loss is important, as in surgery on hemophiliacs.

Experimental Surgery

Stellar treated a limited number of malignant tumors for palliation, beginning in 1969, and while the operations were all technically successful, the laser wounds healed well, and tissue evaporation offered new perspectives as expected, the hoped for dramatic improvement in hemostasis did not occur as it had in small animals. Goldman et al in 1970 excised several hemangiomatous skin lesions with good results.[42] Goodale (1970) treated uncontrollable bleeding from stress ulcers in two young patients who had been prepared for gastrectomy. These operations were successful, the bleeding was controlled with the unfocused CO_2 laser beam and the stomachs of these patients saved (Goodale RL, personal communication, 1970). The need for laparotomy and gastrotomy discouraged the further use of the CO_2 laser for coagulation of gastrointestinal bleeding.

Levine et al in 1972 performed a successful burn debridement operation.[43] Kaplan and Ger, stimulated by the burn debridement work of Stellar et al[22] in 1972 undertook a broad range of experimental surgery trials with an American Optical Model 200 laser system at the Beilinson Hospital, University Medical School, Tel Aviv, Israel.[28] These authors confirmed findings relating to good hemostasis in avascular fields, uneventful take of skin grafts, ease of operating in infected and necrotic areas, benign postoperative course and patients' reports of decreased postoperative discomfort.

While most of the cases were in the area of plastic surgery, Kaplan et al[44] treated several cases of cervicitis and rectal lesions. They stressed the potential advantages of the CO_2 laser in endoscopic surgery. In connection with cancer surgery, they noted with caution that excision of tumorous tissues might take place with decreased spread of malignant cells owing to the property of the CO_2 laser to seal small vessels, including lymphatics.

In subsequent work, Kaplan and his colleagues used the CO_2 laser in many areas of plastic and general surgery including malignant lesions. In this work they used the Sharplan 791 system for surgery shown in Figure 1-4. The rearrangement of the components of the system, a lighter, more slender articulated arm and a thinner handpiece, made this system, in principle, more convenient for clinical surgery.[45]

Fidler et al[46,47] conducted extensive trials of burn debridement in children, while Levine et al[31] did so in adults. Fidler started his clinical work with the AO-100 and continued it with the Sharplan 791. He used the technique consistently for selected cases of burn debridement in children at the Shriners Burn Hospital in Cincinnati; however, the laser method of burn debridement has not been found to offer clear-cut advantages.[48] Stellar et al,[49] using the AO-100, initiated a series of decubitus ulcer treatments.

Using the Sharplan system, a large variety of pathological conditions, benign and malignant, have been treated with plastic, head and neck, orthopedic, chest, urological and neurological surgery.[50-52] In all

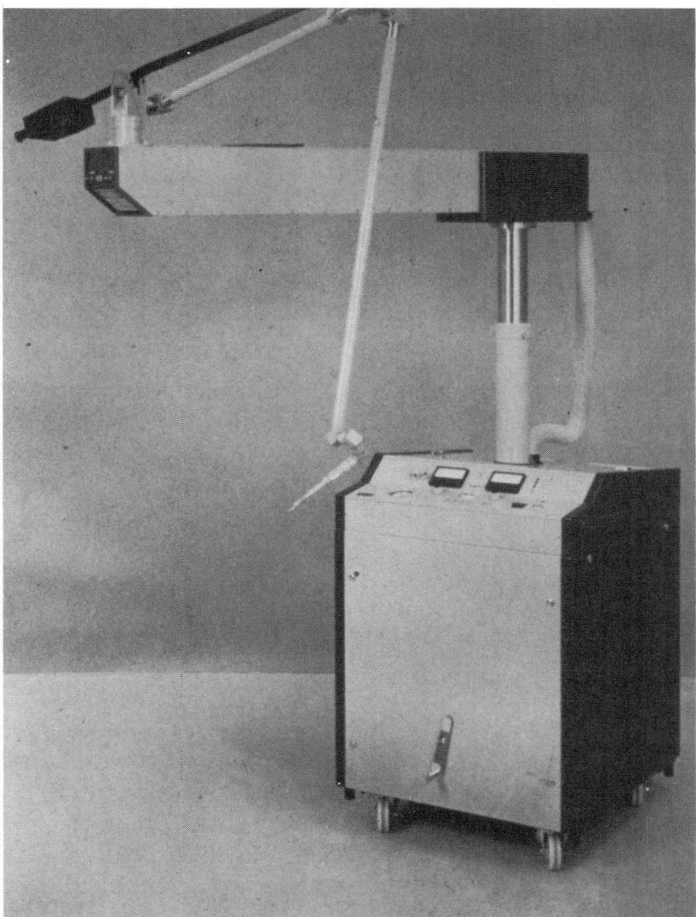

Figure 1-4 The Sharplan 791 carbon dioxide laser instrument for surgery (1972). The horizontally positioned laser leaves ample space between operating table and control box. The beam manipulating arm is slender and has little inertia; the hand-pieces are thin. All these features make this design more adapted for clinical use than the AO-100. (Courtesy: Advanced Surgical Instruments, Chicago, Illinois.)

these applications, the freely movable hand-held focusing pieces are used as light scalpels. Widely accepted major applications have not emerged from this method so far.

In selected areas of microsurgery, however, the CO_2 laser modality has found wide acceptance. Here, the focal spot of the laser beam is positioned indirectly with a micromanipulator, which controls small displacements of a mirror essentially fixed in space. The focal spot is observed with an operating microscope and the operating field is practically blood-free.

MICROSURGERY AND ENDOSCOPIC SURGERY WITH CO_2 LASERS

In 1971, Strong and Jako began using the CO_2 laser in laryngeal microsurgery. The initial results already suggested a superior form of surgery had been found; this conviction only strengthened, as experience accumulated in many hands.

In later years, it was found that the instrumentation and the techniques developed for laryngeal microsurgery could be used in gynecological microsurgery, and the first patients receiving such treatment, did so in ENT operating rooms with the assistance of ENT surgeons.

The experimental, instrumental and clinical development of laryngeal microsurgery and of bronchial endoscopic surgery with CO_2 lasers will now be reviewed in more detail.

Experimental Research

Interest in using the CO_2 laser for laryngeal surgery began in 1967 when it was found, as noted previously, that the focused beam of this laser could produce discrete lesions of any size in a cadaver larynx. Jako, who performed this experiment, was particularly impressed, since he had tried unsuccessfully in 1965 to achieve such results with a Nd-in-glass laser. With this laser, only poorly localized lesions could be made and those, only after painting the laryngeal tissues with copper sulfate.[53] The dramatic difference in these results is a consequence of the strong absorption by biological tissues of electromagnetic radiation at the wavelength of the CO_2 laser and the weak absorption at the wavelength of the Nd laser.

The in vivo experiment was performed by Jako in 1969 with an endoscopic attachment to the beam manipulating arm. He found that discrete lesions of clinically desirable size were produced in the canine larynx by irradiating it for 1/10 to 1/2 sec with a 5 to 30 W CO_2 laser beam focused to a spot size of 2 mm diameter; the operating field was blood free, and healing was excellent. The experimental setup for this work is shown in Figure 1-5.

Further progress in the laryngeal work required a method to deliver the laser beam to the larynx, observed in an operating microscope, trained through a laryngoscope. H. C. Bredemeier developed such an attachment to the beam manipulating arm, thus integrating the CO_2 laser system with a Zeiss operating microscope.[15] This attachment was first called *stereo-endoscope* and later, *micromanipulator*. It is illustrated in Figure 1-6. Using this attachment, Jako[53] studied canine vocal cord surgery in an experimen-

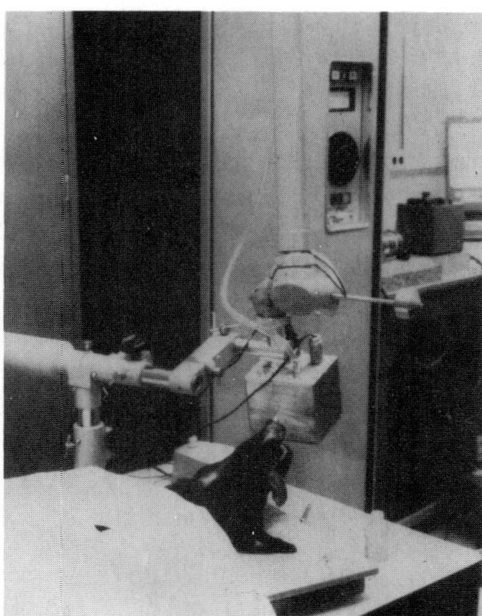

Figure 1-5 In vivo vocal cord surgery with the CO_2 laser (1969). The large cubical box is attached to the laser beam manipulating arm; it contains a lens to focus the laser beam at the distal end of the endoscopic tube and other means that permit viewing the impact site of the focused laser beam. The observation port is on the side of the cube opposite the one to which the large, 15-mm diameter, endoscopic tube is attached. (See also Figure 1-8.)

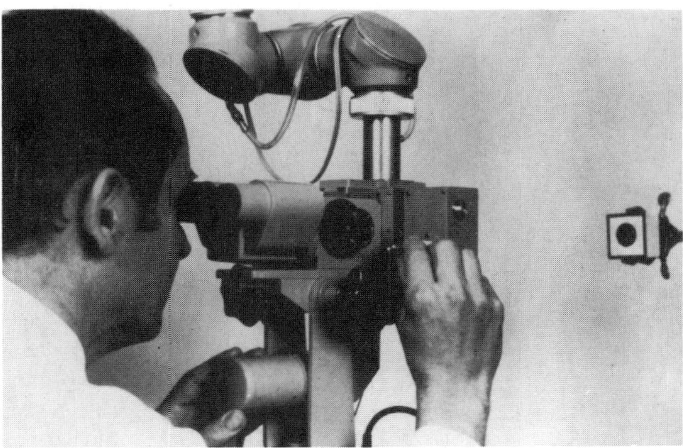

Figure 1-6 H.C. Bredemeier testing the attachment for microsurgery with CO_2 lasers (1970). The micromanipulator attachment is fitted to a Zeiss operating microscope and is joined to the laser beam manipulating arm. A lens and a 45° deflecting mirror focus the laser beam on a distant target at the working distance of the microscope. Motions of the joystick transmitted to the 45° mirror permit precise positioning of the focal spot of the laser within the field of view of the operating microscope.

tal setup similar to that used in clinical practice (Figure 1-7). The study showed that tissue volumes of any desired size could be selectively and rapidly vaporized using appropriate energy dosages of the focused CO_2 laser beam. The depth and extent of tissue removal could be controlled with ease, and the progress of tissue removal seen clearly through the operating microscope. Tissue removal was bloodless and healing uneventful.

Jako concluded the experimental study in 1970 and submitted it as a candidate's thesis to the American Laryngological, Rhinological, and Otological Society. He suggested that vocal cord surgery with the CO_2 laser was ready for clinical trials. These were started soon afterwards. The development of the clinical work will be reviewed in the last part of this section following a review of the instrumentation.

Instrumentation

The micromanipulator attachment to the Zeiss operating microscope was used clinically without any changes. The endoscopic attachment, which was fitted to a 15 mm diameter endoscopic tube for the canine work, was modified in 1973 to accept standard Pilling ventilating bronchoscopes of 3 to 8 mm in diameter (Figure 1-8). A much smaller and lighter bronchoscopic attachment was developed by R. A. Wallace in 1974[54,60] (Figure 1-9). With this and the micromanipulator, the basic instrumentation for endoscopic surgery and microsurgery with CO_2 lasers was completed.

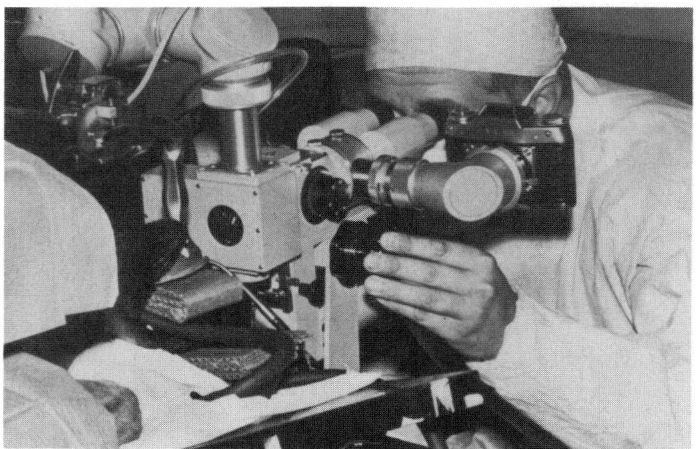

Figure 1-7 Experimental laryngeal microsurgery (1970). Using the attachment shown in Figure 1-6, the CO_2 laser beam is focused on the vocal cords through a Jako laryngoscope. (Reproduced by permission from Jako GJ: Laser surgery of the vocal cords. *Laryngoscope* 82(12):2204–2216, 1972.)

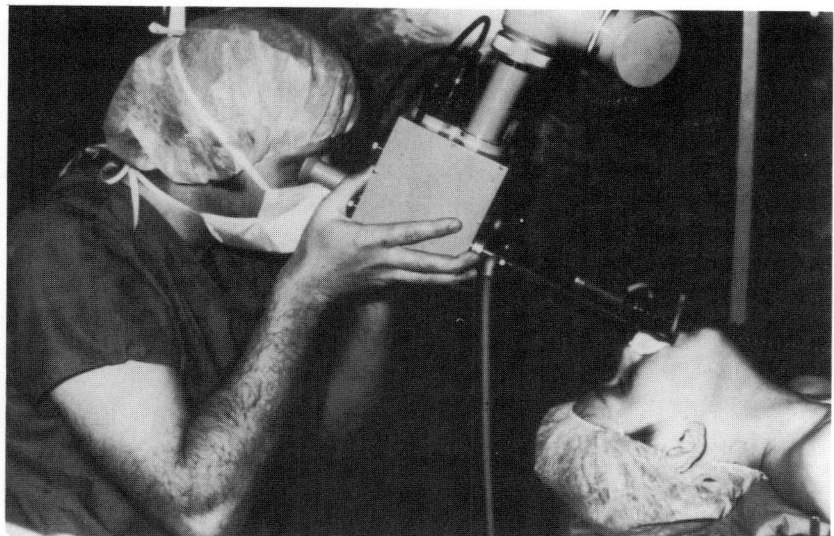

Figure 1-8 Bronchial surgery with the CO_2 laser (1973). This attachment for bronchial surgery is the same as the one developed for the first in vivo experimental surgery on dogs (see Figure 1-5). For clinical use, it was fitted with a standard Pilling bronchoscope. (Reproduced by permission from Strong MS, Jako GI, Polanyi TG, et al: Laser surgery of the aerodigestive tract. *Am J Surg* 126:529–533, 1972.)

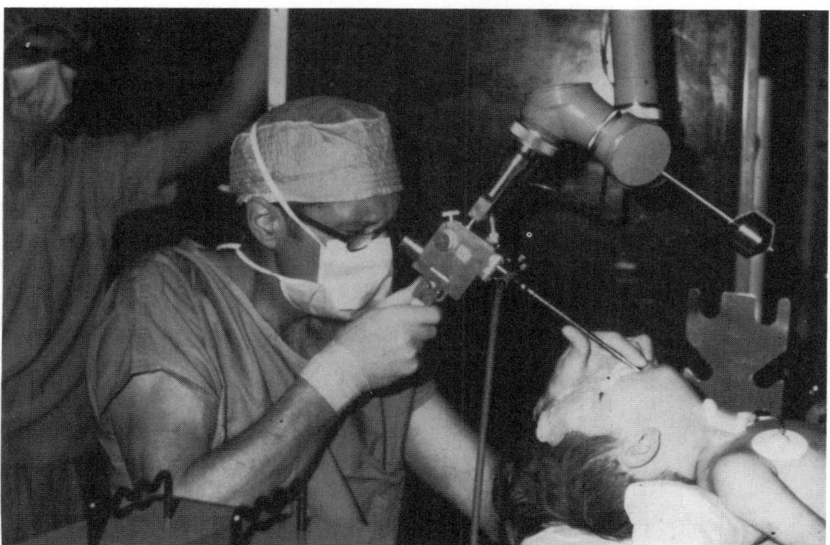

Figure 1-9 Bronchial surgery with CO_2 lasers and the second generation endoscopic attachment (1974). (Reproduced by permission from Berci G (ed): *Endoscopy*. New York, Appleton-Century-Crofts, 1976, p 196.)

A basically different type of CO_2 laser system for microsurgery was developed by Polanyi, Wallace, and Pejchar in 1974.[56] By mounting a CO_2 laser directly on the operating microscope, the need for a beam manipulating arm was eliminated. An instrument of this type, called the AO-300 (Figure 1-10), was the first commercial instrument for microsurgery. This instrument, developed in the laboratories of the American Optical Corporation, was taken over by the Cavitron Corporation who developed it further.

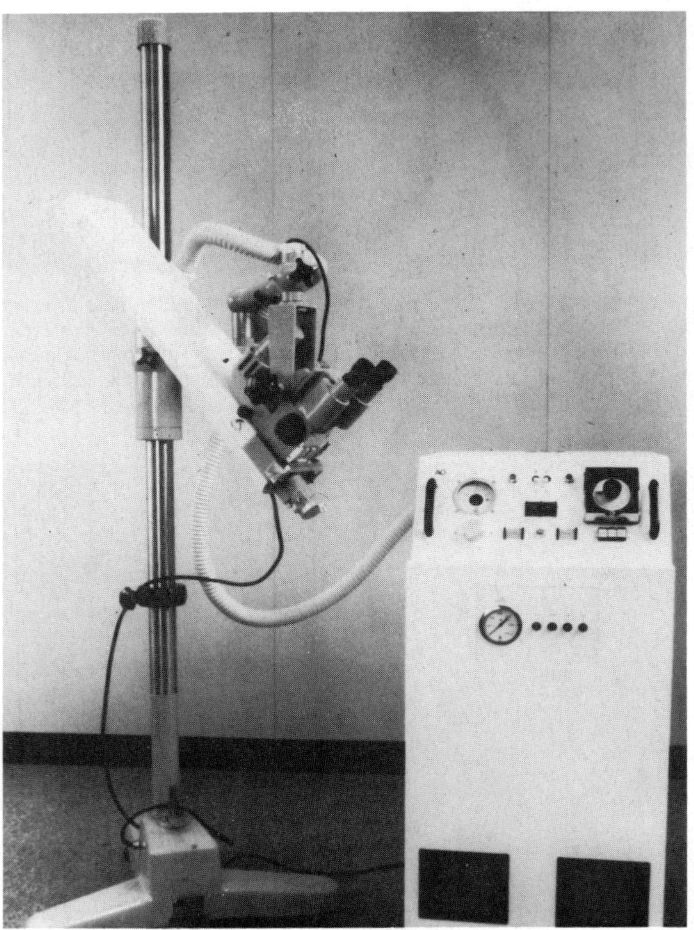

Figure 1-10 A new type of CO_2 laser instrument for microsurgery only, called AO-300 (1974). The laser is attached directly to the operating microscope, and therefore, the laser beam manipulating arm is not needed. (Courtesy: Cavitron Corporation.)

Many commercial systems for microsurgery have become available since 1974. The first to follow the AO-300, in 1975, was Coherent's System 400, shown in Figure 1-11. In 1977, Ferlux Biophysique Medicale introduced their Model FC-25 at the XI World Congress of Oto-Rhino-Laryngology in Buenos Aires, Argentina. This system was patterned after the AO-100. In the same year, the Sharplan 733 (Figure 1-12) was introduced at the meeting of the American College of Ophthalmology and Otolaryngology in Dallas. Merrimack's ML-800 (Figure 1-13) was introduced in 1980 at the meeting of the American College of Obstetricians and Gynecologists in New Orleans, Louisiana. The AO-300 and the System 400 were later supplemented with arms and attachments for bronchial surgery.

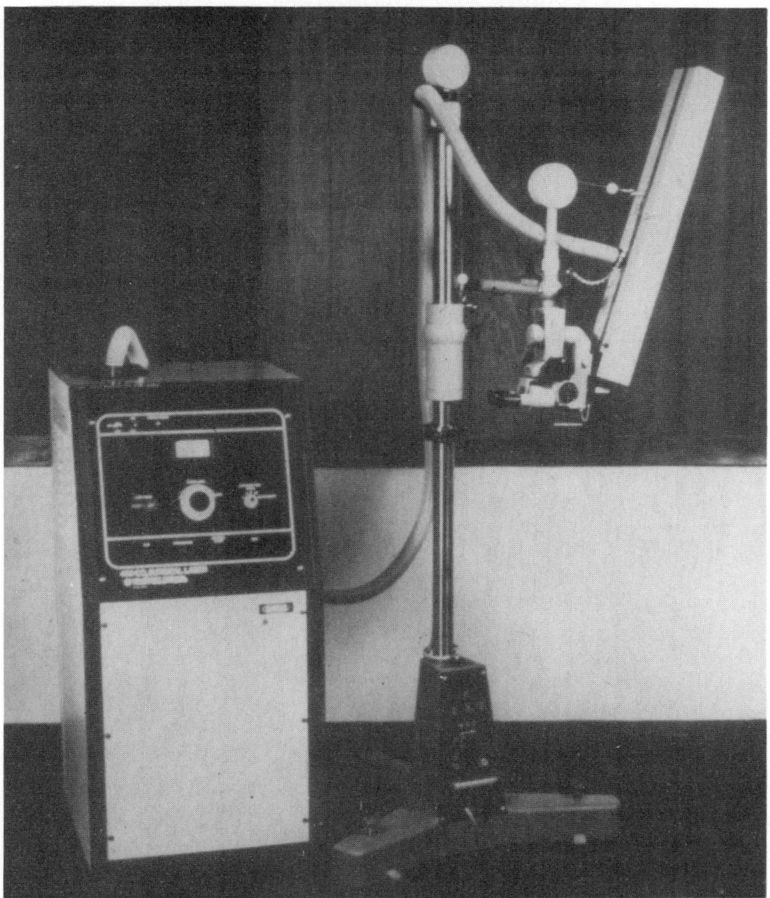

Figure 1-11 System 400, another instrument for microsurgery with CO_2 lasers (1975). (Courtesy: Coherent Medical, Palo Alto, California.)

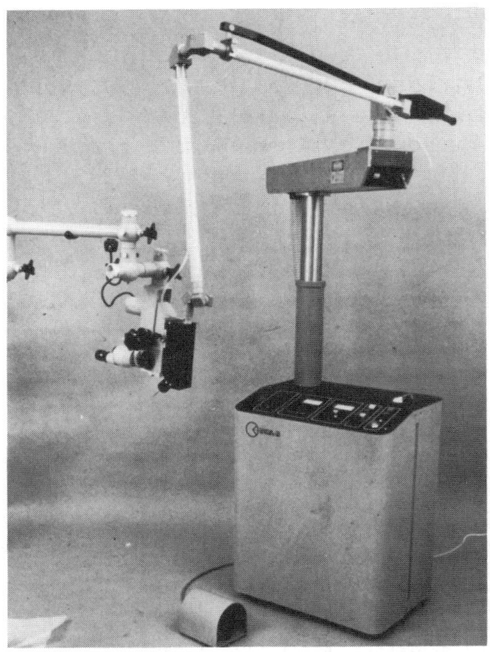

Figure 1-12 Sharplan 733, instrument for surgery and microsurgery with CO_2 lasers (1977). A smaller version of the Sharplan 791 with a micromanipulator attachment to a Zeiss operating microscope. (Courtesy: Advanced Surgical Instrumentation, Chicago, Illinois.)

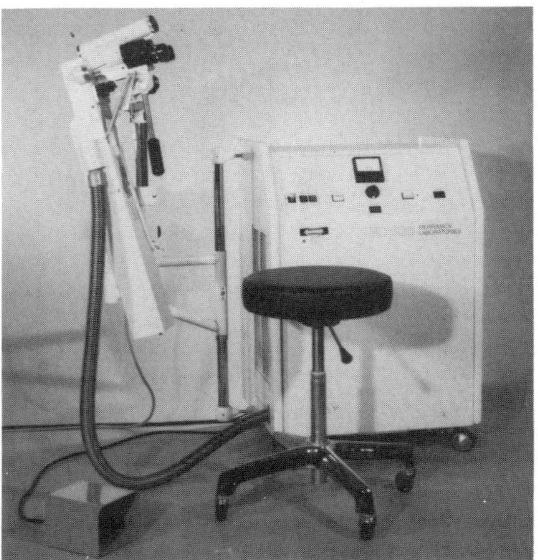

Figure 1-13 ML-800, instrument for gynecological microsurgery in office setting (1980). (Courtesy: Merrimack Laboratories, Inc, Hudson, Massachusetts.)

Clinical Development in Otolaryngology

At the 1972 meeting of the American Broncho-Esophagological Society, Strong and Jako[57] reported on fourteen cases treated with the CO_2 laser. The findings were summarized as follows:

1. The CO_2 laser is a practical instrument for incision or excision of tissue.
2. The microsurgical laser attachment to the operating microscope allows surgery of the vocal cords to be carried out with exquisite precision.
3. Laser surgery has been used successfully in the treatment of vocal cord keratosis, carcinoma in situ, nodules, polyps and papillomas.
4. Following laser surgery, healing is prompt and associated with a minimum of postoperative swelling and scarring.
5. Further application of laser surgery in otolaryngology will be forthcoming as experience and expertise accumulate.

In the same year, A. H. Andrews introduced the use of the CO_2 laser surgical modality at the Department of Otolaryngology of the University of Illinois in Chicago, and in 1973, Ronald French at The Eye, Ear, Nose and Throat Hospital in New Orleans, Louisiana. Both workers confirmed earlier results. Andrews[58,59] initiated the development of instrumentation facilitating exposure of all areas of the larynx to the CO_2 laser beam; French extended the technique to tonsillectomies and to subglottic hemangiomas.[60] In 1973, Strong et al[55] started using the bronchoscopic attachment to the CO_2 laser for the treatment of papillomas and other lesions in the trachea and main stem bronchi. This work was presented to the Society of Head and Neck Surgeons in the same year. Treatment of lesions of the nose and sinuses, oral cavity, pharynx and nasopharynx was also discussed.

At the 1974 meeting of the American Broncho-Esophagological Association, Strong et al[61] reported on 70 bronchoscopic interventions in 15 patients, of which 13 had extensions of papillomas in the main stem bronchi. He concluded: "In the future, it is expected that this method will be given clinical trial in other cases of solid tissue obstructing the trachea and bronchi, including fibrous stenosis without malacia, bronchial adenoma and inoperable carcinoma." At a conjoint meeting with the American Laryngological Association, Andrews[58] discussed his experiences with the use of the CO_2 laser in 41 cases and said, "We have been impressed, like Strong and Jako, with the precision of the surgical procedures, the absence of bleeding and the lack of postoperative reaction in the early and late recovery periods." Andrews concluded: "The laser, by its precision, absence of bleeding, control of depth and area of destruction, reduction of tissue reaction, and preservation of normal tissue, has extended the quality of our operative procedures."

At the Centennial Conference on Laryngeal Cancer, Toronto, Canada, May 1974, Strong[62] reported for the first time on the treatment of selected carcinomas of the larynx with the CO_2 laser modality. In 1974 and 1975, laryngeal microsurgery with CO_2 lasers was introduced at several other centers in the United States and abroad.

In 1975, Strong et al[63] at a plenary session of the meeting of the American Academy of Ophthalmology and Otolaryngology reviewed the combined clinical experience developed in the treatment of 563 patients and over 1,000 operations at Boston University Hospital, the University of Illinois in Chicago and the Eye, Ear, Nose and Throat Hospital in New Orleans. His summary: "The advantages of laser surgery in otolaryngology are so significant that it can be recommended for continued usage. Many applications of this unique surgical instrument have been identified but others need to be explored in the future."

Gynecological Microsurgery with the CO_2 Laser

As noted previously, the first use of the CO_2 laser in gynecology was reported by Kaplan and Ger in 1973.[44] In 1973, R. Upton at the Naval Hospital in Portsmouth, Virginia, started exploring the CO_2 laser microsurgical modality in gynecology with an AO-200 system attached to a Zeiss operating microscope. He wanted to determine whether the CO_2 laser could be used in the treatment of cervical intraepithelial neoplasias. Upton started his clinical experiments on subjects who were slated for hysterectomy for pathologic conditions not related to the cervix. He investigated tissue removal from the cervix, and acute and delayed, up to 12 weeks, tissue reactions. He reported this work to the Society of Gynecological Oncologists meeting in Key Biscayne, Florida in January of 1975.[64] In further work, he treated a group of patients with carcinoma in situ of the cervix (Upton RT, personal communication, 1981).

In 1974, J. Bellina observed R. French performing several laryngeal microsurgical procedures with the CO_2 laser. He felt that the benefits of this modality would apply equally to the treatment of selected cervical, vaginal and vulvar lesions. Within the span of a few months, he treated several cases of vaginal adenosis and of condylomata acuminata at the Eye, Ear, Nose and Throat Hospital in New Orleans, Louisiana. Bellina reported this and subsequent work at seminars, published his initial results in 1974,[65] and held a scientific exhibit at the 1975 Meeting of the American College of Obstetricians and Gynecologists in Boston.

Bellina's initial work took place at a time of peak concern with possible malignant degeneration of vaginal adenosis in young women, whose mothers had ingested diethystilbestrol (DES) during pregnancy.

Bellina showed that vaginal epithelium could be removed with the CO_2 laser beam under microscopic control and that regeneration of the epithelium occurred rapidly without scarring or synechiae, and that after some time, hardly any trace of the operation was left. These and similar results with other lesions spurred on many gynecologists to explore the use of this new modality. Stafl[66] and Friedrich,[67] Medical College of Wisconsin, Krantz and Carter,[68] University of Kansas Medical School, were among the first to undertake clinical investigations following Bellina's reports.

Much clinical research still remains to be done and controversy exists as to the effectiveness of the CO_2 laser method for the treatment of vulvar dystrophies and herpetic infections, or even as to the need for this new modality as opposed to cryosurgery; eg, in the treatment of cervical intraepithelial neoplasias. Clinical evidence, however, is accumulating, which indicates that the modality is highly effective in the treatment of selected lesions in the cervix, vagina, vulva and in the perianal and periurethral regions, and that treatment of these lesions with the CO_2 laser is accompanied by less postoperative discomfort or morbidity and results in maximum preservation of function.

SUMMARY

Lasers have been firmly established in the surgical armamentarium of several specialties within two decades of the discovery of the first laser. In ophthalmic surgery, intense non-laser light sources were used for many years following the pioneering work of Meyer-Schwickerath in the early fifties. Substitution of coherent for noncoherent light sources may appear in retrospect as a logical step. But in other areas of application of lasers to medicine, the road was unchartered; false starts, twists and turns were unavoidable. Early hopes for great advances in the treatment of cancer, and later for the ultimate in bloodless surgery, were not fulfilled.

The unique attributes of CO_2 lasers of importance to surgery became slowly apparent through the work in laryngeal microsurgery. The focal spot of the CO_2 laser, as of all light beams, can be positioned with any degree of accuracy using the fine mechanical motions of a mirror. The high absorption of human tissues for the radiation of the CO_2 laser and the high intensity of this laser permit, by using long focal length lenses, the precise removal of tissues deep within body cavities, and sharp demarcation of the wound margins without mechanical manipulation. The narrow field within which this type of surgery must take place is not limited further by the presence of mechanical instruments; this, in conjunction with a generally bloodless field, preserves the excellent visualization provided by the operating microscope. These unique properties have firmly established the use of CO_2 lasers in laryngeal and gynecological microsurgery. Further such applications can be confidently expected.

Ongoing investigations in freehand surgery, with or without the operating microscope, will most likely lead to other applications.

Work in progress with ion lasers and neodymium lasers will further extend the use of lasers in surgery and may even realize in some areas the most ancient dream of surgeons, bloodless surgery.

ACKNOWLEDGMENTS

First of all, I would like to pay tribute to the memory of Herb C. Bredemeier, a brilliant engineer and a kind human being; he originated the basic instrumentation for surgery with CO_2 lasers. Bredemeier fell victim to an automobile accident in the fall of 1972, just before his 50th birthday. Mr. R. A. Wallace filled the void left by Bredemeier and thanks to his high technical skills, the project continued without interruption. Mr. Wallace's valuable contributions to the field are continuing. I am grateful to him for his devotion to this project and for his loyalty to me throughout our almost thirty years of collaboration.

I want to thank my brother, Dr. Michael L. Polanyi, whose certain judgment has been invaluable to me in the choice of surgical projects. For the over one-decade duration of this project, he gave generously of his time to offer me valuable suggestions, encouragement, and support. The project on surgery with CO_2 lasers owes much to his keen criticism. I am grateful to him for all this and for his faith in me.

I would like to acknowledge gratefully the late Dr. Stephen McNeille, Director of Research of the American Optical Corporation and his successor, Dr. William R. Prindle, for their support and encouragement of the project on surgery with CO_2 lasers.

Finally, I would like to thank my wife, Alice, who lovingly and graciously accepted my endless involvement in this work and who strengthened my faith in it when success appeared doubtful.

REFERENCES

1. Keifhaber P, Nath G, Moritz K: Endoscopical control of massive gastrointestinal hemorrhage by irradiation with a high-power neodymium-YAG laser. *Prog Surg* 15:140–155, 1977.

2. Maiman TH: Stimulated optical radiation in ruby. *Nature* 187:493–494, 1960.

3. Snitzer E: Optical maser action of Nd^{3+} in Ba crown glass. *Phys Rev Letter* 7:444, 1961.

4. Ketcham AS, Hoye RC, Riggle GC: A surgeon's appraisal of the laser. *Surg Clin N Am* 47:1249–1263, 1967.

5. Patel CKN: Selective excitation through vibrational energy transfer and optical maser action in N_2-CO_2. *Phys Rev Letter* 13:617–619, 1964.

6. Yahr WZ, Strully KJ: Blood vessel anastomosis by laser and other biomedical applications. *J Assoc Adv Med Instr* 1(2):28–31, 1966.

7. Polanyi TG, Bredemeier HC, Davis TW, Jr: CO_2 laser zur emperimentellen chirurgie. *LASER und Angewandte Strahlentechnik 4,* 1969.

8. Polanyi TG, Bredemeier HC, Davis TW Jr: CO_2 Laser for surgical research. *Med Biol Eng Comput* 8:549–558, 1970.

9. Pletnev SD, Abdurazakov MS, Karpenko OM: Laser surgery in oncological practice. *Khirurgiia* (2):48–52, 1977.

10. Edlich RF: Personal communication, 1968.

11. Gonzalez R, Edlich RF, Bredemeier HC, et al: Rapid control of massive hepatic hemorrhages by laser radiation. *Surg Gynecol Obstet* 131:198–200, 1970.

12. Goodale RL, Okada A, Gonzalez R, et al: Rapid endoscopic control of bleeding gastric erosions by laser radiation. *Arch Surg* 101:211–214, 1970.

13. Bredemeier HC: 1969, Laser Accessory for Surgical Applications. *US Patent,* 3, 659, 613, issued 1972.

14. Madden JE, Edlich RF, Custer JR, et al: Studies in the management of the contaminated wound. *Am Surg* 119:222–224, 1970.

15. Bredemeier HC: 1973, Stereo Laser Endoscope. *US Patent,* 3, 796, 220, issued 1974.

16. Naprstek Z, Rockwell RJ: Some laser applications in cardiovascular research. *Proceedings of the 8th International Conference of Medical and Biological Engineers,* July, 1969.

17. Goldman L, Rockwell RJ, Naprstek Z, et al: Some parameters of high output CO_2 laser experimental surgery. *Nature* 228:1344–1345, 1970.

18. Fidler JP, Hoefer RW, Polanyi TG, et al: Laser surgery in exsanguinating liver injury, *Surg Forum* 23:350–352, 1972.

19. Mullins F, Jennings B, McClusky L: Liver resection with the continuous wave carbon dioxide laser: Some experimental observations. *Am Surg* 34:717–722, 1968.

20. Stellar S, Polanyi TG, Bredemeier HC: Experimental studies with the carbon dioxide laser as a neurosurgical instrument. *Med Biol Eng Comput* 8:549–558, 1970.

21. Stellar S: The carbon dioxide laser in experimental and clinical surgery for neoplasms. *Panminerva Medica* 16(1–2):32–36, 1974.

22. Stellar S, Ger R, Levine N, et al: Carbon dioxide laser for excision of burn eschars. *Lancet* 5, 1971.

23. Stellar S, Levine N, Ger R, et al: Laser excision of acute third-degree burns followed by immediate autograft replacement: An experimental study in the pig. *J Trauma* 13:45–53, 1973.

24. Hall RR: The healing of tissues incised by a carbon dioxide laser. *Br J Surg* 58:222–225, 1971.

25. Hall RR, Beach AD, Hill DW: Partial hepatectomy using a carbon dioxide laser. *Br J Surg* 60:141–144, 1973.

26. Hall RR, Hill DW, Beach AD: A carbon dioxide surgical laser. *Ann R Coll Surg Engl* 48:181–188, 1971.

27. Hall RR, Beach AD, Baker E, et al: Incision of tissue by carbon dioxide laser. *Nature* 232:131–132, 1971.

28. Kaplan I, Ger R: The carbon dioxide laser in clinical surgery. *Isr J Med Sci* 9(1):79, 1973.

29. Stellar S, Polanyi TG, Bredemeier HC: Lasers in surgery, in Wolbarsht ML (ed): *Laser Applications in Medicine and Biology,* vol II. New York, Plenum Publishing Co, 1974.

30. Levine N, Ger R, Stellar S, et al: Use of a carbon dioxide laser for the debridement of third degree burns. *Ann Surg* 179:246–252, 1974.

31. Levine NS, Salisbury RE, Peteson HD, et al: Clinical evaluation of the carbon dioxide laser for burn wound excisions: A comparison of the laser, scalpel, and electrocautery. *J Trauma* 15:800–807, 1975.

32. Fidler JP, Hoefer RW, Polanyi TG, et al: Laser surgery in exsanguinating liver injury. *Ann Surg* 181:74–80, 1975.

33. Verschueren R: *The* CO_2 *Laser in Tumor Surgery,* Assen/Amsterdam, Van Gorcum, Medical Series, vol 232, 1976.

34. Morein S, Gassner S, Kaplan I: Laser induced epiphyseodesis, in Kaplan I (ed): *Proceedings of the 1st International Symposium of Laser Surgery.* Jerusalem, Jerusalem Academic Press, 1976.

35. Ben-Bassat M, Gassner S, Kaplan I, et al: The healing process in experimental bowel surgery: The surgical knife compared with the carbon dioxide laser, in Kaplan I (ed): *Proceedings of the 1st International Symposium of Laser Surgery.* Jerusalem, Jerusalem Academic Press, 1976.

36. Ben-Bassat M, Ben-Bassat M, Kaplan I: An ultrastructural study of the cut edges of skin and mucous membrane specimens excised by carbon dioxide laser, in Kaplan I (ed): *Proceedings of the 1st International Symposium of Laser Surgery.* Jerusalem, Jerusalem Academic Press, 1976.

37. Ascher PW: *Der* CO_2*-Laser in Der Neurochirurgie.* Wien, Verlag Fritz Molden, 1977.

38. Ascher PW: Neurosurgery Seminar, Ether Dome, Massachusetts General Hospital, Boston, July 13, 1978.

39. Mihasi S, Jako GJ, Incze JM, et al: Laser surgery in otolaryngology: Interaction of CO_2 laser and soft tissue. *Ann NY Acad Sci* 267:263–294, 1976.

40. Oosterhuis JW, Verschueren RCJ, Oldhoff J: Experimental surgery on the Cloudman S91 melanoma with the carbon dioxide laser. *Acta Chir Belg* 74:422–429, 1975.

41. Oosterhuis JW: *Tumor Surgery with the* CO_2 *Laser, Studies with the Cloudman S91 Mouse Melanoma.* Groningen, Veenstra-Visser Offset, Oude Kijk In't Jatstraat 69, 1977.

42. Goldman L, Naprstek Z, Johnson J: Laser surgery of a digital angiosarcoma. *Cancer* 39:1738–1742, 1977.

43. Levine N, Levenson SM, Ger R, et al: Mechanical CO_2 laser and chemical methods for debriding third degree burns. *American Burn Association Meeting.* San Francisco, April 1972.

44. Kaplan I, Goldman J, Ger R: The treatment of erosions of the uterine cervix by means of the CO_2 laser. *Obstet Gynecol* 41:795–796, 1973.

45. Kaplan I, Sharon U, Ger R: The carbon dioxide laser in clinical surgery, in Wolbarsht ML (ed): *Laser Applications in Medicine and Biology,* vol II. New York, Plenum Publishing Co, 1974.

46. Fidler JP, MacMillan BG, Law EJ, et al: Comparative CO_2 laser and Bovie excision of acute burns with immediate autografting. *American Burn Association Meeting.* Cincinnati, 1974.

47. Fidler JP, Law EJ, MacMillan BG, et al: Comparison of carbon dioxide laser excision of burns with other thermal knives. *Ann NY Acad Sci* 267:254–263, 1976.

48. Jackson DM, Cason JS: Burn excision by a carbon-dioxide laser. *Lancet* 5(1):1081–1084, 1977.

49. Stellar S, Meijer R, Walia S, et al: Carbon dioxide laser debridement of decubitus ulcers followed by immediate rotation flap or skin graft closure. *Ann Surg* 179:230–237, 1974.

50. Kaplan I (ed): *Proceedings of the 1st International Symposium on Laser Surgery.* Israel, November 1975, Jerusalem, Jerusalem Academic Press, 1976.

51. Kaplan I (ed): *Proceedings of the 2nd International Symposium on Laser Surgery.* Dallas, October 1977, Jerusalem, Jerusalem Academic Press, 1978.

52. *Proceedings of the 3rd International Symposium on Laser Surgery.* Graz, Austria, September 1980. To be published.

53. Jako GJ: Laser surgery of the vocal cords: An experimental study with carbon dioxide lasers on dogs. *Laryngoscope* 82:2204–2216, 1972.

54. Wallace RA, Pejchar J: 1974, Endoscopic Surgical Laser System. *US Patent,* 3, 906, 953, issued 1975.

55. Strong MS, Jako GJ, Polanyi TG, et al: Laser surgery in the aerodigestive tract. *Am J Surg* 126:529–533, 1973.

56. Polanyi TG, Wallace RA, Pejchar J: 1974, Micro-surgical laser system. *US Patent,* 3, 910, 276, issued 1975.

57. Strong MS, Jako GJ: Laser surgery in the larynx, early clinical experience with continuous CO_2 laser. *Ann Otol Rhinol Laryngol* 81:791–798, 1972.

58. Andrews AH Jr, Moss HW: Experience with the carbon dioxide laser in the larynx. *Ann Otol Rhinol Laryngol* 83:462–470, 1974.

59. Andrews AH Jr, Goldenberg RA, Moss HW, et al: Carbon dioxide laser for laryngeal surgery. *Surg Annu* 459–476, 1974.

60. French RJ: Tonsillectomy with a carbon dioxide laser: Alleviation of bleeding and pain. *National Medical Association,* New Orleans, July 29, 1974.

61. Strong MS, Vaughan CW, Polanyi TG, et al: Bronchoscopic CO_2 laser surgery. *Ann Otol Rhinol Laryngol* 83:769–776, 1974.

62. Strong MS: Laser management of premalignant lesions of the larynx. *Can J Otolaryngol* 3:4, 560–563, 1974.

63. Strong MS, Jako GJ,Vaughan CW, et al: The use of the CO_2 laser in otolaryngology: A progress report. *Trans Am Acad Ophthalmol and Otolaryngol* 82:595-602, 1976.

64. Upton RT: Carbon dioxide laser surgery in the management of CIN, *6th Annual Meeting of the Society of Gynecologic Oncologists.* Key Biscayne, Florida, 1975.

65. Bellina JH: Gynecology and the laser. *Contemp Obstet Gynecol* 4:24–34, 1974.

66. Stafl A, Wilkinson EJ, Mattingly RT: Laser treatment of cervical and vaginal neoplasia. *Am J Obstet Gynecol* 128:128–136, 1977.

67. Friedrich SG, Jr: Treating vulvar dystrophy. *Contemp Obstet Gynecol* 10:19–22, 1977.

68. Carter R, Krantz LE, Hara GS, et al: Treatment of cervical intraepithelial neoplasia with the carbon dioxide laser beam. *Am J Obstet Gynecol* 131:831–836, 1978.

2 Physics of Surgery with the CO_2 Laser

Thomas G. Polanyi, PhD

The first laser was set in operation by Theodore Maiman in 1960.[1] He was the winner in a historic race between physicists in laboratories in all technically advanced parts of the world, who were seeking to realize the predictions of other physicists that it was possible to produce light beams having an intensity far exceeding that of the sun and a spectral purity never before achieved. This had been a dream of physicists, inventors, and science fiction writers.

In the twenty years since the realization of that first laser, the ruby laser, operating in weak millisecond-duration pulses at the red edge of the visible spectrum, great advances have been made in this field. Lasers have been discovered having wavelengths from the ultraviolet to the far infrared; power and energy output of selected types of lasers were increased by many orders of magnitude, and the time domain of operation of others was broadened from the picosecond range (10^{-12} sec) or less to continuous operation (continuous wave or CW lasers). The understanding of the physics of lasers has advanced rapidly, together with the solution of the engineering and technological problems related to the fabrication of laser devices and the control of their characteristics. Major applications of lasers to physics, chemistry, engineering, technology, biology, and medicine have been developed over the past twenty years. Nevertheless, laser technology is still a young and advancing field; new types of lasers, improved laser devices, and advances in the materials needed to utilize the output of lasers, may deeply affect the range of application of lasers in medicine and elsewhere. For these reasons, those interested in utilizing lasers in surgery may profit from insight into the basic physics of lasers and the related technical problems of laser devices.

FUNDAMENTAL CHARACTERISTICS OF LASER LIGHT SOURCES

Lasers are devices that emit light or, more generally, electromagnetic (EM) radiation. The unique characteristic of lasers that sets them apart from any non-laser source, is that all the energy they emit is contained in a narrow, almost parallel beam that is exceedingly monochromatic (Figure 2-1). Parallel monochromatic light is called coherent light. *The unique characteristic of laser devices is that they emit coherent light.* As a conse-

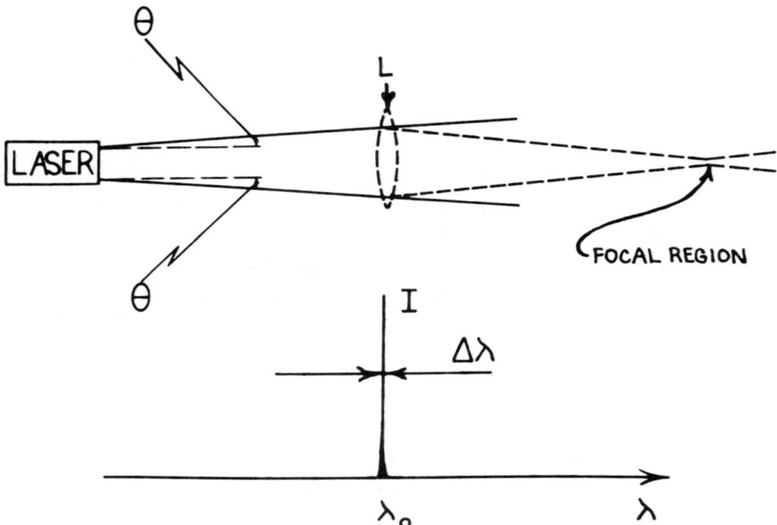

Figure 2-1 Fundamental characteristics of laser light sources are 1) all energy is emitted in a parallel bundle (θ very small). Therefore, the lens L can concentrate all the energy emitted by the laser into its focal region, and 2) wavelength spread $\Delta\lambda$ is much smaller than for any non-laser source.

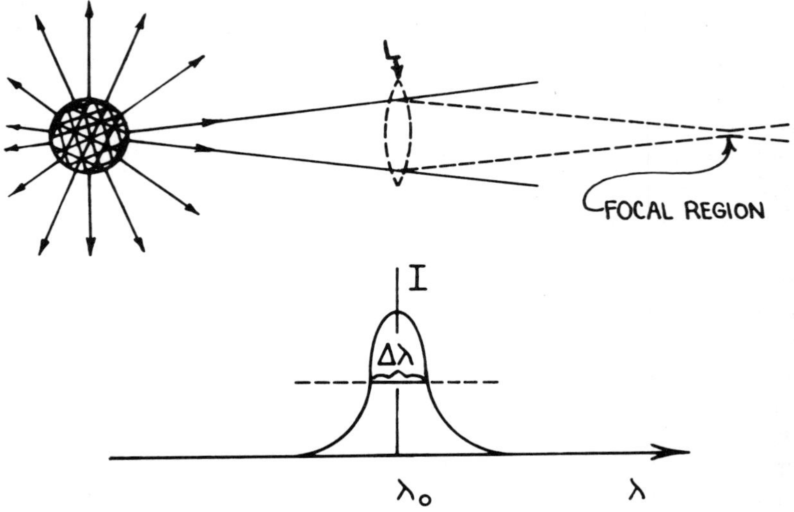

Figure 2-2 Extended light sources (non-laser light sources). Light is emitted from each point into all directions; the lens L can concentrate into its focal region only a small fraction of the energy emitted by this source. The wavelength spread is much larger than for laser sources.

quence of the parallelism, all the energy emitted by a laser can be concentrated in the focal spot of a lens. In this focal spot, whose diameter can be very small, an extremely high power density* can be obtained, of a magnitude higher than that obtainable from any non-laser source. The reason for this is that light from any non-laser source originates from a large assembly of points (extended source), all of which radiate into all directions in space. A lens can concentrate into its focal region only the light reaching it from a vanishingly small region of the source and, therefore, only a small fraction of the energy emitted by non-laser source can be concentrated in the focal region of a lens (Figure 2-2). The novelty and the extraordinary usefulness of laser light sources become even more apparent from the following considerations:

1. Many applications, including surgery, require high radiant power density in selected regions of the EM spectrum.
2. High intensity laser sources exist in regions of the spectrum for which non-laser or natural sources of radiation are not known, eg, in the ultraviolet (UV) or the infrared.

*Power density is measured in such units as calories/sec/cm^2, joules/sec/cm^2 or W/cm^2.

LASER DEVICES AND GENERATION OF LIGHT BY A LASER

Laser Devices, An Overview

Laser light, as any light, originates from a selected assembly of atoms, molecules, or ions. These particles may be in the gaseous phase as is the case in gas lasers, or they may be dispersed in solids of liquids to form other types of lasers. In all cases, to obtain energy output in the form of coherent light, energy must be supplied to the system. This energy is needed to excite the particles to particular energy states. This process is called *pumping* the laser. Gas lasers are generally pumped by producing an electrical discharge in the gas, solid lasers by powerful light sources. When the selected material system, the laser medium, is pumped, it becomes the *active laser medium.* The most important property of the active medium is that it can cause an increase in the intensity of a beam of electromagnetic radiation that is traveling through it—it can amplify light. The active medium, however, can only amplify electromagnetic radiation having a particular wavelength. The wavelength, which can be amplified by the active medium, is determined by the atomic and molecular structure of the medium. Note that in all common experience the intensity of light traversing a medium is either affected very little (the medium is transparent) or is decreased by absorption and scattering in the medium. Laser light is generated when the active laser medium, usually in the shape of a long narrow cylinder, is terminated by two mirrors, one at each end (Figure 2-3). These mirrors have a common axis coincident with the axis of the active medium. The two mirrors, as defined, and the space in between are called the *optical cavity*, or, for reasons which will become more apparent later, the *resonant cavity.* Light waves of the appropriate wavelength propagating along the axis of the cylinder will be amplified as they travel along this axis. The intensity of the wave continues to increase as it is reflected back and forth between the two mirrors until an equilibrium intensity is reached. One of the mirrors is partially transmitting and the laser output is obtained through it. The output is directed along the axis of the system. Further insight into the operation of a laser requires reviewing certain properties of matter and of electromagnetic energy. This review and the additional material presented in Appendix I will clarify further the nature of an active laser medium, and the concept of resonant cavity. Some of the technical problems related to the fabrication of laser devices will also be touched upon in this Appendix. The major objective of Appendix I is to explain the process of light amplification by simulated emission of radiation, which has led to the acronym, *laser.* The assimilation of the concepts presented in Appendix I may present a challenge to many readers, and can be left for a second reading. The factual material needed more directly as a guide to the use of lasers in surgery is presented in the following sections.

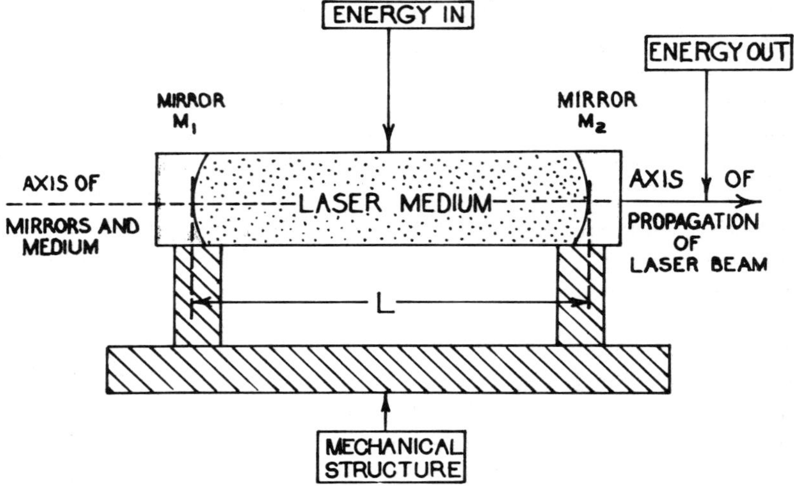

Figure 2-3 The basic components of any laser are 1) a laser medium, 2) a source of energy called the laser *pump*, 3) the optical cavity formed by M_1 and M_2 and the space in between, 4) a mechanical structure to make the axes of mirrors M_1 and M_2 coincident. Laser light leaves the cavity through mirror M_2, which is partially transmitting.

Common Construction Features of Laser Devices

All laser light sources have the following components illustrated in Figure 2-3:

- A laser medium
- A source of energy
- An optical cavity
- A mechanical structure.

The laser medium usually has the shape of a long narrow cylinder. For gaseous media, the length of the cylinder varies from a few tens of centimeters to several meters, with a cross section from a few millimeters to about one centimeter in the longer lasers. A solid laser medium of interest in surgery today is the neodymium ion dispersed in a crystalline rod of yttrium-aluminum-garnet (YAG). The length of such a rod is at most 15 centimeters with a diameter of a few millimeters.

The source of energy activates or pumps the laser medium. Gas lasers are activated by producing an electrical discharge in the gas. The gas pressure of the laser medium and current density through the medium must be carefully controlled to excite the atoms or molecules to certain desired energy states by the pump energy. Solid lasers are generally crystals or glasses and can be pumped only by powerful light sources. The solid absorbs a portion of the output of the light source and is thereby activated.

The optical cavity is formed by mirrors located at both ends of the laser medium. These mirrors can be plane or spherical; the axes perpendicular to the two mirrors must coincide and also be coincident with the axis of the cylindrical laser medium. One of the mirrors is made as reflective as possible, approximating 100%, the other partially transmitting at the wavelength of operation of the laser. The laser beam propagates along the common axis of mirrors and medium, and is emitted through the partially transmitting mirror.

As the length of the optical cavity is decreased from meters to a few tens of centimeters, the length of the cavity must also be rigidly controlled to avoid severe fluctuations of the power output. This implies in varying degrees the use of materials with small coefficients of thermal expansion, control of the ambient temperature and of the operating temperature of the cavity or other means.

The mechanical structure ensures that the mirrors are properly aligned and maintain their alignment during the operation of the laser, when large amounts of power are dissipated within the laser medium. Since only a fraction of the pump energy can be transformed into a coherent laser beam, most of the unused pump energy causes heating of the laser medium. For all lasers used in surgery, the pump energy that must be dissipated as heat is so large that the medium must be cooled by forced circulation of air or water.

Laser Types Used in Surgery

Many types of lasers exist and their number is increasing; the fundamental difference between types is their wavelength of operation. There are lasers at numerous locations in the electromagnetic spectrum, from the vacuum ultraviolet to the submillimeter region in the infrared. Lasers may also differ in the temporal characteristics of their output; some emit continuously (CW lasers), while others characteristically emit energy in pulses lasting less than one millisecond. There is also a great variability in the efficiency of lasers, ie, the fraction of pump energy recovered in the form of coherent light. It will be shown in later sections that for applications to surgery, specifically tissue removal and localized tissue devitalization, lasers are required that operate at a wavelength whose primary effect on tissues is heating. This leads to lasers operating in the visible and in the infrared regions of the spectrum. Lasers are needed, with rare exceptions, that operate in the continuous mode at high power levels from about one-half watt to many tens of watts. At the higher end of this power range, the efficiency of the laser becomes important for practical reasons. These requirements have limited the lasers used in surgery to a very few types; their spectral locations are shown in Figure 2-4 and a short description of each type follows. The carbon dioxide laser is described in detail.

Argon ion laser This is a CW gas laser operating in the blue at 0.48 μ. The active medium is ionized argon. Excitation is obtained by producing an electrical discharge in the gas. A very high current density is needed for pumping this laser. The efficiency of this laser is low, about 0.1%. This laser is used extensively in ophthalmic surgery and is likely to find applications in other areas of microsurgery and endoscopic surgery.

Ruby laser This laser emits at 0.69 μ, at the red edge of the visible, characteristically in the pulsed mode. The laser medium is a dilute solution of chromium ions in a single crystal of alumina. Activation is obtained by high intensity light pulses. This first of all lasers was for many years the only high power laser producing visible light. It was used extensively for the treatment of retinal lesions until about 1970. Experimental surgery in other areas was attempted with this laser with limited success.

Neodymium in yttrium-aluminum-garnet (Nd-YAG) Laser emission from neodymium ions in a solid host takes place at 1.06 μ. When the

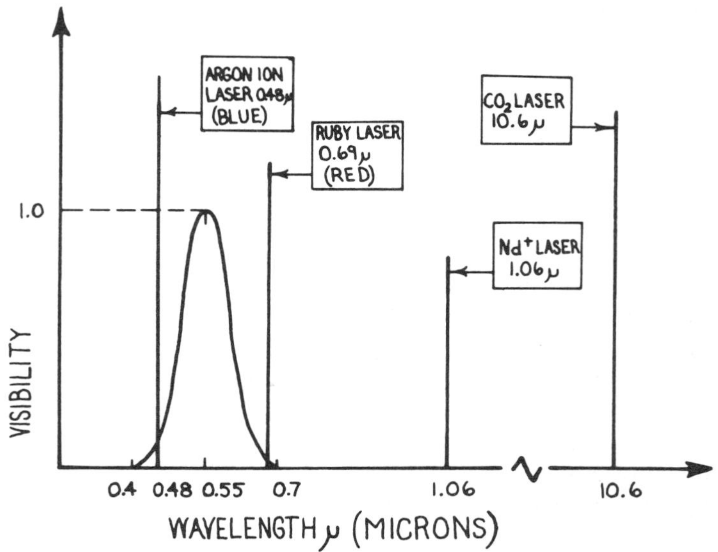

Figure 2-4 Wavelengths of principal lasers used in surgery. The curve is the standard light visibility curve of the eye. It is at a maximum in the green at 0.55 μ and it is zero at 0.4 μ, which is the boundary of the UV and at 0.7 μ, which is the boundary of the infrared (1 μ = 10 cm^{-4}).

host is a single crystal of yttrium-aluminum-garnet, high power, pulsed, or CW emissions up to hundreds of watts can be obtained. If the host is glass, only pulsed emission is obtained. Excitation is obtained by strong light, continuous, or pulsed. Efficiency of this laser is fairly high, around 1%. Radiation at 1.06 μ penetrates several millimeters in tissues, and applications to surgery must be extremely selective.

Carbon dioxide laser This gas laser emits at about 10.6 μ. The laser medium is carbon dioxide with added nitrogen and helium; the optimal proportions of these gases are approximately 0.8:1:7 and depend upon the details of the laser device. Activation of the medium is by an electrical discharge. The pressure of the gas mixture varies from about 10 mm of Hg to a few 100 mm of Hg depending upon the diameter of the tube. The discharge current is typically one or two milliamperes per square millimeter of discharge. Voltage depends upon tube diameter and varies from approximately 5,000 V to 15,000 V/m of discharge, the voltage per unit of length increasing with decreasing diameter of the discharge tube.

The CO_2 laser is the most efficient laser known. Efficiencies of 10% to 15% are common. This high efficiency is associated with two characteristics of this system: 1) the energy levels of the CO_2 molecules giving rise to the emission are very close to the lowest energy state of the CO_2 molecule and can, therefore, be excited very efficiently, and 2) by a fortuitous circumstance, the addition of N_2 selectively and efficiently transfers the pump energy to the energy level of the CO_2 molecule from which laser emission is obtained. There are also some difficulties associated with this laser. In the gas discharge, the CO_2 molecule dissociates into CO and O, thus depleting the active material. To overcome this loss, the gas in the discharge tube is replaced by continuously flowing gas into the discharge tube from high pressure reservoirs and exhausting it into the air by means of a vacuum pump. In the discharge tube, the desired steady state pressure is maintained by balancing the inflow and outflow of gases with pressure-reducing valves and orifices. With increasing volume of gas flow, the output power increases. Rapid gas removal from the discharge region is one of the major engineering problems associated with industrial CO_2 lasers operating at output powers of many kilowatts. Another problem specific to CO_2 lasers is that temperature elevation of the gas decreases the output power of the laser. The He, which is added to the CO_2 and N_2 mixture in large amounts, serves to transfer heat to the walls of the discharge tube, which are cooled by a rapid flow of water or air. A typical CO_2 laser as described is illustrated in Figure 2-5.

Sealed-off CO_2 lasers The desire to operate CO_2 lasers without the complication of reservoirs and circulating pumps, stimulated investigations aimed at reversing the dissociation process taking place in the gas discharge.[2] Several such methods have been developed and sealed-off gas

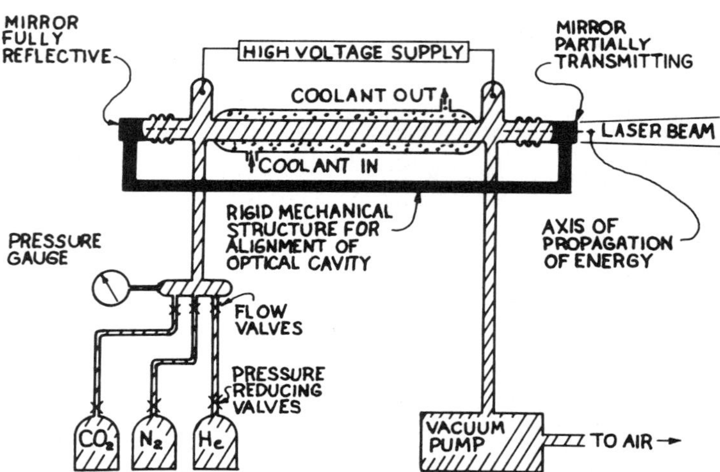

Figure 2-5 Typical carbon dioxide laser. The active medium is a low pressure mixture of carbon dioxide, nitrogen, and helium gases admitted into the laser cavity through pressure-reducing valves from high pressure tanks, and exhausted to air by a vacuum pump. The laser pump is a high voltage supply that provides a gas discharge. Cooling of the discharge tube is accomplished with air or water. The fully reflective mirror is generally a polished metal. Materials such as germanium, zinc selenide, gallium arsenide, etc, with a partially reflective coating, must be used for the partially transmitting mirror.

lasers with long life are becoming commercially available, particularly in the lower, less than 20-watt power range. In this lower power range, the sealed-off lasers are generally of the waveguide type; the discharge takes place in a narrow tube of approximately a few millimeters in diameter and the discharge tube acts as a waveguide. The gas discharge is produced either with DC or with radio frequency voltages.

The efficiency of these lasers is generally less than that of conventional flowing systems. Their use in surgery will be determined by the convenience of the overall system for selected applications.

Pulsed carbon dioxide lasers By using appropriate voltage pulses, carbon dioxide lasers can be made to emit high power pulses lasting a few milliseconds or less.[3] For this mode of operation, the ratio of peak to average power is generally very high. Beckman et al[4,5] have described a rapid pulsed laser, sometimes called a superpulsed laser, for use in ophthalmic surgery. High power and short exposure times limit heat spread to surrounding tissues (see Chapter 28 and Appendix IV, this chapter). Blood loss with pulsed CO_2 lasers is generally more pronounced than with continuous wave CO_2 lasers.[6]

Power Density in the Focal Spot of a Laser Beam

Laser types differ by their wavelength of operation; a qualitative difference. Lasers of the same wavelength still may differ in other characteristics. For the surgical applications of a given type of CO_2 laser, however, the basic characteristics of importance are only two: maximum output power and intensity distribution within the laser beam.

Power The maximum output power of carbon dioxide lasers discussed here depends on essentially only the length of the discharge. For optimized CO_2 lasers, the output power is about 60 W/m. The actual length of the laser can be shorter than the length of the discharge since the optical cavity can be folded with mirrors.

Intensity distribution within the beam All lasers emit a parallel, monochromatic beam of electromagnetic radiation. Nevertheless, there can be profound differences in the detailed structure of the laser beam. These differences are best revealed by investigating the intensity distribution, which is obtained when the laser beam impinges on a surface that is perpendicular to its direction of propagation (Figure 2-6). This would be the situation when a laser beam is directed at a tissue plane "straight on"

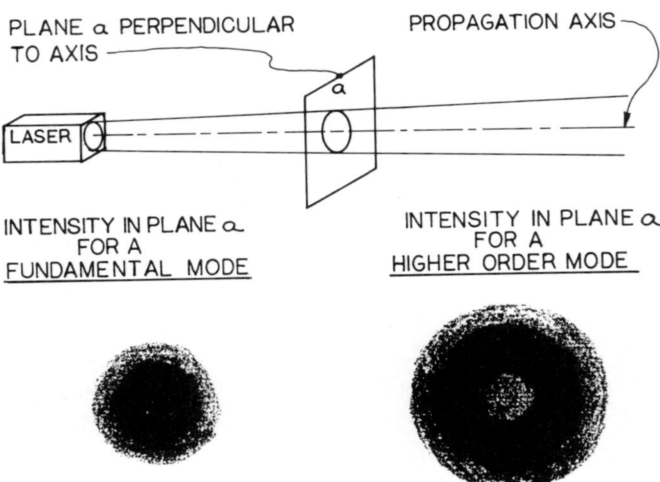

Figure 2-6 Intensity distributions in laser beams. A laser beam is shown passing through a plane perpendicular to its axis of propagation. When the laser beam is composed of visible light and a white sheet of paper is placed in the position of the plane, one of a variety of light intensity patterns can be seen on the paper. The shape of this pattern depends upon the *mode* in which the laser is operating. Two such shapes are shown in this figure. The dark areas are regions of highest intensity. For lasers producing invisible radiation, the intensity pattern can be made visible by other means.

rather than obliquely. Without the benefit of any experience, one would intuitively expect to see, if the laser operates in the visible region of the spectrum, an intense small circular spot of light. One would not be surprised to see a maximum of intensity at the center of the spot, and a more or less gradual decrease to zero of the intensity when moving away from the center of the spot. This intuitive expectation is indeed quite correct,

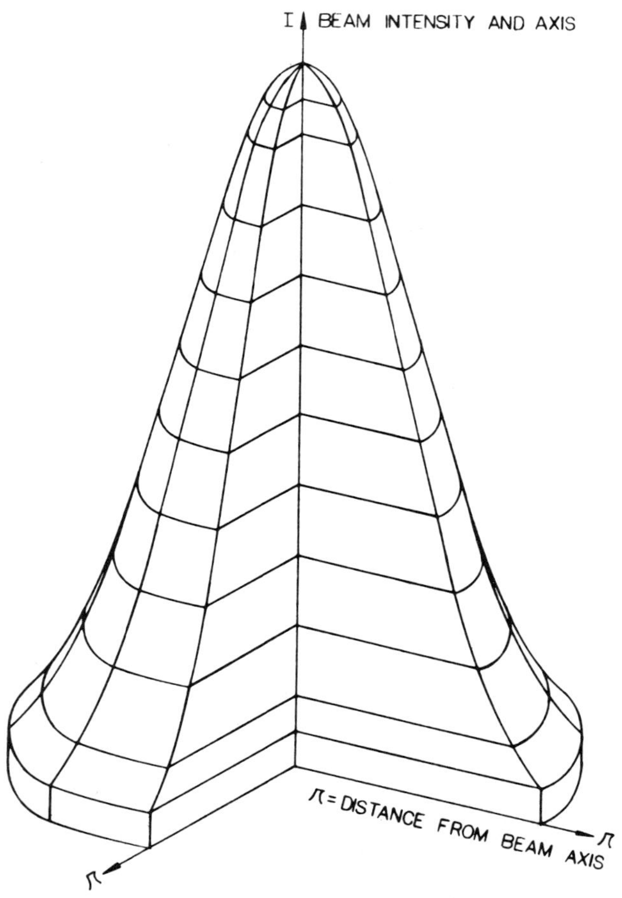

Figure 2-7A Three dimensional representation of the intensity distribution of a (0,0) mode in a plane perpendicular to the axis of the beam. This is a quantitative representation of the intensity pattern shown in the lower left corner of Figure 2-6. The maximum intensity is located along the propagation axis, which is at the center of the beam. In any direction perpendicular to this axis at a distance r from it, the intensity decreases as the error curve shown in Figure 2-7B. The bell-shaped intensity pattern of a (0,0) mode causes the inverted bell-shaped defects often produced when a soft absorbing material or soft biological tissue is exposed to a CO_2 laser beam.

and the only additional insight offered by a mathematical analysis of the problem is an exact description of how the intensity of the spot decreases away from its center where it is at its maximum. The intensity decreases like the Gaussian or error curve and theoretically, is zero only at infinity. A three dimensional diagram of intensity would look like a bell (Figure 2-7A). The intensity distribution shown in Figure 2-7A is advantageous in many applications of lasers; its relevance in surgery will be discussed in the next section. It is not, however, the only possible one.

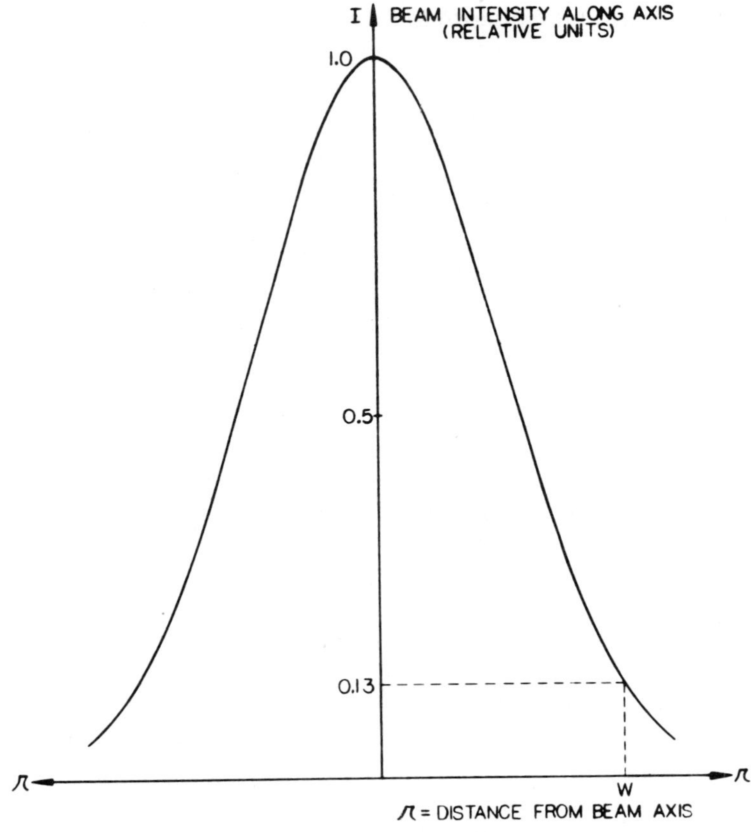

Figure 2-7B Intensity distribution in a (0,0) mode laser beam. This figure shows the intensity distribution along any line which crosses the laser beam axis in a plane perpendicular to the axis. If one cuts the bell-shaped surface of Figure 2-7A with any plane containing the laser beam axis, one also obtains the curve of Figure 2-7B. If the plane on which the laser beam impinges is moved farther away from the laser, the intensity pattern becomes larger because the laser beam spreads. However, the light intensity in a plane perpendicular to the beam axis is still described by Figures 2-7A, B. In any such plane, the distance from the beam axis, *w*, at which the intensity has decreased to 13% of the peak intensity, is called the laser beam radius.

Indeed, many other types of intensity distributions are possible. Their shapes are beyond intuition, but they can be described by mathematical analysis of the physics problem.* The bell-shaped distribution shown in Figure 2-7A and 2-7B is called the fundamental or lowest order mode, or the (0,0) or TEM_{00}† mode.

Another intensity distribution that frequently occurs is shown in- Figures 2-8A and 2-8B. The intensity is zero along the axis, increases as one moves away from the (dark) center of the spot, it reaches maximum some distance away from the center, and then decays to zero in a fashion similar but not equal to the (0,0) mode. This mode or intensity distribution is best designated with the colloquial but highly descriptive word

*One may have an intuitive feeling for the existence of these intensity distributions, or *modes* as they are called, by thinking of the optical cavity as a resonator for electromagnetic waves—a resonator whose dimensions are extremely large compared to the wavelength of light. Inside the resonator, the field must be stationary since we have a constant output from the cavity; but since the wavelengths are so small, one can well imagine that the standing wave configurations can assume a variety of shapes or modes.

†TEM stands for transverse electromagnetic field; transverse because the intensity variations take place in a direction transverse to the direction of propagation.

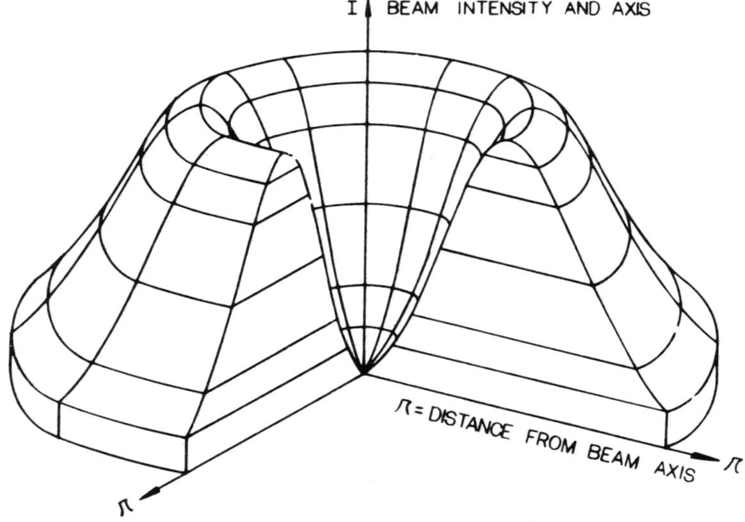

Figure 2-8A Three dimensional representation of the intensity distributions of a donut mode in a plane perpendicular to the axis of the beam. This is a quantitative representation of the intensity pattern shown in the lower right corner of Figure 2-6. This figure has the same significance for a donut mode as Figure 2-7A does for a (0,0) mode. Figures 2-7 and 2-8 may be used to compare the intensity distribution of (0,0) and donut modes of laser beams that contain the same total power and have propagated the same distance from a particular laser. The donut mode of Figure 2-8 has zero intensity along the beam axis, and a lower peak intensity than the (0,0) mode of Figure 2-7.

"donut" mode.‡ Figures 2-7B and 2-8B are drawn to scale for two laser beams generated in the same optical cavity and having the same total power. Some other types of intensity distributions are shown in Figure 2-9. A few of the simpler ones are sometimes seen in commercial carbon dioxide lasers.

Operation of a laser in one transverse mode or another depends on a multitude of parameters, principally: the length and the diameter of the optical cavity, the radii or curvature of the mirrors, and the uniformity of

‡It is sometimes, not quite correctly, designated as a (0,1) or $TEM_{0,1}$ mode.

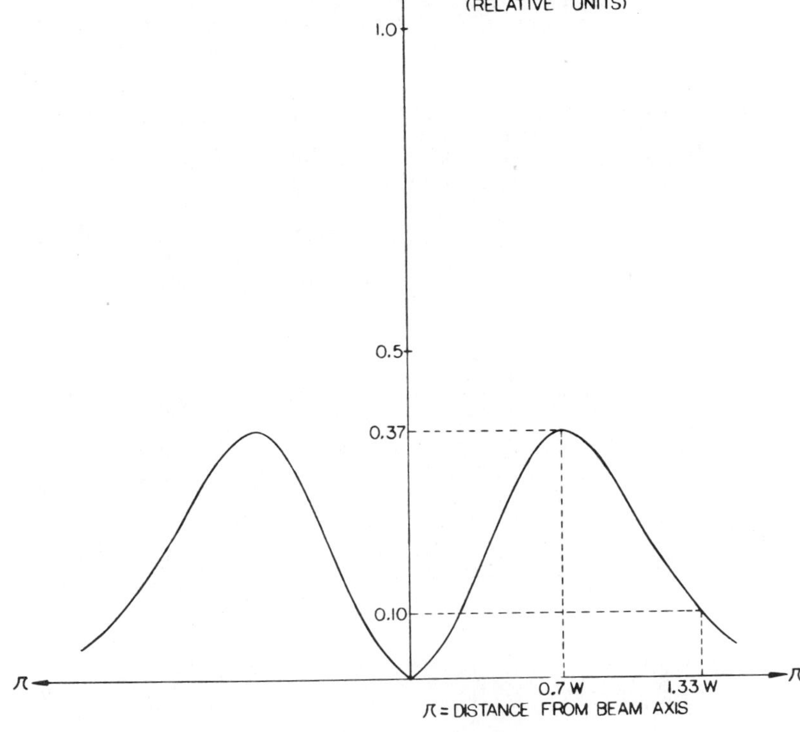

Figure 2-8B Intensity distributions in a donut mode laser beam. This figure is related to Figure 2-8A as Figure 2-7B is related to Figure 2-7A. Figures 2-8B and 2-7B are drawn to the same scale in order to make it easy to compare the intensity distributions of sets of figures. Note that the peak intensity of the donut mode is 0.37 times less than that of the equivalent (0,0) mode, but that the intensity of the donut mode is appreciably higher than that of the (0,0) mode at distances greater than 0.7 *w* from the beam axis. The distance 1.33 *w* from the beam axis at which the intensity of the donut mode has decreased to 27% of its peak intensity is called the radius of the donut mode. The value of *w* is the same as that used in Figure 2-7B to describe the (0,0) mode.

the active medium. Any of the modes shown and many others are "legitimate" laser modes; however, one mode may be more useful than another for a given application. It is quite possible for one laser to operate in several modes at the same time, or to switch modes in rapid or slow succession as a consequence of thermal changes in the cavity. If the cavity mirrors are not in good alignment or there is lack of uniformity of the ac-

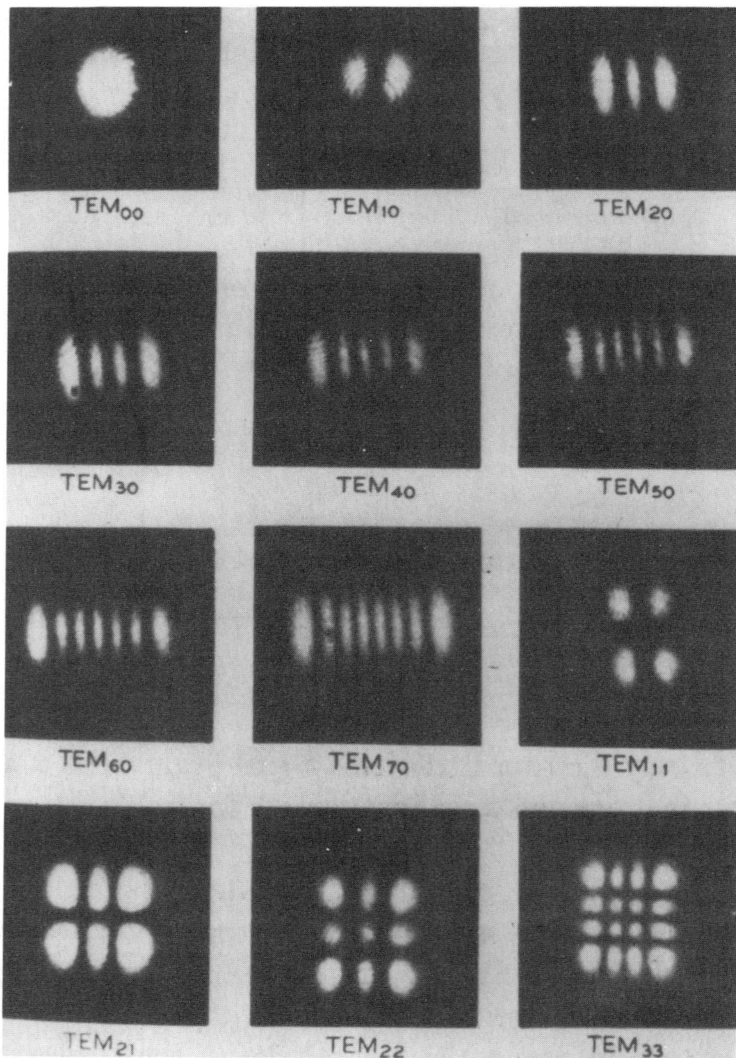

Figure 2-9 Mode patterns. Some of the many possible modes of a laser with their designations. Copyright © 1966 IEEE. (Reproduced by permission from Kogelink H, Li T: Laser beams and resonators. *Proc of the IEEE* 54(10):1312–1329, 1966.)

tive medium, the laser beam may exhibit intensity distributions quite different from the ones illustrated. These modes generally lack symmetry and can be called anomalous or "pathologic." They are generally less useful in applications than modes with good symmetry, and sometimes even unusable.

Intensity and power density It is important to discuss in more detail the meaning and implications for surgery of the intensity distribution curves. As shown in Figures 2-7A and 2-7B, the beam intensity is the highest at the center of the spot and decreases further away from it. The reason for this is that the energy impinging per unit time on a small circular area *a* surrounding the center of the beam is larger than the energy impinging per unit time on an equal circular area *b* located within the spot further away from the center (Figure 2-10).

The beam intensity measures the amount of energy per unit time, or power, impinging on the small area *a*. The ratio of the power *P* to the area *a* on which it impinges is, by definition, the *power density* and is numerically equal to power per unit area. It is important to realize that the intensity distribution in the laser beam and the total power *P* are

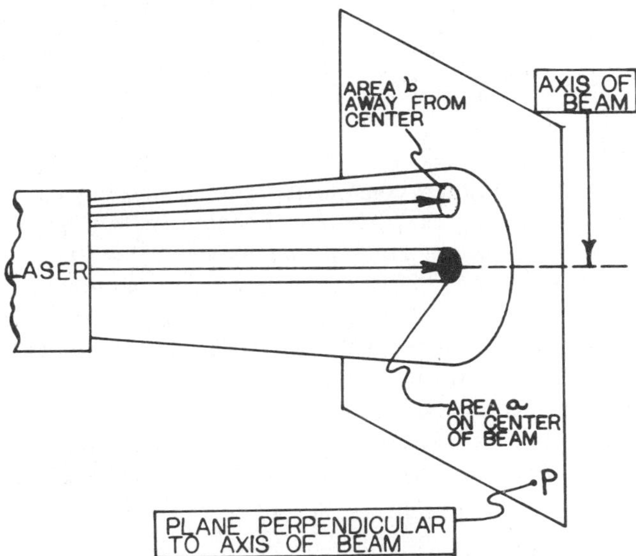

Figure 2-10 Intensity and power density. Figure 2-10 shows the beam from a laser operating in the (0,0) mode striking a plane *P*, which is perpendicular to the axis of the beam. Within the beam on plane *P* are two equal small areas, *a* and *b*. Area *a* is centered on the axis of the beam, while area *b* is at some distance from the axis of the beam. The laser beam is more intense in area *a* than it is in area *b*. The energy arriving at either *a* or *b* per unit time divided by the area is called the power density at *a* or *b*. The power density and the intensity in a (0,0) mode laser beam are both at maximum on the beam axis and decrease to zero at the edge of the beam.

characteristics of the laser and of the mode in which it operates. When the laser beam impinges on a surface (perpendicular to the direction of propagation of the beam), the total energy of the laser will be contained in the spot thus formed, while the energy distribution within the spot will mirror the intensity in the beam. In this sense, beam intensity and power density have similar meanings. The power density is inversely proportional to the area of the spot; if an optical system is used to focus the laser beam, the power density in the focused spot is inversely proportional to the square of the working distance, as is shown in later sections.

When electromagnetic energy is applied to tissues for a short period of time (the exposure time), the effect depends on the amount of energy interacting with *unit volume* of tissue per unit time. The volume interacting with the laser beam has a shape that is approximately cylindrical with a circular cross section of area A equal to the laser beam spot size and depth d related to the absorptive properties of tissues (see the section on quantitative interaction). The energy E delivered to this volume penetrates into the volume through its face A and equals the total power P in the beam multiplied by the exposure time t. The energy E_o delivered to the *unit volume* of tissue is given by:

$$E_o = \frac{P \times t}{V} = \frac{P \times t}{A \times d} = \frac{P}{A} \times \frac{1}{d} \times t$$

Thus, the energy interacting with unit volume of tissue is proportional to the power density in the beam and not to the total power P in the beam.

Surgery with CO_2 lasers consists of vaporizing rapidly and with control, selected tissue volumes. The energy required for vaporization is supplied by the laser beam. The formula above indicates that the power density in the beam is one of the parameters determining the energy supplied to the unit volume of tissue. Both peak and average power density in a laser beam are different for different modes; hence, the relevance to surgery of the modal properties of laser beams.

A more detailed analysis of the power density distributions in the (0,0) and donut modes is presented in Appendix II. In summary: in a (0,0) mode, the peak power density is on the axis of the laser beam and equals $\frac{2P}{\pi w^2}$ where P is the total beam power and w is the spot size of the laser beam. In a donut mode, the peak power density is on a circle centered on the axis of the beam and is zero on the axis. The peak power density of the (0,0) mode is 2.7 times that of the donut mode produced by the same laser and of equal total power. The average power density of the (0,0) mode is 1.8 times higher than that of the donut mode, the average being taken over the beam spot sizes, which are appropriate for each of these modes.

Laser beam spot size As Figures 2-7A, B and 2-8A, B indicate, the power density in a plane perpendicular to the axis of propagation of the laser beam reaches a maximum on the axis (for a [0,0] mode) and is zero theoretically only infinitely far from the axis of the laser beam; for a donut mode, there is another zero of power on the axis of the beam. It is clear, therefore, that a definition of spot size is needed. A generally accepted definition is the circular area centered on the axis of the beam that contains 86% of the total power in the beam. The radius of this circle w is called the beam radius (see Appendix III for more details).

Focusing of laser beams Tissue removal with a CO_2 laser requires that the laser beam be focused on the tissue site to be operated on. The power density distribution in the focal spot is a replica in smaller dimension of the power density distribution that is obtained in any plane perpendicular to the laser beam axis. It follows that the power density distribution in the focal spot is still given by Figures 2-7A, B for a (0,0) mode or Figures 2-8A, B for a donut mode. The smallest spot size w_0 attainable by focusing a (0,0) mode laser beam is given by:

$$w_0 = 0.6 \frac{\lambda}{D} f_w, \qquad \text{where:}$$

λ = wavelength of operation
D = laser beam diameter
f_w = working distance

Formally stated: The smallest spot size w_0 is directly proportional to the wavelength of the laser and to the distance f_w from the lens to the focal point; it is inversely proportional to the diameter of the cross sectional area of the beam at the focusing lens (see Figure 2-11). This formula gives the theoretically smallest possible value of w_0. Any non-ideality in the system will make w_0 larger. If the same optical system is used to focus a donut mode, from the same laser, the minimal spot size is $1.33 \times w_0$ (see Appendix II).

Example: A laser beam in the (0,0) mode is focused by appropriate lenses at the working distances f_w of 50, 200, 300 and 400 mm. In each case, the diameter of the beam at the lens is 1 cm.

The smallest possible radii w_0 at these working distances for a CO_2 laser and an argon ion laser are obtained from this formula using the indicated values of f_w in mm, setting $D = 10$ mm and $\lambda = 10.6 \times 10^{-3}$mm for the CO_2 laser and $\lambda = 0.48 \times 10^{-3}$ mm for the A^+ laser. The results are given in Table 2-1.

Table 2-1
Radii w_0 (mm) of laser beams focused at the distance f_w:

f_w(mm)	50	200	300	400
CO_2 laser	0.03	0.13	0.19	0.254
A^+ laser	0.0013	0.006	0.008	0.01

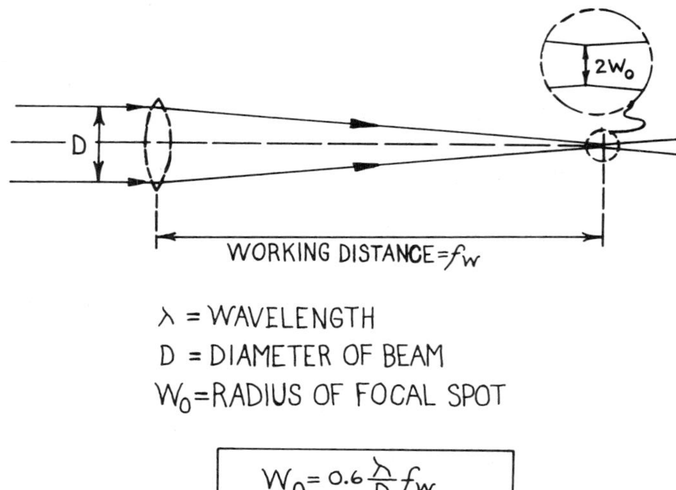

Figure 2-11 Focusing of a laser beam.

If the laser operates in the donut mode, all other conditions being unchanged, the above values of *w* must be multiplied by 1.33.

INTERACTIONS OF ELECTROMAGNETIC ENERGY WITH MATTER

Qualitative Interaction

Electromagnetic radiant energy stretches over an immense range of frequencies (wavelengths). At the high frequency end are the x-rays having wavelengths down to 0.01 Å or less; at the low frequency are the radio waves with wavelengths of kilometers. The diverse interactions that take place when radiant energy impinges on matter depend exclusively on the frequency of the electromagnetic energy. This can be made plausible intuitively with the following considerations:

1) Electromagnetic radiant energy can be thought of as composed of photons whose individual energies E are given by the expression:

$$E = h\nu,$$

where:

h = Planck's constant = 6.63×10^{-34} joule-sec
ν = frequency, cycles per sec

2) The effect of electromagnetic energy on matter is a result of interactions of individual photons with individual atoms or molecules. If the photon has sufficient energy to ionize an atom, eg, ionization can take place, the number of ionizations will be proportional to the number of photons having the required energy. If the photon energy is not sufficient to ionize a given atomic species, however, no ionization will take place irrespective of the number of photons present in the electromagnetic field.

A portion of the electromagnetic spectrum extending for eight decades in frequency (wavelengths) is shown in Figure 2-12. Broad regions of the spectrum have traditionally been assigned names: x-rays, ultraviolet, visible, infrared, etc. These are indicated in the figure. The prevalent types of interaction of radiation with matter are also shown. The frequency limits of these interactions are not sharply defined and may overlap. The locations in the spectrum of the lasers most often used in surgery are indicated. They are all in the visible and in the infrared. Many

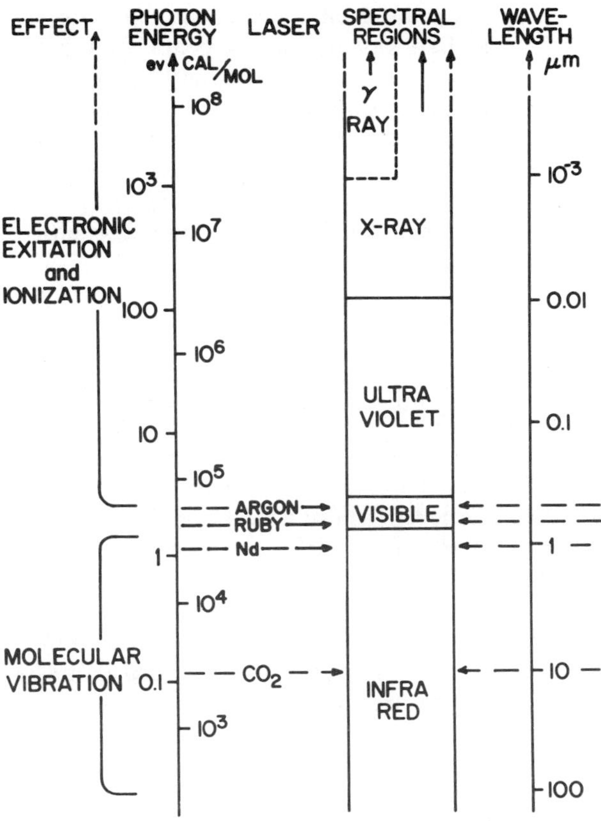

Figure 2-12 A portion of the electromagnetic spectrum showing location of the wavelengths of the lasers most used in surgery.

photochemical effects essential to life take place in the visible portion of the spectrum. Nevertheless, the major effect of electromagnetic radiation on biological materials in this region, and further in the infrared, is thermal in nature; ionization and radical formation are absent. Heating of biological materials follows the excitation of molecular vibrational and rotational energy levels.

Quantitative Interaction

The quantitative interactions of electromagnetic energy with matter, ie, the interactions that depend on the intensity of the radiation, or the number of photons in the electromagnetic field, is discussed best by introducing the two related concepts of coefficient of absorption and extinction length. In Figure 2-13, a beam of radiant energy of intensity I_0 impinges on a thin slab of material of thickness x. The slab need not be physically isolated; it can be mentally isolated from a larger volume. In general, the following happens: part of the beam is reflected, part is absorbed in the material and interacts with it, and part is transmitted. The reflected portion does not interact with the material. For simplicity, we will ignore the reflected beam in our considerations. I_0 in Figure 2-13 denotes the incident beam less the reflected beam.* If the transmitted beam has the intensity I, the amount of energy interacting with the material is $I_0 - I$. In general, the intensity of the transmitted and of the incident beams are related by Beer's law:

$$I = I_0 e^{-\alpha x}$$

e = base of natural logarithm (2.7 . . .)

The coefficient of absorption is denoted as α. If x is measured in centimeters, α must be expressed in reciprocal centimeters, cm^{-1}; if x is measured in millimeters, α is expressed in reciprocal millimeters; $e^{-\alpha x}$ gives the ratio of I to I_0. The coefficient of absorption is a measure of the effectiveness of the thickness x of material to attenuate electromagnetic radiation. It also indicates the strength of the interaction between electromagnetic radiation and the selected material. The coefficient α is a function of the wavelength λ of the incident radiation, and the chemical composition and physical state of the material (denser material absorbs more strongly since there are more molecules per unit volume, liquid water, eg, absorbs more than water vapor even though the chemical composition of the two substances is the same).

---

*Electromagnetic energy of the wavelength of the CO_2 laser (10.6 μ) is minimally reflected by biological tissues. Metals reflect very strongly at this wavelength (see Chapter 3, Hazards and Safety Considerations).

It is useful to introduce the quantity L called extinction length, which has an immediate physical meaning. It is defined here as the thickness L of material that absorbs 90% of the incident energy. If a slab of material of thickness L is followed by a second slab of the same thickness, the intensity incident on this second slab is 10% of the initial intensity I_0 incident on the first slab. Since the second slab will also absorb 90% of the radiation incident on it, the total radiation transmitted by the thickness $2L$ of material is therefore 1% of the radiation incident on the first slab. Equivalently, one can say that a thickness $2L$ of material absorbs 99% of the incident energy. The extinction length is related to the coefficient of absorption by the simple relation $L = 2.3/\alpha$; the larger the α, the thinner is the thickness of material that absorbs 90% of the incident energy.

The absorptive properties of tissues have a fundamental role in the applications of lasers to surgery. In principle, the coefficient of absorption of a material is determined by measuring the intensity, at the wavelength λ, of the beam I_0, which impinges on the thickness x of

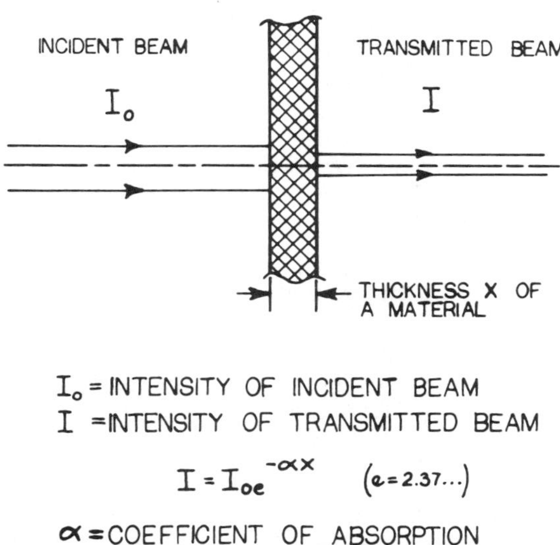

Figure 2-13 Absorption of electromagnetic energy. The beam I exiting from the thickness x of material is shown thinner to symbolize the fact that it is less intense than the incident beam I_0. The coefficient α depends on the wavelength of the incident radiation and on the chemical composition and physical state of the material slab whose thickness is x.

material and that of the beam I that is transmitted (Figure 2-13). *It is assumed that the intensity of the radiation is sufficiently low so as not to alter the physical and chemical properties of the material.*

Coefficients of absorption of biological tissues in vivo are generally not known and, at best, difficult to measure. They are inferred from in vitro measurements and other considerations. The diffuse reflectance of the skin for visible light has been measured extensively.[7] At the wavelength of the CO_2 laser, it is approximately 5% at very low intensities. For visible light only, the color of an organ is a good indication of absorptive properties. White fatty tissue, for example, which diffusely reflects all visible light, will absorb only little at the blue wavelength of the argon ion laser; blood, on the other hand, which is red and because it strongly absorbs in the blue green, will strongly absorb the radiation of the A^+ laser. Cornea, crystalline, vitreous humor, are obviously transparent to visible light, while the retina strongly absorbs it. For these reasons lasers operating in the visible can be used for surgery of the retina without affecting the tissues in front of it. This is the only case in which electromagnetic radiation can be used to operate on a remote organ leaving intact the tissues surrounding it. This, of course, is the uniqueness of the organ of vision.

In general, it is necessary to investigate experimentally the effect of a laser on tissues not only because the coefficients of absorption are not known, but, more importantly, because at the high intensities of radiation used in surgery, tissues may undergo modifications that cause strong changes of the coefficient of absorption during irradiation. As an example, white fatty tissue (or a white piece of paper) has a very low but not zero coefficient of absorption for the blue radiation of the argon laser. At very high intensities the small fraction of energy absorbed may be sufficient to form a thin layer of carbonized tissue, thereby increasing dramatically and irreversibly the absorption properties of white tissue or paper. These intensity-dependent phenomena must be studied experimentally.

In the infrared at the wavelengths of Nd^+ laser (1.06 μ) and of the CO_2 laser (10.6 μ), few in vivo or in vitro measurements have been made.[8-12] Since biological soft tissues contain 80% to 90% of water,[13] the absorption coefficient of water as a function of wavelength is a useful guideline for the absorption properties of tissues.

The absorption coefficient for pure water in the wavelength region from 0.7 to 10 μ is shown in Figure 2-14. For this wavelength change, the absorption coefficient varies by more than four orders of magnitude from .001 mm^{-1}. At the wavelength of the Nd^+ laser, $\lambda = 1.06\ \mu$, the extinction length is 60 mm and at that of the CO_2 laser, $\lambda = 10.6\ \mu$, it is 0.03 mm. Recalling the definition of extinction length, this means that 90% of the radiation of a Nd^+ laser is absorbed in a 6-cm layer of water, while 0.03 mm of water are sufficient to absorb 90% of the CO_2 laser radiation.

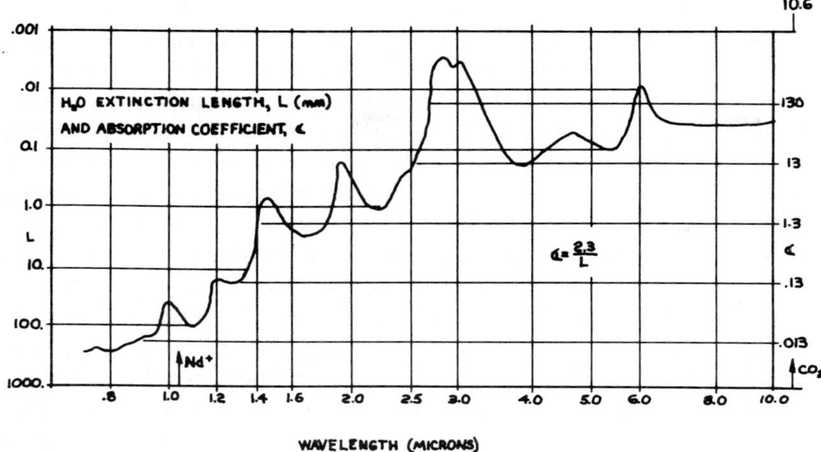

Figure 2-14 The absorption coefficient of water α and extinction length L, between 0.7 μ and 10.0 μ. Adapted from Bayly JG, Karta VB, Stevens WH: *Infrared Physics* 3:211, 1963. Courtesy of Infrared Spectrum, Pergamon Press.

Tissues, of course, are not water and variations in density in chemical composition and structural inhomogeneities alter the coefficients of absorption. As an example, the extinction length of the Nd-YAG radiation in the stomach wall of dogs has been measured experimentally and found to be about 2.3 mm. The few measurements that have been made on tissues for the wavelength of the CO_2 laser and the actual practice of surgery confirm the extremely high absorption of biological tissues to the wavelength of this laser.

Mechanisms of Tissue Removal with the CO_2 Laser

In the surgical applications discussed in this book the focused beam of a carbon dioxide laser of appropriate power is used to vaporize tissues. An incision similar to a scalpel incision is produced by moving the finely focused beam of the laser along a line. A thin surface layer of an extended area can be removed with the laser beam by tracing adjacent lines separated by a distance equal to the focused beam diameter (larger spot diameters are preferable for such use). A defect of almost any depth and width can be produced in a small region by applying the beam to it for an appropriate length of time. The basic process is always the same: tissue vaporization in depth along a thin line, or cutting, or tissue vaporization to a shallow depth of an extended thin volume (as in the removal of a leukoplakia), or vaporization of a volume (as in the removal of a papilloma or a plantar wart).

Tissue removal by vaporization takes place as follows: a tissue site is exposed to the radiation of the CO_2 laser beam; this radiation is strongly absorbed by tissues and by their high water content; the absorbed electromagnetic energy is essentially instantaneously transformed into heat energy, and as soon as sufficient energy is accumulated in a tissue volume, vaporization takes place. Effective use of this surgical tool requires a few additional considerations. The increase in tissue temperature, which takes place immediately upon absorption of electromagnetic radiation, causes heat to flow from hotter to cooler areas due to the thermal conductivity of tissues. Therefore, tissues not directly exposed to the beam and not vaporized by it may suffer thermal damage. It will be recalled that the conduction of heat between two regions at different temperatures increases with time, is proportional to the heat conductivity of the medium and to the temperature difference. Since the heat conductivity of tissues (which is low) cannot be influenced, and the temperature difference can generally be kept at 63°C, but not lower,* the speed of tissue evaporation is the only variable at the disposal of the surgeon to minimize heat transfer to the tissues to be preserved. Fortunately, the high output powers available from CO_2 lasers and the high absorption of biological tissues at the wavelength of this laser permit rapid accumulation of energy in tissues and their rapid evaporation.

A numerical example will illustrate this. The energy required to transform into steam at 100°C one cubic millimeter of water-like tissue initially at 37°C, is about 0.606 calories, equivalent to 2.5 joules. A CO_2 laser with an output of 25 W will deliver this amount of energy (2.5 joules) in one tenth of a second (joules = watts × seconds). If the laser beam is focused to a cross-section of 1 mm^2, a depth of tissue of one millimeter is removed in one tenth of a second. Tissue removal is rapid under these conditions, it depends only on the energy delivered to the unit of volume per unit time, and the time available for heat transfer by diffusion (1/10 of a second) can be short.

The numbers derived from the example should not be taken literally, since tissues are not exactly water-like and there are variations from tissue to tissue. The example, however, indicates that with a power density of 2500 W/cm^2 (25 watts in a one square millimeter spot), tissue vaporization is rapid and small tissue defects can be produced comfortably with much lower power densities. Clearly, as the power density in the beam is progressively decreased, by any combination of lowered output power and increased spot size, a value will be reached where the energy supplied to unit volume of tissue balances the energy lost by heat conduction. At this lower limit of power densities, tissues exposed directly to the beam can be heated to 100°C or less without significant vaporization; tissue

---

*Tissue vaporization takes place essentially at 100°C. Experimentally this was demonstrated by Hall[13] and by Mihasi.[14]

volumes below the surface are heated by conduction and thermally denatured. Pletnev[15] used this method for the treatment of large skin tumors. The denatured tissue sloughs off in time. Theoretical calculations[16] and some experimental evidence[15,17] indicate that this lower limit of power densities is in the neighborhood of 10 W/cm^2. Additional considerations on the mechanism of tissue removal with a CO_2 laser are presented in Appendix IV.

It is comfortable to know there is such a wide range between the power density at which evaporation essentially does not occur, and the power densities suitable for rapid tissue vaporization (readily available from the CO_2 laser systems used in surgery). A question may be asked: Is there an upper limit to the power that can be utilized in surgery? In fact such a limit is set by the ability to control comfortably tissue removal, and this will depend on the surgical application.

To summarize these considerations, I would like to quote R.J.C. Verschueren[18] who has made extensive investigations related to the use of CO_2 lasers in surgery:

> Using a CO_2 laser for incising tissues, the viability of the margins can be optimally preserved by cutting with a high power output. This will shorten the required contact of every fraction of the incision with the beam, reduce the time factor, and consequently lessen the tissue damage at the edges.
>
> While using a CO_2 laser to vaporize a tumor, it is advisable to use short bursts of high power output, thus obtaining the desired vaporized volume while optimally preserving the viability of the margins. It is obvious that the choice of output has to be made in accordance with the local tissue situation. Using a high output for skin incision in a small animal, compels the surgeon to move the handpiece quickly in order to avoid the incision being too deep. The speed of this movement will decrease the accuracy of the incision. When vaporizing a rectal tumor, the use of high output entails the risk of perforation of the rectal wall, even with short exposures. Here again, the local tissue situation claims an appropriate choice of output. It is, however, impossible to give precise technical data for the safe use of the CO_2 laser in different tissues, just as it is impossible to tell an intern how much pressure to apply to the scalpel for incising tissues. Before using this new tool, the surgeon should acquire some experience in the animal laboratory, in order to get used to this new technique and have an idea of the relationship of the vaporized volume with power output and exposure time. Only this practical experience will enable the surgeon to make judicious choice of output for every individual situation.

ACKNOWLEDGMENTS

The author gratefully acknowledges many suggestions by Dr Thomas Brocki in the preparation of this manuscript and the critical review of several sections by Mr William Strouse. Both are his colleagues at Merrimack Laboratories, Inc.

APPENDIX I:

BASIC PHYSICS OF LIGHT

Matter and Electromagnetic Radiation

Light is generated in processes occurring in atoms, molecules, or ions. These submicroscopic systems are called quantum systems. The behavior of quantum systems can be described only by the newer mechanics, quantum mechanics, and not by the more familiar classical mechanics, which applies only to larger bodies such as planets, sun, stars, and baseballs. One of the more important results of the new mechanics is that the energies a quantum system can have are discrete; they cannot assume a continuum of values as can, for example, a body (ie, a stone or a car) whose energy (kinetic or potential, or a sum of these two) can be varied smoothly between wide limits.

The atom is composed of a positively charged nucleus and one or more negatively charged electrons. The atomic species differ by the charge of the nucleus and the number of electrons. The more electrons there are, the more are the possible discrete energy values the system's nucleus and electrons can assume. An analogy, which permits one to visualize the energy levels, E_0, E_1, E_2....E_n, is the (potential) energy of a ball located on steps having the heights, h_0, h_1,h_2,...h_n (Figure 2-15a). The (potential) energy of the ball on ground level (h_0) is called ground state energy E_0. By redrawing the diagram of Figure 2-15a with the energy levels E_0...E_n, one above the other (Figure 2-15b), the energy level

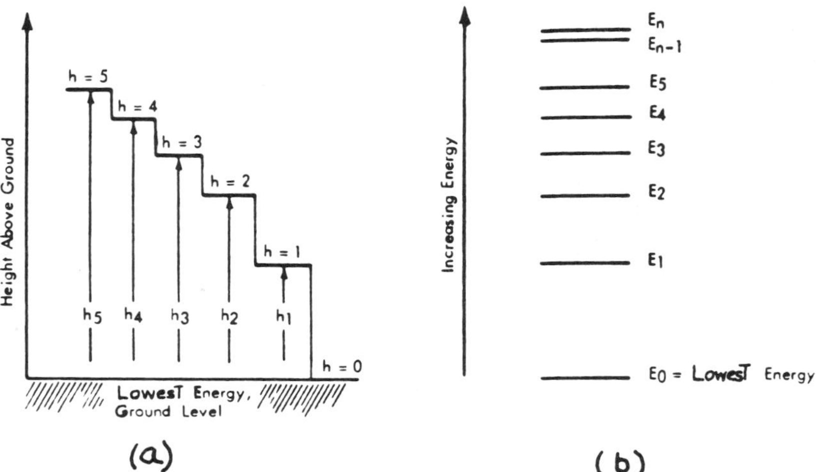

Figure 2-15 Energy levels of an atom. (a) An analogy: If a stone can be located only on one of the steps, its potential energy can assume only discrete values. (b) The standard representation of a simplified energy level diagram of an atom.

diagram generally used in atomic physics textbooks is obtained. As a rule, atoms are in their lowest energy level E_0; energy must be supplied to the atom to take it to a higher energy level or an excited state.

Generation of Light

The production of light is closely connected with the energy levels of quantum systems, atoms in particular. Atoms can only generate light of a frequency close to ν_{ab}, which is related to two possible energy levels E_a, E_b of the atom. The frequency, ν_{ab} of the light that is generated is connected to the energy levels E_a, E_b by the Bohr relationship:

AI. 1
$$\nu_{ab} = \frac{E_a - E_b}{h}$$

where: h is Planck's universal constant.

Emission and Absorption

The processes leading to emission of light from atoms and the basic interactions of light with atoms were described at the beginning of this century by Einstein. He showed that three distinct processes occur; these are spontaneous emission, absorption, and stimulated emission.

Spontaneous emission The atom is in one of its excited states E_a (Figure 2-16a). In returning to the lower state, the atom loses the energy $E_a - E_b$. The entire energy lost in this transition reappears in the form of light energy having the frequency given by (AI. 1) Bohr's relationship (see Figure 2-16b). This is the process of *spontaneous emission.*

Absorption The atom is initially in its lower energy level E_b, generally the ground state (Figure 2-16c). Electromagnetic energy of frequency ν_{ab} irradiates it. The atom is capable of removing light energy from the irradiating beam. After some time of irradiation, the atom will be in the higher energy level E_a and an amount of energy equal to $E_a - E_b$ has been removed from the light beam (Figure 2-16d). Some of the energy of the light beam has been *absorbed.* Absorption is a phenomenon observed in daily experience. Stained glass appears red, green, or blue in white light, because of certain substances that absorb all the other colors contained in the white light while passing red, green, or blue. Material objects absorb some of the colors of white light and the reflected light is *colored*; it has the *color* of the object. Filters often used in photography absorb a portion of the incident light to which the film may be much more sensitive than to other colors, thus distorting the photographic image.

SPONTANEOUS EMISSION

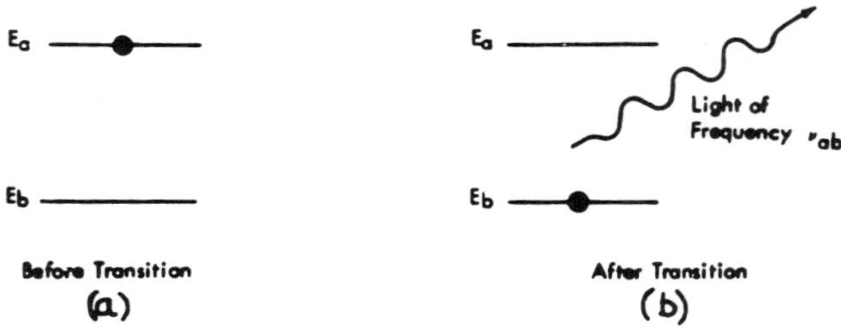

ABSORPTION

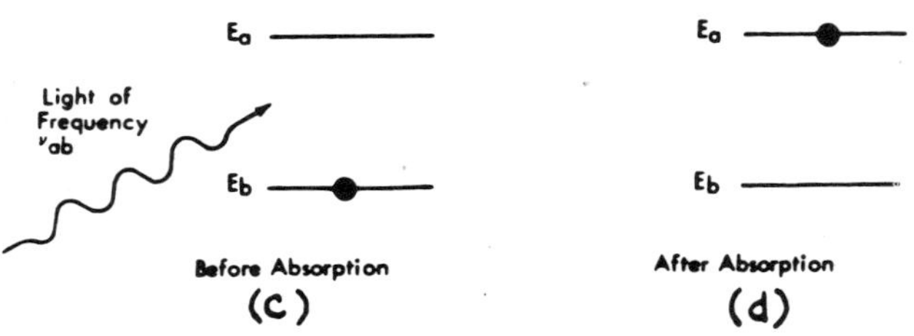

STIMULATED EMISSION

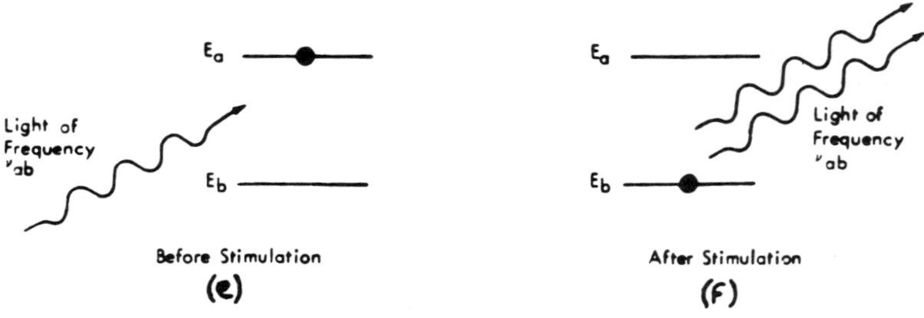

Figure 2-16 Light emission and absorption by atoms. (a,b) Spontaneous emission of light; (c,d) Absorption of light; (e,f) Stimulated emission of light. The two parallel lines symbolize two energy levels of the atom; when the black dot is on the upper line it means that the atom is in its excited state, when on the lower line the atom is in the lower level. The wavy line with the arrow symbolizes an electromagnetic field and its direction of propagation. Note that in the stimulated emission case the stimulating field and the field produced by stimulated emission add together since they have the same phase and the same direction.

Goggles used by welders and glass blowers absorb the UV radiation, which would cause erythema and painful irritation of the cornea.

Stimulated emission The last process predicted by Einstein is stimulated emission. This occurs (Figure 2-16e) when an atom in the excited state E_a is irradiated with light having the frequency ν_{ab}; we know already that the atom at some time will decay to the lower energy state by spontaneous emission. The addition of the irradiating light strongly increases the probability for this transition to take place. This is the process called *stimulated emission.* The light energy that stimulates the emission is not decreased in the process of stimulation; the energy decrease of the atom is *added* to the stimulating light energy (Figure 2-16f).

Characteristics of Spontaneous Emission, Absorption, and Stimulated Emission

Light emitted through spontaneous emission propagates with equal probability in *any direction;* the frequency of the emitted light may differ slightly from ν_{ab}, but is contained in a narrow range of frequencies $\Delta\nu_{ab}$, centered at ν_{ab}; $\Delta\nu_{ab}$ is called the width of the transition and ν_{ab} the center frequency. Equally in the absorption process, the irradiating light need not have exactly the frequency ν_{ab}, but the probability of stimulating the atom to make a transition to the higher level E_a is greater when the stimulating light frequency is closer to ν_{ab}. Equally in the process of stimulated emission, the probability of stimulating a downward transition increases when the frequency of the stimulating light approaches ν_{ab}. For equal frequencies, the probability to stimulate the excited atom to emit is equal to the probability to stimulate the atom in the ground state to absorb. Further, light from stimulated emission increases the intensity of the stimulating light and has *precisely the frequency and the direction of the stimulating light.*

Absorption and Amplification of Light

The elementary processes of light emission, absorption, and stimulated emission lead one to understand why a medium can absorb light of a given frequency, amplify it, or be transparent to it. For simplicity, let us consider a medium containing many atoms all in the ground state (or lower level) and a beam of light having a frequency close to ν_{ab}, which propagates in the medium (Figure 2-17a). Some atoms of the medium will be stimulated to absorb the radiation and the light beam will therefore be weakened. *Absorption of the light has taken place.* Assume next that all the atoms are in upper level E_a; some atoms will be stimulated to emit radiation of the frequency ν_{ab} in the direction of propagation and in the proper phase to strengthen the light beam. Hence, *amplification* takes place (Figure 2-17b). If the number of atoms in the upper level is equal to the number of atoms in the lower level, stimulated absorption will equal stimulated emission and the medium will be *transparent* to the radiation. Absorption of light at frequency ν_{ab} takes place if there are more atoms in the lower level E_b than in the upper level E_a, and conversely, amplification takes place when there are more atoms in the upper level E_a than in the lower level E_b.

Population inversion In the overwhelming majority of all cases, when energy is applied to a material and the atoms of the material are made to populate the energy levels above the ground state, the population of the energy levels *decreases* with *increasing* energy of the level. Using the example of the atom having energy levels E_a and E_b, there will be fewer atoms in the higher level E_a than in the lower level E_b and the medium will absorb light of the frequency, $\nu = \frac{E_a - E_b}{h}$. But this is not a universal law.

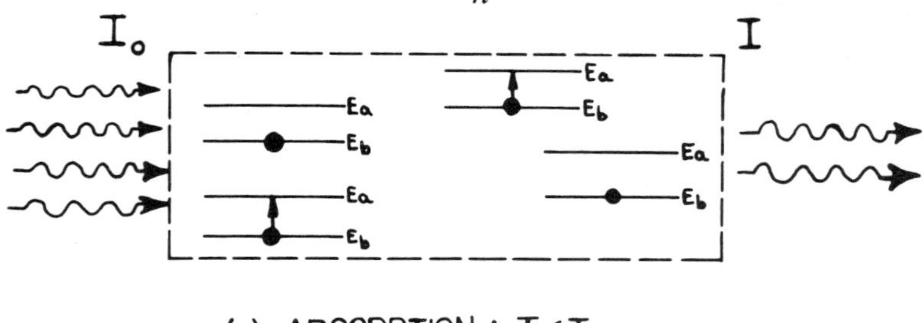

(a) ABSORPTION : $I < I_0$

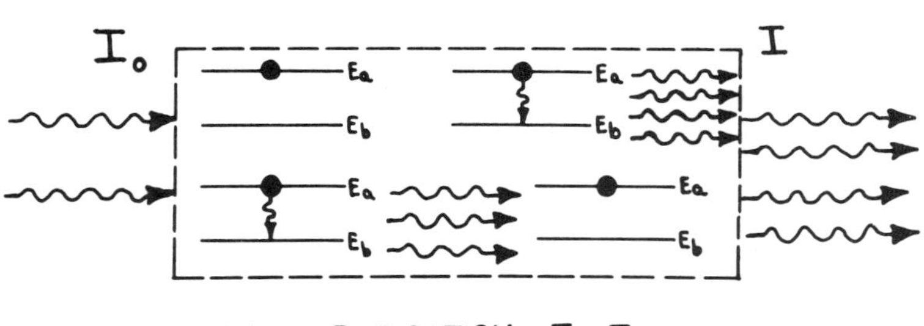

(b) AMPLIFICATION : $I > I_0$

Figure 2-17 Absorption and amplification of light. The dotted lines symbolize a region containing a gaseous medium. In (a) all atoms are in the lower level. They absorb some energy of the incident beam I_0; hence, the incident beam is weakened and I is less than I_0. In (b) all atoms are in the upper level; the incident beam I_0 stimulates some of the atoms to emit light, which is in phase with and in the direction of the incident light. The emitted light adds to the incident light and the beam is strengthened making I larger than I_0.

One can, by special means in selected materials, produce a situation in which there are more atoms in a higher energy level than in a lower one. This is called establishing a *population inversion.* A medium with population inversion will amplify a light wave of the appropriate frequency. *Such media are the essential prerequisite of lasers.*

Generation of Coherent Light by Means of (L)ight (A)mplification of (S)timulated (E)mission of (R)adiation (LASER)

The generation of laser light can be described as follows: an excited laser medium is present in the optical cavity, ie, between mirrors M_1 and M_2 (Figure 2-18); let E_a and E_b be the upper and the lower energy levels of the quantum systems, atoms, or molecules of the active medium. An atom in the upper level E_a will at some time decay spontaneously to the lower level E_b with emission of a light wave. Of the many atoms which emit spontaneously in all directions, one ([1] in Figure 2-18) will emit light along the axis of the cavity. The light emitted by this one atom is capable of stimulating other atoms in the upper energy level to emit light and, owing to the properties of stimulated emission, the light emitted in this way is in the proper phase to double the intensity of the stimulating light, and this enhanced wave propagates along the axis of the optical cavity.

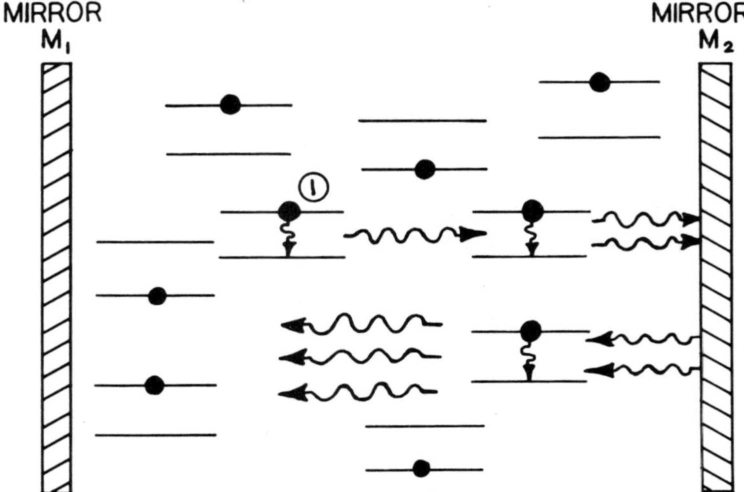

Figure 2-18 Generation of laser light. In the region between mirrors M_1 and M_2 there is a medium with more atoms in the upper level than in the lower level. One of the atoms, 1, in the upper level by chance emits spontaneously in the direction of the common axes of the two mirrors. The light field generated by atom 1 can stimulate other atoms to emit in the same direction and the process of laser light generation is continued by multiple reflections at the mirrors.

As this process continues, a wave of continuously increasing intensity is propagated along the axis of the optical cavity. The wave encounters the mirror, which reflects it back into the cavity, and the growth process of the wave continues as it travels back and forth between the mirrors. With increasing intensity, the light wave stimulates the emission of more and more atoms that are in the upper energy level. An equilibrium intensity is reached when as many atoms per unit time are stimulated to emit radiation as are excited to the upper level by the pump supplying energy to the active medium. If one of the mirrors, eg M_2, is made partially transmitting, some of the light existing in the cavity is transmitted through the mirror along the axis of the optical cavity. Clearly, the gain in energy of the wave for each round trip in the cavity must equal the amount of energy emitted through the mirrors as useful output, plus the unavoidable losses due to imperfections of the mirrors, spontaneous emission, etc. The coherence of laser light is inherent in the characteristics of stimulated emission. All the atomic systems of the active medium are made to emit in phase and in the same direction; hence the parallel and narrow beam. Since the probability of stimulated emission is higher as the frequency of the stimulating field is closer to ν_{ab}, in a short time, emission at ν_{ab} will prevail; hence the extreme monochromaticity of laser light.

The resonance condition A further consideration is needed to complete the picture. It should be clear from this discussion that a standing light wave exists in the optical cavity between the two mirrors (Figure 2-19). A standing wave can exist only if the wave has a *node* or a zero of intensity at each mirror surface. For this to happen, the length of the cavity L must contain an integral number m of half-wavelengths, or:

AI. 2 $$m\frac{\lambda}{2} = L$$

Because of this relationship, which must be satisfied, the optical cavity is more properly called optical resonant cavity as an analogy to sound phenomena.

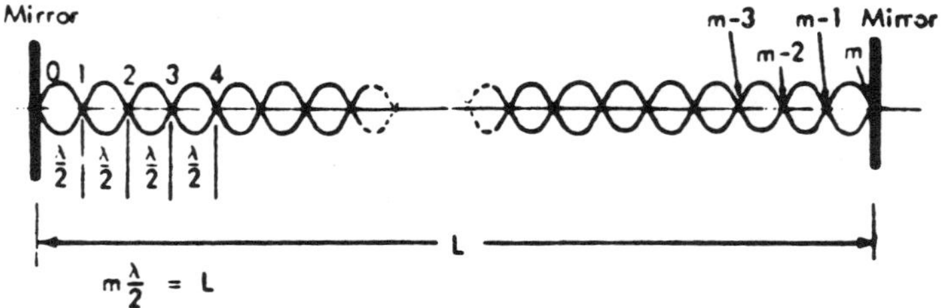

Figure 2-19 Standing waves inside a laser cavity. For a standing wave to exist within the laser cavity there must be a node, or zero of intensity, at each mirror. This gives rise to the resonance condition that an integral number m of half-wavelengths, $\lambda/2$, must equal the length L of the cavity.

Consequences of the resonance condition A discussion of the consequences of the resonance condition $m\lambda = 2L$ leads to an insight into some of the characteristics that may be exhibited by laser devices and also, into some of the engineering problems related to these devices.

It is clear to start with, that the integral number m is very large; eg, if the wavelength of operation of a laser is 0.5 μ (the argon ion laser operates at 0.48 μ) and the laser cavity is 50 cm long, the number of half-wavelengths fitting in the cavity are two million, ie, $m = 2 \times 10^6$. (This is obtained by rewriting AI. 2 under the form $m = 2L/\lambda$ and substituting for L and λ, 50 cm and 0.5×10^{-4}cm respectively.) If the same cavity length of 50 cm is used for a CO_2 laser operating at about 10 μ, then $m =$ 100,000.

In practice, however, unless special precautions are taken, the length of a cavity is only approximately constant; ambient temperature variations alone are sufficient to change it by many half-wavelengths. Each time the change in length equals one half-wavelength, the effect is not noticeable since the resonance condition is fulfilled and a change in length of the cavity of even many thousands of wavelengths has negligible effect on the output power. When the cavity length changes *less* than one half-wavelength, however, interesting phenomena can take place, ie, the laser stopping to operate or the intensity of the output changing. This will be discussed in the next section.

Longitudinal modes of a cavity The resonance condition, $m \dfrac{\lambda}{2} = L$, can be rewritten in terms of the frequency of the electromagnetic wave using the formula below:

AI. 3 $\lambda\nu = c =$ velocity of light $= 3 \times 10^{10}$ cm/sec.

One then obtains:

AI. 4 $$\nu = \frac{mc}{2L}$$

the frequencies $\nu_1 = \dfrac{c}{2L}$, $\nu_2 = \dfrac{2c}{2L}$, $\nu_m = \dfrac{mc}{2L}$ (Figure 2-20) which are the resonant frequencies of the cavity and are called the *longitudinal modes* of the cavity. The modes encountered previously in this chapter, ie, the (0,0) or (0,1) modes were called *transverse* modes. The frequency difference, $\Delta\nu$ between adjacent longitudinal modes for which the integer m changes by one unit, is given by:

AI. 5 $$\Delta\nu = \frac{mc}{2L} - \frac{(m-1)c}{2L} = \frac{c}{2L}$$

In Figure 2-21 the longitudinal modes for two cavities are shown: one cavity (a) is 2 m long and the other (b) is 25 cm long; for the

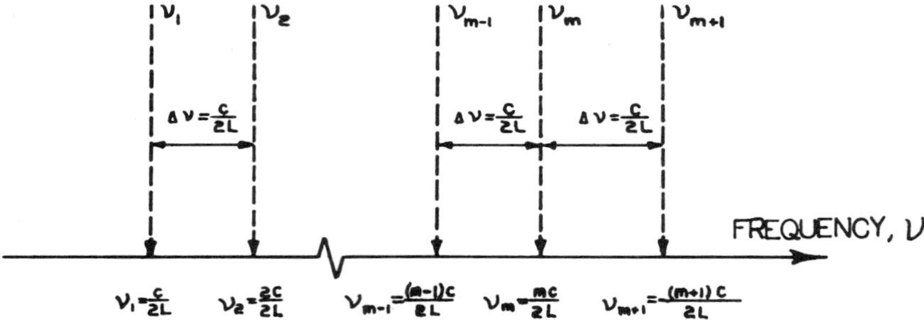

Figure 2-20 The optical cavity is resonant at the frequencies $\nu_1 \ldots . \nu_m$; the frequency difference $\Delta\nu$ between adjacent resonances is always the same: $\Delta\nu = \frac{c}{2L}$. The frequency axis is interrupted to permit representation of low frequencies and high frequencies ($m = 1,2,\ldots$ and m very large).

first $\Delta\nu = \dfrac{c}{2L} = 3 \times 10^{10}/2 \times 200 = 75$ Mhz,* for the second $\Delta\nu = 3 \times 10^{10}/2 \times 25 = 600$ Mhz. The center frequency of the atomic transition giving rise to the laser is denoted with ν_{ab}, and the width of the transition $\Delta\nu_{ab}$ is assumed to be 400 Mhz for the laser medium illustrated.

It is apparent from the figure that in the situation depicted in (a), at least three longitudinal modes overlap the frequency range $\Delta\nu_{ab}$†, while in case (b) no more than one longitudinal mode can overlap the frequency range $\Delta\nu_{ab}$ over which laser emission can take place. It is interesting to analyze what happens when the length L of the cavity changes by one half-wavelength. We use equation AI. 4 and find the difference in frequencies $\delta\nu$ of the longitudinal modes corresponding to the lengths L and $L + \dfrac{\lambda}{2}$ belonging to the same value of m. We obtain:

AI. 6
$$\delta\nu = \frac{mc}{2L} - \frac{mc}{2L + \frac{\lambda}{2}} = \frac{mc}{2L} \times \frac{\lambda}{2} \times \frac{1}{L + \frac{\lambda}{2}} .$$

Since $\dfrac{\lambda}{2}$ is extremely small with respect to L, we can neglect $\dfrac{\lambda}{2}$ in the denominator of (AI. 6) and rewrite this formula, by rearranging terms, as:

AI. 7
$$\delta\nu = \frac{mc}{2L} \times \frac{\lambda}{2L}$$

*1Mhz = 10^6 cycles/second

†In these conditions, the laser may oscillate at several frequencies separated by the frequency interval $\Delta\nu$.

and, recalling formula AI. 2: $m\frac{\lambda}{2} = L$ or $\frac{\lambda}{2L} = \frac{1}{m}$, we conclude that: $\delta\nu = \Delta\nu$.

We can interpret this result as follows: as the cavity length increases in length, the longitudinal modes change in frequency in such a way that when the cavity has increased by *one half-wavelength,* the longitudinal mode corresponding to the number m coincides with the original mode of

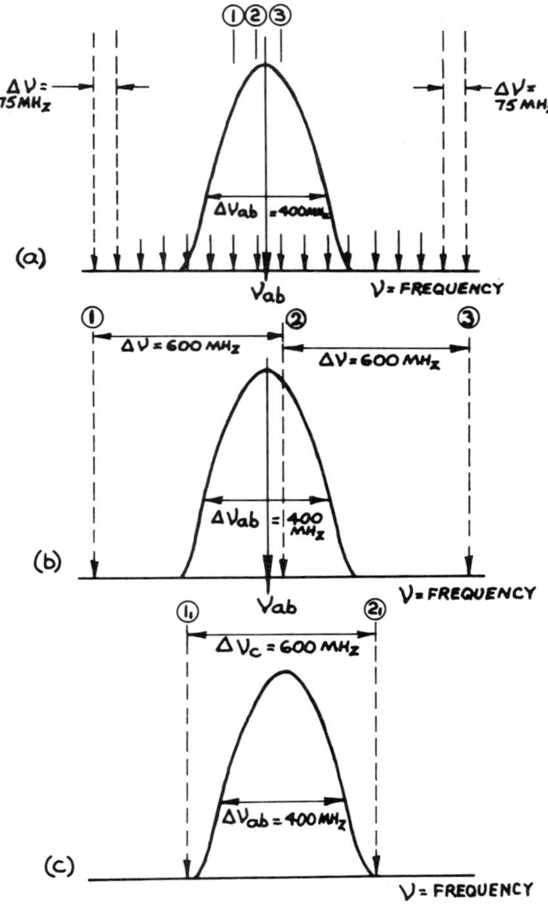

Figure 2-21 Cavity resonances and the laser transition. (a) Long cavity—the resonant frequencies are close to each other and several such frequencies 1, 2, 3, overlap in frequency with the laser transition of width $\Delta\nu_{ab}$. (b) Short cavity—the resonant frequencies are spaced much further apart; they may or may not overlap with the frequency span of the laser transition. In (b) one overlaps. (c) The cavity length has changed by less than one half-wavelength from (b) and has stabilized at a length at which no resonant frequency overlaps the laser transition. There is no laser output.

number $m - 1$. In other words, the longitudinal mode frequencies slide over the frequency scale and at the end of the half-wavelength change of the length of the cavity, the frequencies of the longitudinal modes coincide again with the original ones. What happens to the laser output while this length change of one half-wavelength takes place?

In Figure 2-21 (a), mode (2) moves from 2 to 1, mode (3) from 3 to 2, etc; in the meantime, the frequency of the laser output changes over the frequency range $\Delta\nu_{ab}$. In case (b) the same events take place but during the motion of mode (2) into position 1 and of mode (3) into 2 there will be an interval of time in which modes (1), (2), (3) will be outside the frequency range $\Delta\nu_{ab}$ over which the laser can operate. Hence, the laser output will first decrease in intensity while its frequency changes over the interval $\Delta\nu_{ab}$, then stop oscillating all together for some fraction of the time interval during which the half-wavelength change of the resonator takes place. Should the resonator stabilize in length at the new mode positions 1_1 and 2_1 (Figure 2-21c) there will be no laser output.

The profound difference between cases (a) and (b) is the cavity length, which determines the frequency difference $\Delta\nu = \frac{c}{2L}$ of the longitudinal modes. This difference is inversely proportional to the cavity length L; when the frequency interval $\Delta\nu$ becomes comparable to the frequency range $\Delta\nu_{ab}$ over which the laser can operate; one half-wavelength change in the cavity length can cause severe intensity fluctuations as mentioned in the section entitled, Common Construction Features of Laser Devices.

Summary The resonance condition is a fundamental characteristic of laser devices which can be stated as follows: constancy of wavelength (or frequency) of the output of a laser requires that the optical cavity length L be kept constant within a small fraction of one-half-wavelength. Since for most construction materials, ambient temperature variations are sufficient to cause a length change greatly exceeding one half-wavelength, a constant frequency output implies engineering challenges. Fortunately, extreme wavelength stability is not required in many areas of laser application including all those that are based on the intensity of laser sources, ie, surgery.

The engineering problems imposed by the resonance condition become progressively more complex in the following two situations: 1) when high frequency and output power stability are required as is the case in selected communication and physics applications; and 2) when the physical size of the laser is progressively decreased for convenience of usage, eg, in surgery. Decreasing the cavity length L implies a progressively larger shift in wavelength of operation for small changes in cavity length, and this implies in its turn that the stimulated emission takes place further and further away from where it has a maximum of probability to occur and from where the output power is the greatest. To offset the intensity variations that take place in such short lasers when the cavity length changes, it becomes necessary to use for the laser cavity materials with low coefficients of thermal expansion, and to employ additional means to compensate for the temperature variations.

APPENDIX II

POWER, POWER DENSITY, MODES AND SPOT SIZES

Power density $\overline{P}$ is defined by the formula:

AII. 1 $$\overline{P} = \frac{P}{A},$$

ie, the ratio of the power impinging on an area A to the area itself; it is usually expressed in W/cm^2 and is equivalent to power per unit area since, for a beam of uniform intensity, halving the area reduces the power to one half and the ratio $\frac{P}{A}$ remains unchanged. It was shown in Figures 2-7A, B and 2-8A, B, however, that laser beams have nonuniform intensity distributions. Power density is then defined for each point of the plane on which the beam impinges as the power P impinging on a small area a surrounding the point as illustrated in Figure 2-10. For nonuniform intensity laser beams, the average power density $\overline{P}_{av}$ is a useful quantity. The average is usually taken over the beam spot size (see Appendix III), which is the area containing ~ 86% of the total beam power.

Power Density in the Fundamental (0,0) Mode

The intensity and its associated power density $\overline{P}$ in a fundamental mode vs distance r from the axis of the laser beam is shown in the curve of Figure 2-7B; the power density reaches its maximum on the axis where $r = 0$. The distance r at which the intensity or power density has decreased to ~ 13% of the peak intensity is generally the definition of spot radius and is often designated with the letter w (Figure 2-7B). As mentioned, ~ 86% of the beam power is contained in the circle of radius w centered on the axis.

It can be shown that the peak power density, $\overline{P}_{max}$ for a laser beam of power P is given by the formula:

AII. 2 $$\overline{P}_{max} = \frac{2 \times \text{total power in beam}}{\text{area of spot size}} = \frac{2P}{\pi w^2}\ .$$

The average power density P_{av} over the spot size is given by:

AII. 3
$$\overline{P_{av}} = \frac{0.86P}{\text{area spot size}} = \frac{0.86P}{\pi w^2}.$$

The ratio of peak to average power densities is given by:

AII. 4
$$\frac{2P}{\pi w^2} \div \frac{0.86P}{\pi w^2} = 2.33.$$

Power Density in the "Donut" Mode

The intensity and its associated power density for the donut mode is shown in Figure 2-8B. The units on the two axes and the total power P, are the same as for the (0,0) mode; the two curves are comparable since it is assumed that the (0,0) mode and the donut mode originate from the same cavity. In this mode, 86% of the total power is contained in a circle of diameter 1.33 w, where w is the spot size of the (0,0) mode. The power density is zero on the axis, increases to a maximum of 0.37 of the peak power of the (0,0) mode at 0.7 spot radii and gradually decreases to zero. Using the same symbols as in the (0,0) mode case, one can show that the power densities for the donut mode are the following:

AII. 2a
$$\overline{P_{max}} = 0.37\ \frac{2P}{\pi w^2}$$

AII. 3a
$$\overline{P_{av}} = 0.86\ \frac{P}{\pi(1.33w)^2}$$

AII. 4a
$$\frac{\overline{P_{max}}}{\overline{P_{av}}} = 1.52$$

Summary of Power Densities in (0,0) and "Donut" Modes

Table 2-2

Mode	(0,0)	"Donut"	Ratio
$\overline{P_{max}}$	$\frac{2P}{\pi w^2}$	$0.37\ \frac{2P}{\pi w^2}$	2.7:1
$\overline{P_{av}}$	$\frac{0.86P}{\pi w^2}$	$\frac{0.86P}{\pi(1.33w)^2}$	1.78:1
$\overline{P_{max}}:\overline{P_{av}}$	2.33	1.52	1.53:1

Considerations Related to Power, Power Density, Spot Size, Mode, and their Relative Usefulness in Surgery

The only directly measurable quantity in a laser is the total beam power P. Determination of the peak power density $\overline{P}_{max}$, or of the average power density $\overline{P}_{av}$, requires knowledge of the spot size w. This depends on the details of the laser cavity and the focusing system. The ratio of $\overline{P}_{max}$ to $\overline{P}_{av}$, however, is independent of the spot size for a given mode.

Some manufacturers supply the spot size of the focused laser beam. These are generally calculated spot sizes and may closely represent the actual spot size. They may bear little relationship, however, to the area of tissue that is affected by exposure to the laser beam.

In practice, the term spot size is frequently used to describe the size of the *imprint* obtained when a material, ie, a wooden tongue depressor or a tomato, is exposed to the laser beam. The value of the spot size obtained in this manner can differ substantially from the actual spot size, which does not depend on the beam intensity or on the exposure time. Such measurements have practical utility, however, if imprints are compared that are obtained under controlled conditions (power, exposure time) on closely equivalent and meaningfully selected materials.

Power densities are generally calculated either from the value of the spot size supplied by the manufacturers or from the size of the imprint. The limitations of both methods should be clear in view of the above. *In describing surgical results, therefore, both total power and method of describing the spot size need to be reported.*

Lasers used in surgical systems may change from the (0,0) to the donut mode or to other modes. Table 2-2 indicates that when this happens substantial changes take place in $\overline{P}_{max}$ and $\overline{P}_{av}$.

The question: Which mode is "better"?, naturally arises. It cannot be answered simply.

1. Table 2-2 indicates that the peak power density of a (0,0) mode is 2.7 times that of a donut mode. Hence, the (0,0) mode removes tissues more rapidly than the donut mode, but over a smaller area.
2. The peak power density is closer to the average power density in the donut mode than in the (0,0) mode: 1.52 vs 2.33. It is conceivable, therefore, that tissue removal is more uniform with such a mode resulting in less marginal tissue damage.
3. The power densities in Table 2-2 are based on the assumption that the two laser beams (one in the (0,0) mode and the other in the donut mode) originate from the same optical cavity and have the same total power. It is interesting to

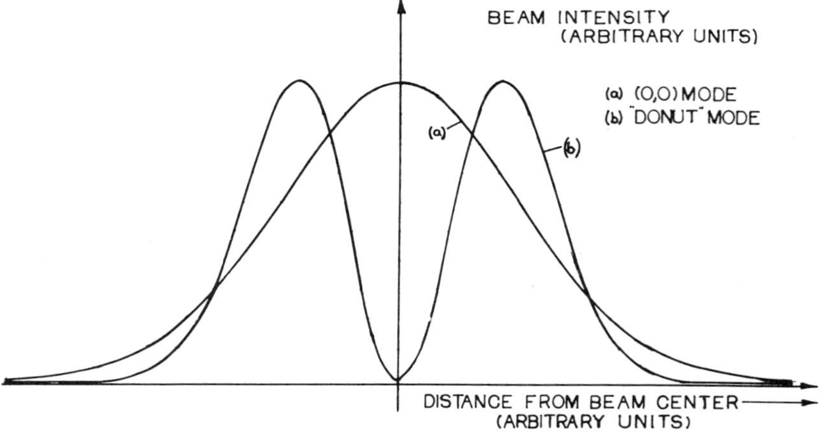

Figure 2-22 Comparison of the intensities of a (0,0) mode and a donut mode of equal peak and total power.

compare (0,0) and donut modes of *equal* peak power densities, as can be done by using different focusing systems for each. The resulting power density distributions are shown in Figure 2-22. The sharper cut off of the donut mode is obvious.

4. It appears from the foregoing that in using the appropriate optical system, both modes are equally *good* and that the donut mode could have advantages.

In summary, the question of which mode is better cannot be fully answered in the absence of adequate experimental surgical data comparing (0,0) mode operation with that of a donut mode. The point, however, can be made that more reproducible surgical results will be obtained if the laser operates either in one mode or the other and without switching modes.

APPENDIX III

DEFINITION OF SPOT SIZE

A generally accepted definition of spot size, meaningful only for intensity distributions with circular symmetry, is obtained in the following way (Figure 2-23): a power detector with a large sensitive area, whose center is on the axis of the laser beam, measures the beam power. In front of the detector, there is an adjustable circular diaphragm whose center coincides with the axis of the laser beam.

When the area A of the diaphragm is very large, the detector measures essentially the total beam power P_0. Closing the diaphragm at first has practically no effect. As it is closed further and further, the power reading decreases rapidly. The radius w of the diaphragm opening, which allows 86% of the beam power to fall on the detector, is defined as the spot size w. At this distance w from the axis, the intensity in a (0,0) mode has decreased to 13% of its maximum value and that of a donut mode to 10%.

This method of measuring the spot size cannot be used in practice to measure the spot size of laser beams focused to small dimensions. For this reason, spot sizes are either calculated theoretically or an *imprint* is used as mentioned in Appendix II.

APPENDIX IV

MECHANISM OF TISSUE REMOVAL

When a laser beam in the visible or the infrared impinges on tissues, two distinct phenomena take place:

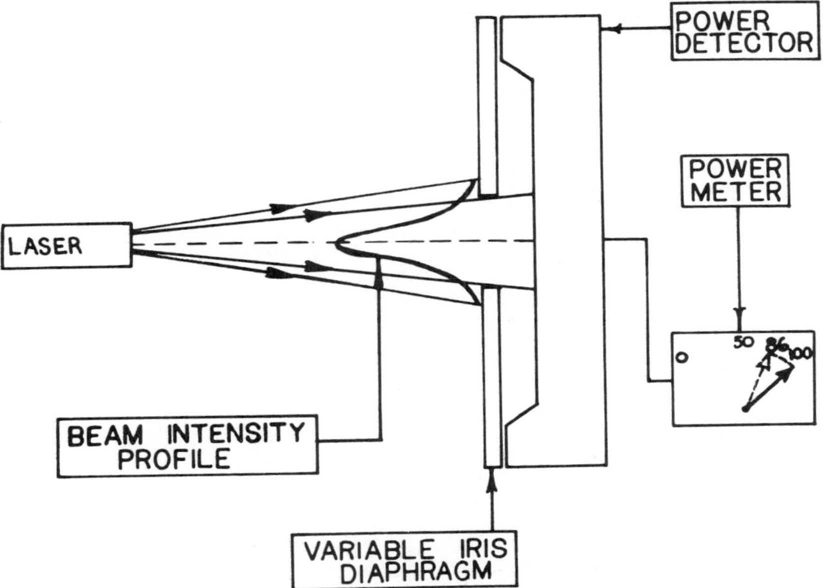

Figure 2-23 Measurement of spot size. A variable diaphragm is centered on the axis of the laser beam in front of the power detector. When the diaphragm opening is very large, the entire beam falls on the detector; as the diaphragm is closed, less energy reaches the detector. When the power detector meter reads 86% of maximum power, the opening of the diaphragm is measured. The radius of this opening is generally called the laser beam spot size.

1. Radiant energy is transformed almost instantly into heat energy and, initially, tissue temperature increases at a rate limited only by the rate of supply of energy.
2. Heat flows from hotter tissues to cooler ones, by diffusion, as a consequence of the heat conductivity of tissues. The amount of heat flowing into adjacent tissues is initially zero and increases with time.

The essential features of the phenomena that take place can be understood using a simplified model, illustrated in Figure 2-24. The CO_2 laser beam of power P and spot size w_0 is assumed to have uniform intensity over its cross section, to impinge on a tissue having water-like thermal properties, and to propagate for a small distance into tissues as a parallel beam. We fix our attention on the cylindrical volume $V = \pi w_0^2 \times L$, whose base is the cross section of the laser beam, of area πw_0^2, and of length L. The length L of the cylinder is the tissue thickness that absorbs 90% of the incident energy. In the section, Quantitative Interaction, this was called the *extinction length* and shown to be about 0.03 mm for radiation at 10.6 μ wavelength incident on water.

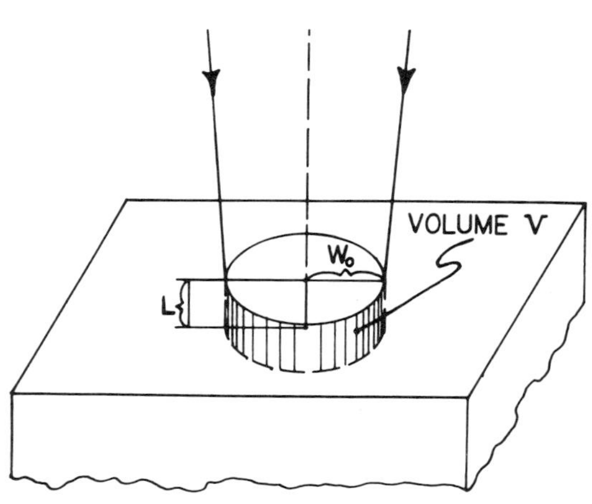

Figure 2-24 Tissue removal with a CO_2 laser beam. A laser beam with power P and spot size w_0 impinges upon tissue that has the thermal properties of water. In the text is the derivation of a formula for calculating the time necessary to vaporize the volume V shown in this figure. For radiation at the wavelength of the CO_2 laser, the length L is 0.03 mm. This justifies the assumption made in the text that the radiation propagates as a parallel beam over this short distance.

We want to find the amount of energy delivered to this small volume by the laser beam, and the time needed to vaporize it, neglecting conduction. If P is measured in watts, time t in seconds, and energy E in joules, then:

AIV. 1 $$E = P \times t$$

When this energy equals that necessary to transform into steam at 100°C a volume V of water originally at 37°C, the volume V will have been vaporized. This energy, one finds, is 0.6 calories ~ 2.5 joules (1 calorie = 4.18 joules) per cubic millimeter; calling this unitary energy E_0, the energy required to vaporize the volume V equals $E_0 \times V$ joules. One obtains from A IV. 1, neglecting the factor 0.9:

AIV. 2 $$E_0 V = E_0 \pi w_0^2 L = Pt \quad \text{and}$$

AIV. 3 $$t = \frac{\pi w_0^2}{P} \times L \times E_0 = \frac{1}{\text{power density}} \times L \times E_0,$$

as the time needed to vaporize tissue to a depth L. As an example, if:

$$P = 15 \text{ watt}$$
$$w_0 = 0.5 \text{ mm},$$

and with $E_0 = 2.5$ joules and $L = 0.03$ mm, we obtain from A IV. 1

$$t = \frac{\pi \times (0.5)^2 \times 0.03 \times 2.5}{15} = 0.004\,s$$

Under the conditions of the example, tissue removal is rapid. In 4 msecs the CO_2 laser beam vaporizes to a depth of 0.03 mm; note that the time required to vaporize tissues to a depth L is inversely proportional to the power density. When tissues are exposed to the beam for one-tenth of a second, eg, the depth of tissue removed will be $0.1 \times \frac{0.03\text{mm}}{0.004} \times 0.03$ $= 0.75$ mm.

The laser beam vaporizes tissues in depth at a rate of $0.1 \times \frac{0.03\text{mm}}{0.004}$ $= 7.5$ mm/sec.

In reality the process of tissue removal is more complex in its details. With the conditions assumed ($P = 15$ W, $w_0 = 0.5$ mm), vaporization of a tissue layer of a thickness, which is a small fraction of the extinction length L, takes place almost immediately after start of the exposure. A moving steam-solid boundary is formed that recedes into the depth of the tissue for the duration of the exposure; the intensity of the beam is not uniform over its cross section. If the laser operates in the fundamental or

(0,0) mode, eg, the depth of tissue removal will be greatest in the center of the beam and will decrease toward the edges. The lesion that is formed will have a crater-like shape mirroring the bell shaped intensity distribution of the beam (Figure 2-7).

Notwithstanding the complexity of the phenomena that takes place in detail during thermal tissue removal, the simple model, which leads to equation A IV. 3, gives results that are in comfortable agreement with experience (in the sense that a CO_2 laser beam, with characteristics well within the range of those used in surgery, produces a tissue defect similar to that found in practice in a time interval well controllable by the surgeon, a fact again confirmed by extensive experience).

The reasonable agreement encourages one to use equation A IV. 3 to make further deductions. Substituting for L in A IV. 3, the depth d in mm of tissue defect produced in time t and solving the equation for d, one obtains, setting $\pi w_o^2 = A$,

A IV. 4 $$d = \frac{P}{A} \times t \times \frac{1}{E_0}.$$

Recalling that P/A is the power density, the equation reads: the depth of the lesion is proportional to the power density and to the exposure time and is inversely proportional to the energy required to vaporize a unit of volume tissue. *Power density alone does not give any information on tissue volume removed.* For this, it is necessary to know the total beam power, the spot size, and the exposure time. It should be noted that the diameter of the lesion appears in the formula only through the spot size of the laser. If one doubles the spot size, four times the power is needed to produce a lesion of the same depth d. The power density in a laser beam varies over its area and, therefore, the depth of the lesion depends upon the details of the intensity distribution.

The depth of the lesion on the axis of a laser beam in the (0,0) mode will be approximately 2.7 times the maximum depth of a lesion produced with a laser operating in the donut mode for otherwise equivalent beams; however, the total area of the lesion with the donut mode will be approximately $(1.33)^2 = 1.8$ times that produced with the (0,0) mode distribution (see Appendix II).

A major limitation of this simple model is that the heat conductivity of tissues is not taken into consideration. As a consequence, it is not meaningful to use equation A IV. 4 except for short periods of time, ie, a few seconds, and with power densities above at least 100 W/cm^2 for which tissue vaporization dominates over heat conduction.

The problem of unwanted damage caused by heat conduction was discussed in the section on the mechanism of tissue removal, and it was mentioned that tissue vaporization is rapid with the power densities generally used in surgery, and that this minimizes the time available for heat conduction. It is extremely difficult to predict tissue damage by heat conduction owing to the complexity of the concrete problem, and the variability of the thermal characteristics of tissues. Several experimental investigations[14,19] and extensive surgical experiences indicate that tissue damage can be kept as low as 100 μ or less by minimizing exposure time, ie, using the higher ranges of the power density generally available. Experience also indicates that if, for any reason, one operates with too low power densities, tissues are dessicated rather than rapidly evaporated. Continued exposure to the CO_2 laser beam causes carbonization with temperature elevation to as high as 300° C, thus increasing heat conduction and tissue damage.

To summarize, tissue damage by heat conduction is controllable and can be kept within acceptable limits provided that tissue removal is as rapid as practicality and precision permit, and that the surgeon minimizes dwell time of the laser beam in one fixed position.

REFERENCES

1. Maiman TH: Stimulated optical radiation in ruby. *Nature* 187:493, 1960.
2. Carbone RJ: Continuous operation of a long-lived CO_2 laser tube. *IEEE Quantum Electronics*, 3:10, 1968.
3. Hill AE: Multijoule pulses from CO_2 lasers. *Appl Phys Lett* 12:9, 1979.
4. Beckman H, Rota A, Barraco R, et al: Limbectomies, keratectomies, and keratostomies performed with a rapid-pulsed carbon dioxide laser. *Am J Ophthalmol* 71(6):1277–1283, 1971.
5. Beckman H, Fuller TA: Carbon dioxide laser scleral dissection and filtering procedure for glaucoma. *Am J Ophthalmol* 88:73–77, 1979.
6. Goldman L, Rockwell RJ, Naprstek Z, et al: Some parameters of high output CO_2 laser experimental surgery. *Nature* 228:1344, 1970.
7. Buettner KJK: The effects of natural sunlight on human skin, in Urbach F (ed): *The Biologic Effect of Ultraviolet Radiation.* Elmsford, New York, Pergamon Press, 1969.
8. Yahr W, Polanyi ML: American Optical Research Laboratory Report, 1965.
9. Kiefhaber P, Nath G, Moritz K: Endoscopical control of massive gastrointestinal hemorrhage by irradiation with a high-power neodymium-YAG laser. *Prog Surg* 15:140–155, 1977.
10. Rother WW, Haldorsson T, Langerholc J, et al: Present status of the Nd-YAG laser in endoscopy and surgery, in Kaplan I (ed): *Laser Surgery, Proceedings of the 2nd International Symposium on Laser Surgery,* Dallas, Texas, October, 1977. Jerusalem, Jerusalem Academic Press, 211–222, 1978.
11. Bucholz J, Haverkampf K, Meyer HJ, et al: Scattering effects in laser surgery, in Kaplan I (ed): *Laser Surgery, Proceedings of the 2nd International Symposium on Laser Surgery,* Dallas, Texas, October, 1977, Jerusalem, Jerusalem Academic Press, 299–307, 1978.
12. Karlin DB, Patel CKN, Wood OR, et al: CO_2 lasers in vitreoretinal surgery. *Lasers Surg Med* 1:123–132, 1980.
13. Hall RR, Beach AD, Baker E, et al: Incision of tissue by carbon dioxide laser. *Nature* 232:131, 1971.

14. Mihasi S, Jako GJ, Incze JM, et al: Laser surgery in otolaryngology: Interaction of CO_2 laser and soft tissue, *Ann NY Acad Sci,* 267–263, 1976.

15. Pletnev SD, Abdurazakov MS, Karpenko OM: Laser surgery in oncological practice, *Khirurgiia* (2):48–52, 1977.

16. Johnson JR: Research Report, American Optical Corporation, Southbridge, MA and Personal Communication, 1973.

17. Gonzalez R, Edlich RF, Bredemeier BS, et al: Rapid control of massive hepatic hemorrhage by laser radiation. *Surg, Gynecol Obstet* 8:198–200, 1970.

18. Verschueren R: The CO_2 laser in tumor surgery, Assen/Amsterdam, Van Gorcum, Medical Series, NR232, 1976.

19. Strong MS, Jako GJ: Laser surgery in the larynx, early clinical experience with continuous CO_2 laser, *Ann Otol Rhinol Laryngol* 81:791, 1972.

3 Hazards and Safety Considerations When Using the CO_2 Laser

Albert H. Andrews, Jr., MS, MD
Thomas G. Polanyi, PhD

When surgery with carbon dioxide lasers first began, Strong and Jako,[1] and Andrews and Moss[2] recognized the importance of the hazards of this new modality and the imperative need to institute safety procedures. Because of this early emphasis, there have been no serious fire complications with the CO_2 laser. Nevertheless, this in no way lessens the importance of stressing the hazards and possible complications of this new surgical technique.

Sharp tools and hot utensils have been handled by most people since childhood, and their hazards are not thought of as such; safety procedures are ingrained and almost natural. The carbon dioxide laser produces heat in such concentrated form that it is beyond anyone's experience. This not only creates fear but requires rigid adherence to the principles of safety.

The U.S. government, recognizing the hazards and safety requirements of lasers, has set various regulations to help insure the safety of patients as well as physicians (see Chapter 4). The hazards associated with lasers can be divided into three types, namely, mechanical, electrical, and fire.

HAZARDS

Mechanical Hazards

The laser apparatuses are heavy and present a hazard to feet and fingers if not handled with appropriate care. The cylinders of gas are also hazardous; even though nonflammable, opening a cylinder that is not attached to a suitable connection may result in injection of gas into the skin. While the laser equipment is rugged, it is still susceptible to damage from rough handling. This is particularly true of the laser chamber itself and its housing, which should be treated with respect. Umbilical cords and cables should also be handled carefully, without kinks, and kept out of the way to avoid running equipment over them. Furthermore, setting up and taking down the laser apparatus should be done gently and in strict accordance with the manufacturer's directions.

Electrical Hazards

Most of the CO_2 lasers operate on 115-volt, 60-cycle house and operating room current. This current presents a definite hazard if allowed to pass through the human body, and must be carefully avoided. The laser equipment is enclosed in cabinets, which have automatic interlocking switches that open when a cover or a door is opened. This is a safety device that should not be bypassed. The laser tube itself operates on extremely high voltages and fairly high currents, and the connections to the laser chambers which contain this high voltage are protected from accidental touching. Again, the safety features must not be bypassed. The electrical connections in the laser machines are to be worked on only by individuals well-acquainted with the equipment and well-trained in the safety procedures.

Fire Hazards

Fire hazard facts and principles of the CO_2 laser can be divided into three categories, namely, reflection, absorption of the beam, and biological absorption.

Reflection The beam is reflected by shiny metallic surfaces. The laser beam is a focused beam, but its reflection from a concave surface (and from a convex surface under certain circumstances) may result in a high-power density that must be avoided. The blackening of instruments exposed to the laser reduces this reflection, but at the same time, they absorb the beam and become hot. This is the primary function of the tonsil hemostat described in Chapter 14. The inside of a nonblackened laryngoscope can reflect the beam, and when this occurs, it may inadvertently hit unplanned areas.

Absorption of the beam The beam is absorbed by glass, ceramics, and plastics. When this occurs, heat is produced, and melting or shattering of the substance may occur, along with fire. Therefore, plastic endotracheal tubes are extremely dangerous, and should never be used. Ordinary glass and plastic, which absorbs the CO_2 beam, will provide adequate protection to the eyes.

Biological absorption The CO_2 laser beam is absorbed by all biological tissues composed of water, and organic and mineral substances. Because the carbon dioxide beam is absorbed efficiently by water, the beam response of tissue with a high water content will be great. In tissue with a low water content, ie, bone, the response will appear slower, but the final temperature will be much higher. When considering a mass of solid elements, excluding hard bone, the response rate will be rapid. When the beam is absorbed, its energy is transformed into heat, the amount of heat being related to the power and the area over which the power is distributed, ie, the *power density*. This quantity is difficult to determine unless the size of the beam at its point of impact is taken into consideration.

SAFETY PROCEDURES

Eyes

Eye protection from the laser for everyone concerned is important. The patient's eyes must be protected; even a relatively small exposure of the cornea to the laser beam will result in permanent corneal damage. The patient's eyes should be covered by moistened eye pads, cloth adhesive tape, and head covers for protection. When under local anesthesia, it is important for the patient to wear glasses or otherwise have his eyes covered. Operating room personnel must also wear glasses. Current knowledge suggests there has been no eye damage; nevertheless, such protective measures should be rigidly enforced (Figure 3-1). For the operating surgeon's further protection, he too should wear glasses; his eyes are protected only while looking into the microscope.

Face

In addition to the eyes, the patient's face also may be exposed to the laser beam. When a small laryngoscope is used, there is danger the beam might not go down the tube, and this danger is increased when a virtual image is used as an aiming marker. There is less danger when the aiming light is a helium-neon laser. As a wise precaution, wrap moistened gauze around the laryngoscope to protect the patient's lips. Dry gauze will burn; use only gauze that is soaking wet, and moisten it from time to time, to prevent it from drying out.

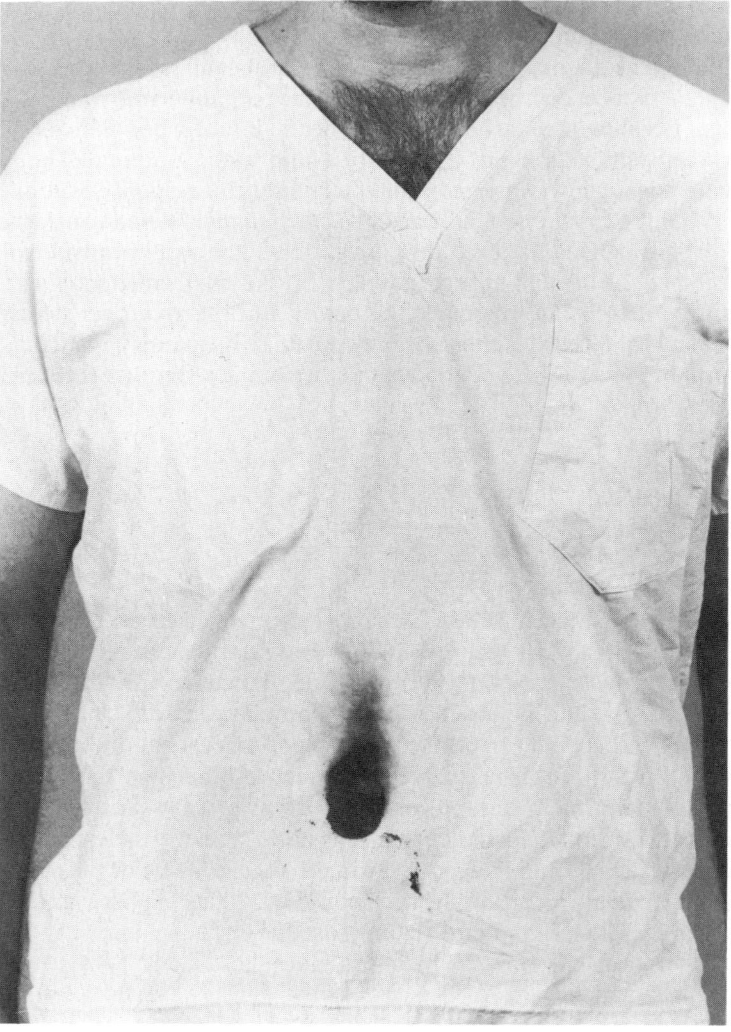

Figure 3-1 Fire in assistant's shirt, caused by inadvertent reflection of the beam. It illustrates the importance of guarding against accidental reflection and eye injury of everyone in the operating room.

Trachea and Endotracheal Tubes

When working in the larynx, there is always a possibility the beam might pass down the larynx and impinge on the wall of the subglottic larynx and trachea, or hit the cuff of the endotracheal tube. If the latter occurs, a hole is invariably made in the cuff, which destroys the seal, and necessitates replacement of the endotracheal tube. A superficial burn of the mucosa of the trachea may still occur even when the beam is out of focus. Although this may do no ultimate harm, it is prudent to protect against it.

As noted previously, the beam is readily absorbed by plastic endotracheal tubes and should not be used with the CO_2 laser.[3] Red rubber tubes are more resistant to the laser beam than are plastic tubes. Additional protection against the laser beam is accomplished easily by wrapping the tube with thin aluminum adhesive tape, overlapping the layers by one-half to one-third of the width, and applying it only in the area potentially exposed to the beam. Wrapping the tube above this area may cause kinking when the tube makes the curve from the pharynx into the mouth. Although the aluminum tape provides protection, it should not be relied on heavily, to the extent that the beam is allowed to hit the endotracheal tube unnecessarily. The tape is only a safety factor and is not absolute.

Norton and de Vos[4] have described a nonflammable, flexible endotracheal tube, which solved the problem of fire with red rubber tubing. These tubes do not have a built-in cuff. When an airtight seal with the trachea is needed, a separable balloon cuff must be slipped over the distal end. This adds a balloon filling tube through the larynx to an already crowded lumen. The metal endotracheal tubes are not completely airtight because of flexibility between the spirals of the tube.

Occasionally, debris from lasing ignites and produces a flare. This is apt to occur when the gas in the area has a high oxygen concentration, as can occur with a leak around the cuff of the endotracheal tube and positive inspiratory pressure used for controlled respiration. A flare of this type was fortuitously recorded in two adjacent frames of a 16-frame-per-second film. Although this flare was of short duration and no visible harm resulted, it is considered poor technique and may cause indirect ignition of any flammable material present.

Recently, Hirschman and Smith[5] demonstrated how flammable endotracheal tubes can be ignited by particles of hot debris caused by lasing char material from a previous lasing. (Strong[6] confirmed this report.) The reported accident occurred while lasing through a tracheal stoma, with the endotracheal tube delivering gases in the trachea above the stoma. An accident like this can be avoided by adherence to the principles of safety and good laser techniques, as follows: 1) avoid lasing char; 2) use local anesthesia when lasing through a tracheal stoma with a nasal speculum;

and 3) administer anesthesia through a bronchoscope or nonflammable endotracheal tube when the tube cannot be sealed below the lesion. Caution: metal endotracheal tubes will not catch fire, but sparks might still burn the tracheal mucosa or even set fire to flammable connections.

Neurosurgical Sponges

Cottonoids, or folded strips of gauze, soaking wet with normal saline solution, are placed below the vocal cords to prevent hitting the trachea or the cuff of the endotracheal tube with the beam. These Cottonoids must be soaking wet and kept wet throughout the procedure. If they dry out, they may catch fire, which may quickly spread to the cuff on the endotracheal tube as well as burn the patient (Figure 3-2). The surgeon should bear this in mind and moisten the Cottonoids from time to time as required. A 10-ml syringe, filled with normal saline, should be available on the operating table at all times to extinguish any fire that might occur during the procedure.

Cottonoids are usually on a thread to facilitate retrieval at the conclusion of the lasing. Even when these threads are soaked in saline, they may still have enough stiffness to protrude into the lumen of the laryngoscope. Occasionally, a thread may be cut by the laser beam, and retrieval of the Cottonoids sometimes requires the passage of a bronchoscope and forceps to remove them from the trachea. This problem can be eliminated by passing a fine jeweler's chain through the Cottonoids and cutting off the thread.[7] The chain lies posteriorly, is highly flexible, and rarely interferes with lasing. The chain can reflect the laser beam, but

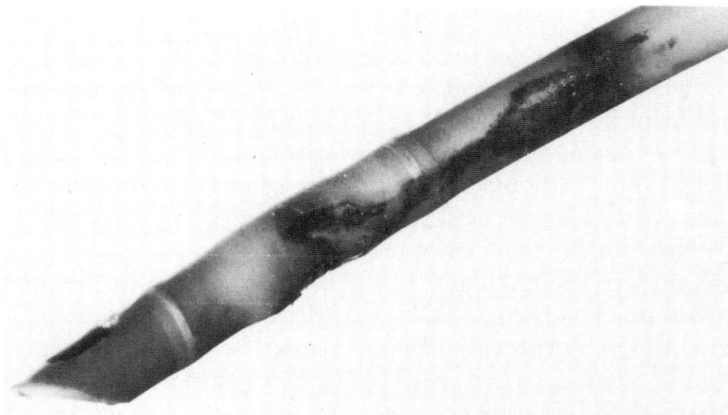

Figure 3-2 Fire occurring when Cottonoids above inflated cuff dried. Although the patient was not harmed, it illustrates the importance of keeping Cottonoids wet at all times.

testing has failed to show this presents a hazard (see Chapter 8, Figure 8-7).

Instruments

Instruments for use with the CO_2 laser have handles at 45° to keep the surgeon's fingers well out of the path of the beam. Occasionally, a surgeon concentrating on the problem at hand may allow his fingers to get in the way. Two different types of burns result. If the beam hits the rubber glove tangentially, it will heat the rubber to a point where he finally notices it. The burning sensation will continue for several seconds, and a blister may result. If the beam hits his glove and finger directly, a small hole will be burned into the glove and skin. This causes immediate pain, but will stop as soon as the laser beam is shut off. The burn is usually larger in the first, rather than the second, instance. Remember, only instruments designed not to reflect the laser beam should be used to prevent reflection inside the laryngoscope. If they are not used, the beam may reflect back and forth, emerge from the end of the laryngoscope, and burn the surgeon, or reflect off an instrument onto a bystander. This has been described by Marhic et al.[8]

Drapes, gowns, and linens must also receive consideration. All such materials absorb the laser beam and may ignite. Disposable paper materials are more susceptible than regular linen.

FLAMMABILITY TESTS

Every laser user, including the anesthesiologist dealing with otolaryngologic patients, should test for flammability. The equipment used to do so is simple. Four bricks serve as a base, sides, and backstop (Figure 3-3). Catheters, tubes, and almost any material can be tested. A tin can, open at one end and with a 1/4-inch brass or copper tube soldered in the side, can be flooded with different concentrations of oxygen and anesthetic gases (Figure 3-4). Small pieces of moist paper make good targets. Endotracheal tubes of different materials and wrapping and with different gases flowing through them can be tested destructively. Common sense demands a bucket of water or a fire extinguisher be close at hand.

SUMMARY

When not in use, the laser should be off, or on standby, or its timer switch shut off. Although the foot switch is guarded, it is still possible to activate the switch inadvertently.

Carelessness is the greatest hazard a surgeon faces. When a fire has occurred, it is almost always possible to identify the error. It is usually caused by thoughtlessness and by not following the principles of hazards and safety. To avoid this, the surgeon must train himself always to be alert to the hazards and to conscientiously follow the safety procedures. The laser beam is just as dangerous as a knife, scissors, or hemostat, but of a different type. When the danger is identified, recognized, and compensated for, the CO_2 laser becomes a safe and valuable addition to the armamentarium of the surgeon.

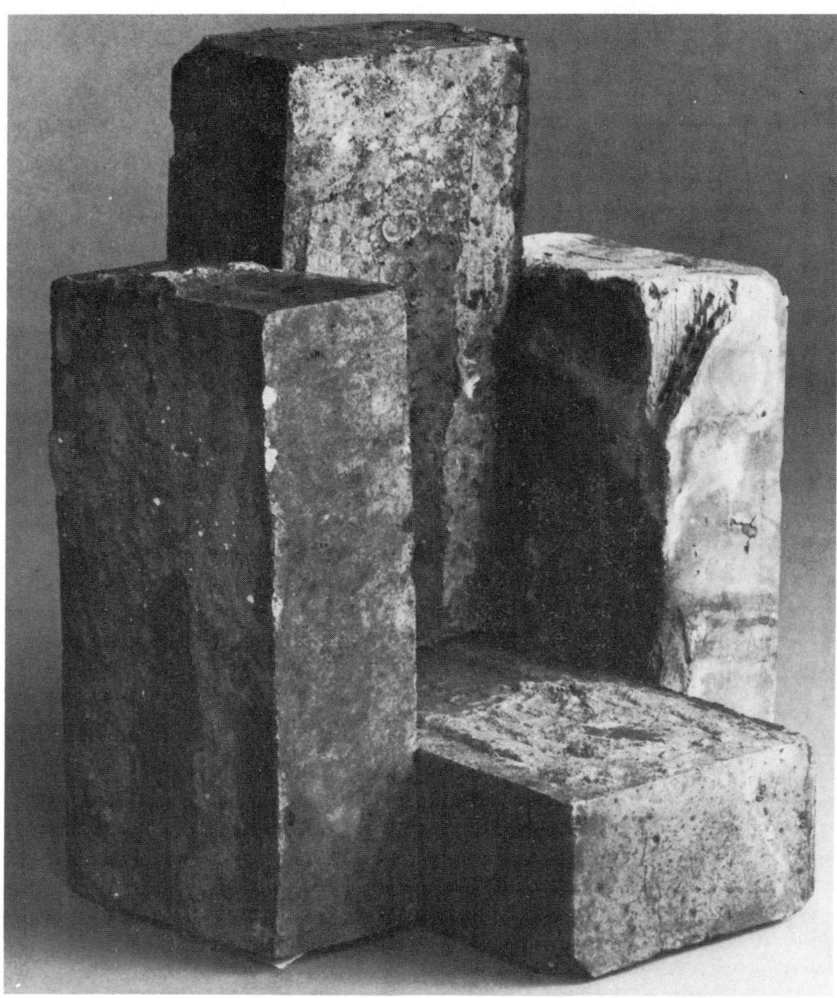

Figure 3-3 Brick enclosures for safety testing of materials for flammability. A fire extinguisher or pail of water should be close at hand.

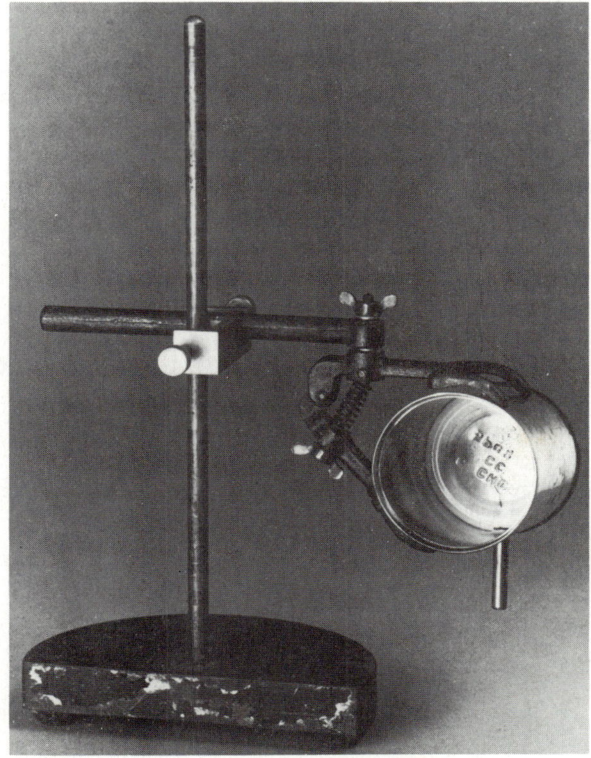

Figure 3-4 Small tin can with side arm for testing flammability of materials in the presence of various concentrations of oxygen and anesthetic gases, which are applied through the side arm.

REFERENCES

1. Strong MS, Jako GJ: Laser surgery in the larynx. *Ann Otol Rhinol Laryngol* 81:791–798, 1972.

2. Andrews AH Jr, Moss HW: Experience with the carbon dioxide laser in the larynx *Ann Otol Rhinol Laryngol* 83:462–470, 1974.

3. Burgess GE III, LeJeune FE Jr: Endotracheal tube ignition during laser surgery of the larynx. *Arch Otolaryngol* 105:561–562, 1979.

4. Norton ML, de Vos P: A new endotracheal tube for laser surgery of the larynx. *Ann Otol Rhinol Laryngol* 87:554–558, 1978.

5. Hirshman CA, Smith J: Indirect ignition of the endotracheal tube during carbon dioxide laser surgery. *Arch Otolaryngol* 106:639–641, 1980.

6. Strong MS: Editorial comment. *Arch Otolaryngol* 106:641, 1980.

7. Andrews AH Jr: Jewelry chain on Cottonoids for CO_2 laser surgery. *Ann Otol Rhinol Laryngol* 88:827, 1979.

8. Marhic ME, Kwan LI, Epstein M: Invariant properties of helical-circular waveguides. *Appl Phys Lett* 33:874–876, 1978.

4 Laser Regulation by Government

William M. Strouse, MS

The U.S. Food and Drug Administration established and enforces regulations concerning lasers under two federal laws. One law is the 1968 Radiation Control for Health and Safety Act,[1] which is concerned with radiation emissions from electronic products, ie, microwave ovens, television sets, x-ray units, lasers, and other devices. The regulations promulgated by the FDA's Bureau of Radiological Health (BRH) under this law require manufacturers to certify that their products are designed and made so that users are not subject to unnecessary radiation and that they meet applicable BRH-promulgated standards (if any). There is a standard for lasers. Among various specific mandates of this standard are certain requirements for labels on a laser system. One label which often elicits queries is shown in Figure 4-1.

The format, content, colors and, laser class are all specified in the BRH standard. All CO_2 lasers for surgery are Class IV, the highest power category of lasers.

No laser system, for medical or any other use, can be legally offered for sale in the United States unless the system is in conformance with the standard.

The other law, enacted in 1976, amends the Federal Food, Drug and Cosmetic Act to bring medical devices under its purview.[2] The purpose of this law is to ensure that all medical devices marketed are safe and effective. The FDA places devices in one of three classes: I.) General Controls, II.) Performance Standards, III.) Premarket Approval.

If a device is put in Class III, this indicates that insufficient information exists about its use. Before it can be marketed, the manufacturer must have submitted and had approved by the FDA an application for premarket approval. Although characterized by some observers as similar to the new drug application (NDA) procedure for drugs, there is greater involvement of outside experts because the classification panels are involved directly in the review of premarket approval applications.[3] For a device in Class II, there is believed to be enough information to establish a performance standard to assure safety and effectiveness. The Class I General Controls apply to all devices, but such classification for a device demands neither of the more stringent requirements of standards or premarket approval.

The FDA's Bureau of Medical Devices (BMD) is guided in its classification by the judgments of 18 advisory panels in various fields of medical specialization. Each panel has seven professional members plus one industry and one consumer representative. CO_2 lasers used for surgery in gynecological practice are in the Performance Standard classification; the standard to be met is the previously cited BRH standard. As of September 1980, no official classification was assigned by the FDA for CO_2 lasers for use in otorhinolaryngology. However, there is strong assurance that these also will be given the Performance Standard classification, following the recommendation of ENT panel, according to the people at the FDA.

The regulations established under these laws apply to manufacturers; they are to protect all users, whether they be physicians, patients or cooks using microwave ovens. Manufacturers are further required to have

DANGER
VISIBLE AND INVISIBLE LASER
RADIATION-AVOID UNINTENDED EYE
OR SKIN EXPOSURE TO DIRECT,
REFLECTED OR SCATTERED RADIATION
HE-NE LASER
MAX POWER 0.5 mW CW
CO2 LASER
MAX POWER 25 W CW
Class IV Laser Product

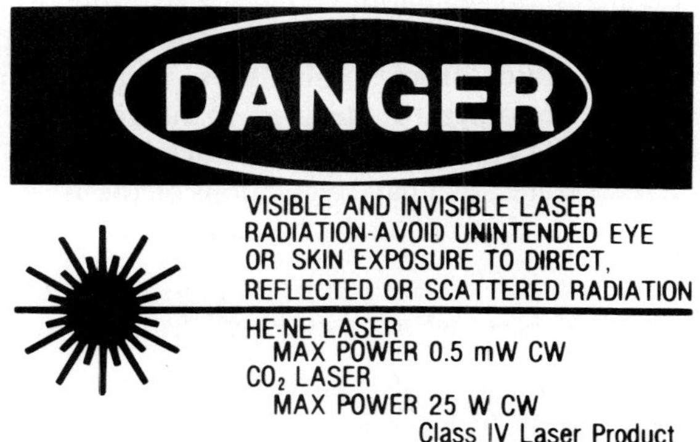

Figure 4-1 FDA-required label for laser systems.

quality assurance programs, good manufacturing practices, and must maintain user records to permit product recalls if necessary. Their premises are subject to government inspection and their products, for cause, can be forced from the market by FDA actions under the 1976 Amendments Act or the 1968 Radiation Safety Act.

For further information regarding the 1968 Radiation Control Act and the regulations under it, direct inquiries to:

Department of Health and Human Services
Public Health Service
Food and Drug Administration
Bureau of Radiological Health
Rockville, Maryland 20857

Concerning the 1976 Amendments Act, inquire of:

Department of Health and Human Services
Public Health Service
Food and Drug Administration
Bureau of Medical Devices
Silver Spring, Maryland 20910

There is one radio-frequency-powered CO_2 laser system for surgery now on the market. The Federal Communications Commission must have evaluated the radio-frequency components to be sure that their requirements are met regarding such matters as interference and frequency stability. The obligation to assume such compliance rests with the manufacturer. The purchaser of such a system should check the product literature and labeling to be certain that FCC requirements have been met.

Six states currently have regulations regarding lasers. These are Alaska, Georgia, Illinois, Massachusetts, New York, and Texas. The State Department of (Public) Health is the cognizant agency in all but New York, where it is the Department of Labor.

In all these states, the regulations require registration by laser owners and the reporting of accidents. There are widely varying other requirements among these states, from nothing more than accident reporting and registration (two states) to detailed mandates for "laser safety officer," marking and control of spaces in which lasers are used, etc. In the four of these six states, that have regulations on the use of lasers, there are specific statements that the use by licensed physicians is not limited.

REFERENCES

1. Public Law 90–602, 90th Congress, H.R. 10790, October 18, 1968.
2. Public Law 94–295, 94th Congress, S. 510. May 28, 1976.
3. HEW Publication No. (FDA) 77–5006, Silver Spring, Maryland, October 1977.

5 Tissue Reaction to the CO_2 Laser in General

R.C.J. Verschueren, MD

The CO_2 laser emits at 10.6 μ and thus its beam is strongly absorbed in water.[1] Moreover, this absorption is not color dependent and follows Beer's exponential law:

$$I = I_0 e^{-\alpha z}$$

I_0 = intensity of the incident beam
I = intensity of the beam z cm beneath the tissue surface
α = absorption coefficient (cm^{-1})
z = tissue depth (cm)
e = base of natural logarithm (2.71...)

Since living tissues contain about 80% or 90% water and since the absorption of the CO_2 laser beam is independent from the color, any tissue will strongly absorb the 10.6 μ beam. This characteristic permits the CO_2 laser to be used as a light knife.

EFFECT OF THE FOCUSED CO_2 LASER BEAM ON TISSUES

The Mechanism of the Action of the Focused Beam

In order to be of use as a surgical tool, the beam of the CO_2 laser should be focused by a lens. Using an appropriate lens, the beam can be focused to a spot with a diameter of a few millimeters or less, thus achieving a considerable energy density. As soon as the focused beam impinges on the surface of a tissue, the incident light is absorbed in an approximately 200-μ tissue layer at the surface. While passing through this superficial tissue layer, the intensity I of the beam decreases exponentially (Figure 5-1), and the amount of light energy I absorbed in a layer Δz will also decrease exponentially.

The small layer at the surface will absorb the highest amount of energy and immediately transform it into heat. The tissue temperature suddenly increases to the extent that intra- and extracellular fluids instantaneously boil and are transformed into steam, provided, of course, that the laser beam supplies the required energy. This is generally the case with focused, CW CO_2 laser of a few watts or more. The volume expansion caused by this transformation entirely disrupts tissue architecture. Some cells explode and are transformed into steam and dust; others remain more or less intact. Mihashi et al[2] investigated the airborne tissue particles originating from the epithelium of the tongue and found a considerable number of squamous cells among the carbonized tissue particles. Most of the cells were partly carbonized; some preserved their original size. No growth was observed when an attempt was made to culture these cells.

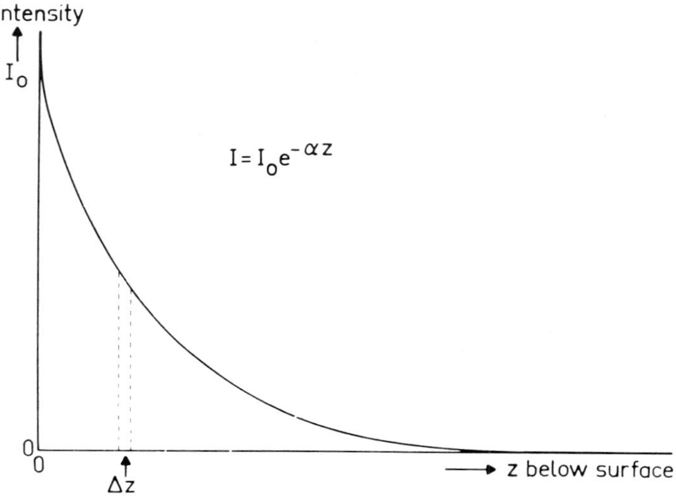

Figure 5-1 Exponential decrease of the beam intensity I in the tissue.

Similar observations were made by Oosterhuis[3] when investigating the effect of the CO_2 laser on the Cloudman S_{91} melanoma. Although only tissue fluids vaporize, while dehydrated tissue particles are taken away in the smoke, *explosive tissue evaporation* nevertheless is an appropriate name for this process.

With the handpiece of the laser positioned so as to focus the beam on the surface of the tissue, a crater is formed on exposure. Since the distribution of the power density in the focal spot is Gaussian and has more or less the shape of a bell, the power density is maximal in the center of the spot and decreases toward the edges (Figure 5-2). Because evaporation of a certain tissue volume is due to the evaporation of the corresponding amount of water contained in it, the tissue volume vaporized per unit of time is determined by the local energy density. Therefore, the tissue defect created at the focus of the laser beam will be conical since the energy density and, hence, the vaporized volume is larger in the center of the focal spot. Mihashi[2] carried out electron microscopic investigations of tissue defects created with the CO_2 laser and, indeed, found that "the general appearance of the crater closely resembles the crater of a volcano."

Moving the focus of the beam over the surface of the tissue makes an incision. The depth of this incision is determined by the speed of the movement and by the power output of the laser. Increasing the speed decreases the exposure time and, consequently, lessens the depth of the cut. Moving the focused beam with the same speed, but with the laser delivering less power, the incision is shallower. The CO_2 laser thus can be used as a tissue-cutting and a tissue-vaporizing instrument.

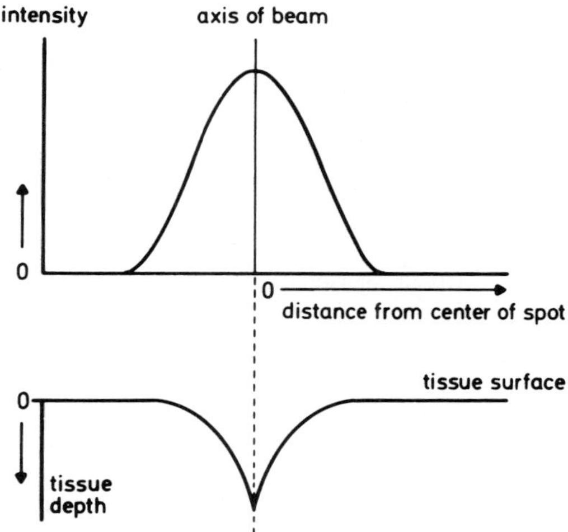

Figure 5-2 Relationship between the intensity distribution in the spot and the configuration of the crater.

Thermal Damage Caused by the Focused Beam of the CO_2 Laser

Hall,[4] reporting about research carried out at the Royal College of Surgeons, stated that the ablation temperature of tissues when incised with the CO_2 laser is about the boiling point of water. The vaporization of tissue fluids has a thermostatic influence and keeps the temperature at about 100°C during evaporation. It is obvious, therefore, that some extent of thermal damage should be expected in the edges of a CO_2 laser incision. As was already stressed, the light energy impinging on the surface is entirely absorbed in a thin layer of tissue about 200 μ thick. The most superficial part of this layer (Δz_1) instantaneously vaporizes, and a temperature of 100°C is soon maintained at the newly created surface (Figure 5-3). From this surface layer downwards, the temperature decreases exponentially, since the locally absorbed light energy is decreasing the same way. The most superficial part of this layer (Δz_{2a}) may be expected to be thermally damaged beyond repair, the local temperature being higher than 70°C. This critical temperature of 70°C is the threshold above which even short exposures cause irreversible tissue damage.[5] The layer Δz_{2b} absorbs energy and transforms it into heat, but the temperature thus generated is not high enough to cause cell damage. The light energy

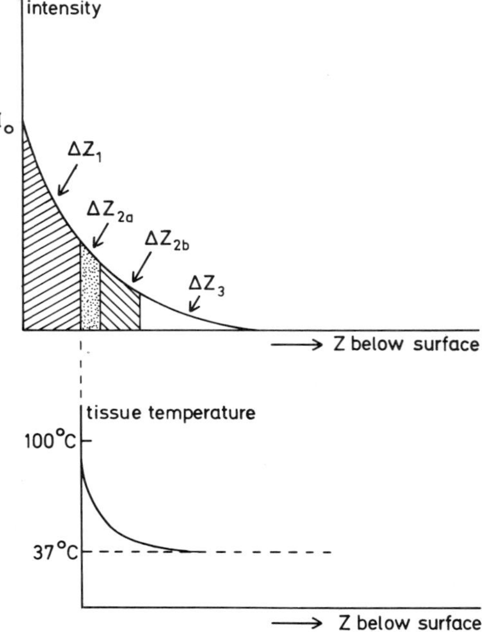

Figure 5-3 The slope of the beam intensity in the tissue, the zones of thermal damage (top) and the corresponding temperature distribution.

absorbed in the layer Δz_3 is not sufficient to raise the local temperature. This explanation is a simplification, merely a "snapshot" of what is happening. The relative thickness of the three layers Δz_1, Δz_2, and Δz_3 as schematically depicted in Figure 5-3 is relevant, but does not claim to be exact.

Morphologically, the thermal damage can be divided in three zones. The first layer closest to the surface has been completely removed by evaporation. The next zone has a rim of carbonized tissue particles, dehydrated cells interspersed with empty spaces originating from steam formation. The third zone looks morphologically normal on H and E stain, but has nevertheless been damaged beyond repair by heat (Figure 5-4). This becomes obvious on the section of Figure 5-5 processed for the determination of glucose-6-phosphatase activity. Below the layer with the morphologically changed cells and the empty spaces lies an uncolored zone where the cells did not take the specific staining since the glucose-6-phosphatase was destroyed by heat.

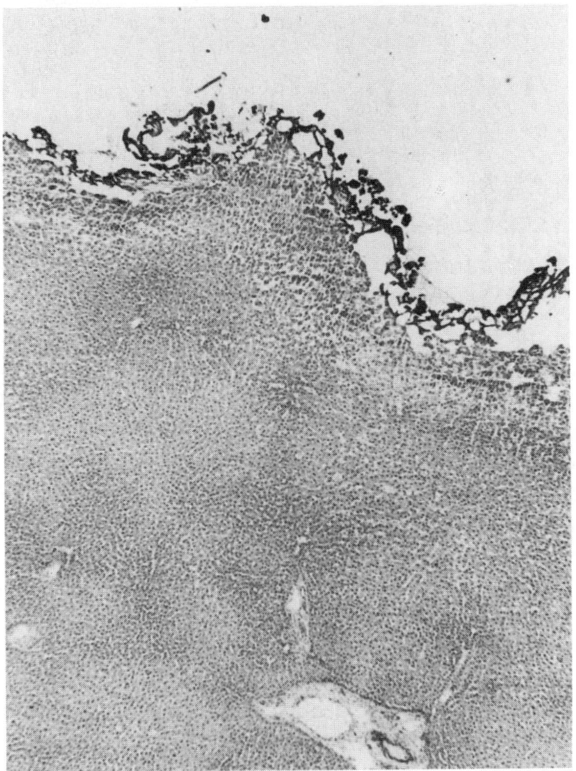

Figure 5-4 Section from a CO_2 laser incision in rabbit liver (H + E stain) showing the carbonized rim and empty spaces (50 ×).

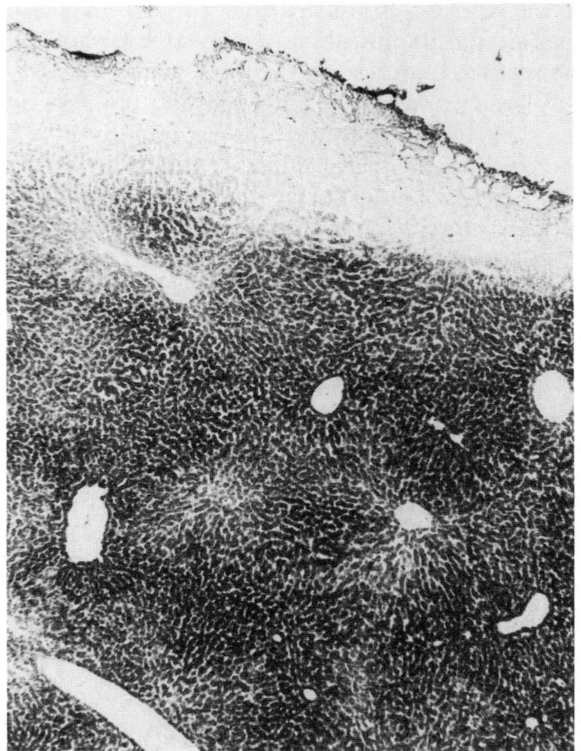

Figure 5-5 Section from a CO_2 laser incision in rabbit liver. The slice has been processed for the determination of glucose-6-phosphatase activity (50 ×).

When incising tissues at a relatively high speed, the thermal damage in the edges of the incision is about 100 μ thick. When the laser beam is moved with a relatively slower speed, the thermal phenomena become more complex since every fraction of the incision is exposed to the beam for a longer period of time. The surface layer kept at a temperature of 100° C during the evaporation acts as a heat source for thermal conduction toward underlying tissues. This thermal damage caused by heat conduction is superimposed on the damage caused by beam absorption.

For practical reasons we can summarize that three different processes are taking place while incising tissues (Figure 5-6):

1. Tissue evaporation deepens and widens the incision.
2. Energy absorbed in the underlying layer causes thermal damage.
3. Heat conduction from the edges causes additional thermal damage.

The depth of this thermal damage in the wall of a crater was investigated by means of enzyme-histochemical methods and proved to be caused mainly by heat conduction and, hence, was time related.[6] Changes in power output affected only the size of the crater without influencing the penetration of thermal damage in the edges.

EFFECT OF THE DEFOCUSED BEAM ON TISSUES

When using the CO_2 laser beam for incising or vaporizing tissue, a slight hemorrhage may occur. The defocused beam will arrest such bleeding. By using a handpiece defocusing can be effected by increasing the distance between the handpiece and the tissue. When performing microsurgery with the laser, the beam can be defocused by switching lenses or by moving the lens away from the target.

With the defocused beam the power density is insufficient for explosive tissue evaporation to take place. The tissue fluids slowly vaporize and when the superficial tissue layer has become dehydrated, the temperature, lacking the thermostatic effect of boiling tissue fluids, rises far above 100°C. The tissues in the beam obviously shrink and soon carbonize, and even start glowing. It can be assumed that the surface temperature of the tissue is at least 300°C, the level required for tissue carbonization and combustion to occur.[7]

During tissue evaporation, the heat conduction surrounding tissues originated from a layer with a temperature of about 100°C. In contrast, when a defocused beam is used, the surface has a temperature at least three times higher. Thermal damage generated by heat conduction consequently will penetrate deeper into the underlying tissues than with a focused beam. Therefore, caution is required when using the defocused beam for hemostatic purposes since overenthusiastic use may lead to considerable thermal damage and delayed healing.

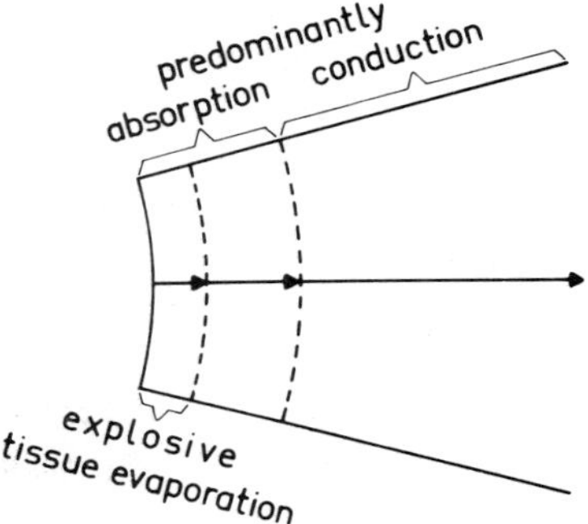

Figure 5-6 Schematic drawing of the three processes determining the extent of thermal damage.

SUMMARY

The CO_2 laser generates relatively simple thermal processes. Knowing what the laser does, the surgeon can increase the reliability and the safety of his procedures by taking into consideration the factors which determine thermal damage.

REFERENCES

1. Bayly JG, Kartha VB, Stevens WH: The absorption spectra of liquid phase H_20, HDO and D_2O from 0.7 μm to 10 μm infra-red. *Physics* 3:211–223, 1963.
2. Mihashi S, Jako GJ, Incze J, et al: Laser surgery in otolaryngology: Interaction of CO_2 laser and soft tissue. *Ann NY Acad Sci* 267:263–294, 1976.
3. Oosterhuis JW: Tumor surgery with the CO_2 laser: Studies with the Cloudman S_{91} mouse melanoma. Thesis—State University, Groningen, The Netherlands, 1977.
4. Hall RR, Beach AD, Baker E, et al: Incision of tissue by carbon dioxide laser. *Nature* 232:131–132, 1971.
5. Moritz AR, Hendriques FC: Studies on thermal injury: II. The relative importance of time and surface temperature in the causation of cutaneous burns. *Am J Pathol* 23:695–720, 1947.
6. Verschueren R: *The CO_2 Laser in Tumor Surgery*. Assen, Van Gorcum, 1970.
7. Moritz AR: Studies of thermal injury: III. The pathology and pathogenesis of cutaneous burns: An experimental study. *Am J Pathol* 23:915–937, 1947.

6 Tissue Reaction to the CO_2 Laser in Malignant Disease

J. Wolter Oosterhuis, MD

The focus of CO_2 laser beam, as pointed out in previous chapters, is a spot of intense heat. The main effect of the CO_2 laser on tissues therefore is thermal destruction.[1] The tissue in the area of the focus is immediately vaporized, leaving a crater lined by a narrow zone of devitalized cells. The width of this zone depends mainly on the exposure time and much less on the output of the laser beam.[2]

The sudden vaporization of tissue from the surface generates a mechanical impulse propagated into the tissue at the impact site, based on conservation of momentum. Measurement of the velocity at which the steam expands from the point of action of the CO_2 laser indicates that the pressure waves due to this mechanism are small.[3]

The CO_2 laser beam has exactly the same effects on normal and malignant tissue. It is the nature of malignant tissues, ie, its capacity to give rise to new tumor foci after spread of viable tumor cells, that requires further discussion of its interaction with a CO_2 laser beam.

ONCOLOGICAL ASPECTS OF CO_2 LASER SURGERY

Removal of a malignant tumor can be accomplished by excision with the laser or by vaporization. When excising a tumor one should leave the same margins as with the conventional scalpel because of the very narrow zone of thermal necrosis. Vaporization requires the same margins. The CO_2 laser has *no oncolytic* effect beyond the zone of thermal devitalization. Incomplete removal of a tumor will result in recurrence. Nevertheless, the zone of coagulation necrosis lining a CO_2 laser incision may have some significance in tumor surgery. The capillaries and larger vessels up to 0.5 mm in diameter are sealed,[3] resulting in reduced bleeding, even when compared to a diathermy incision.[4] It is reasonable to assume that the lymphatics in the cut edge are also sealed. This might reduce spill of tumor cells from the surgical specimen into the operative wound and also reduce iatrogenic, distant tumor spread via blood vessels and lymphatics.[3] The "no touch" removal of tumor tissue by vaporization might also add to the reduction of iatrogenic tumor spread.

On the other hand, it is conceivable that the CO_2 laser promotes iatrogenic tumor spread. The waste material originating during laser vaporization can be divided in two fractions: 1) the steam expanding from the surface, which contains fine tissue particles called *smoke* and 2) the coarser particles, which fall downward called *debris.* Both fractions may contain viable tumor cells and hence cause airborne tumor spill in the operative field. In addition, the pressure effects may force viable tumor cells into adjacent tissue slits, blood vessels, and lymphatics, thereby increasing local recurrence rate and iatrogenic distant tumor spread. The conceivable adverse and beneficial effects of the CO_2 laser on iatrogenic tumor spread are schematically listed in Table 6-1.

Table 6-1
Possible Effects of the CO_2 Laser on Iatrogenic Tumor Spread

	Promoting	Reducing
Local spread	smoke, debris pressure effect	no touch sealing of vessels
Distant spread (blood vessels, lymphatics)	pressure effect	no touch sealing of vessels

These theoretical considerations clearly demonstrate the need of experiments to determine the actual influence of the CO_2 laser on iatrogenic tumor spread, before introducing the instrument on a large scale in tumor surgery. Such experiments are even more desirable in view of the fact that Ketcham and his associates[5] have shown that pulsed lasers cause airborne and local spread of viable tumor, which results in local recurrences.

EXPERIMENTS ON IATROGENIC TUMOR SPREAD WITH THE CO_2 LASER

We performed a series of experiments using the American Optical CO_2 laser[1] and the Cloudman S_{91} mouse melanoma[6] in CD/2 F_1 or DBA_2 female mice.[7] The Cloudman melanoma is an almost black tumor, which metastasizes exclusively to the lungs. The black metastases are easily recognizable.[8] The four experiments are listed in Table 6-2. In the first experiment, we investigated the morphology and viability of the smoke and debris originating during laser vaporization of Cloudman melanomas. In the following three experiments, designed to study the influence of the CO_2 laser on local and distant tumor spread using the parameters listed, we compared the CO_2 laser with conventional surgery. The results of these experiments will be presented. The details of the materials and methods have been published.[9-12]

Table 6-2
Experiments on Iatrogenic Tumor Spread by the CO_2 Laser

Experiments	Parameters	Related to
Investigation of "smoke" and "debris"	{ morphology viability }	airborne spread
radical removal of tumor*	{ local recurrences	—local spread
	lung metastases	hematogenous spread
incisional biopsy of tumor*	—tumor emboli in lungs	hematogenous spread
incision of labeled tumor*	{ radioactivity in lungs	hematogenous spread
	radioactivity in lymph nodes	—lymphatic spread

*randomized studies comparing CO_2 laser surgery with conventional surgery.

Investigation of Smoke and Debris

Cytological smears of harvested smoke and debris showed mainly carbonized particles and apparently thermally damaged cells, but also some morphologically intact cells (Figures 6-1, 6-2, 6-3). Viability was tested with the trypan blue test, culture in vitro, and inoculation in CD_2/F_1 mice, both intramuscularly and intraperitoneally. No dye-excluding cells were found in the trypan blue test. No growth was noted in vitro in 24 culture flasks seeded with 5.10^5 smoke or debris particles per flask. Similarly, no takes were observed in 127 mice injected with 10 -5.10^5 smoke or debris particles, and killed four weeks after inoculation. Viable cells derived from a Cloudman melanoma cell line and added to the smoke and debris suspensions remained viable. Thus, a toxic influence of smoke and debris particles on viable tumor cells, rendering the viability tests meaningless, was excluded (Figure 6-4). It was concluded that it is highly unlikely that viable tumor cells occur in the waste products of tumor vaporization. One would expect this in view of the physical characteristics of the CO_2 laser beam. Its wavelength of 10.6 μ is strongly absorbed in living tissues; 95% of the energy of the beam is absorbed in the first 150 μ of tissue.[2] The continuous delivery accounts for an even distribution of the power density in the target area in a certain period of time. The power densities are high enough to vaporize tissue, but no important pressure effects occur. Within the steam arising from the surface some morphologically intact cells are transported, but these have already been thermally devitalized.

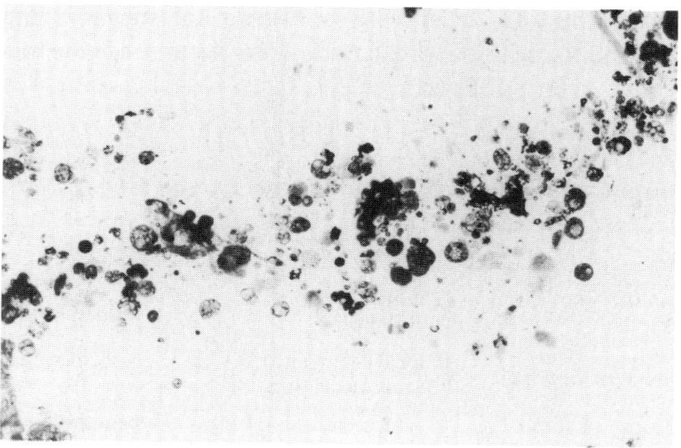

Figure 6-1 Smear of smoke suspension. The cell-sized carbonized particles, consisting of closely packed "steam bubbles," are in the majority (May-Grünwald-Giemsa, × 140).

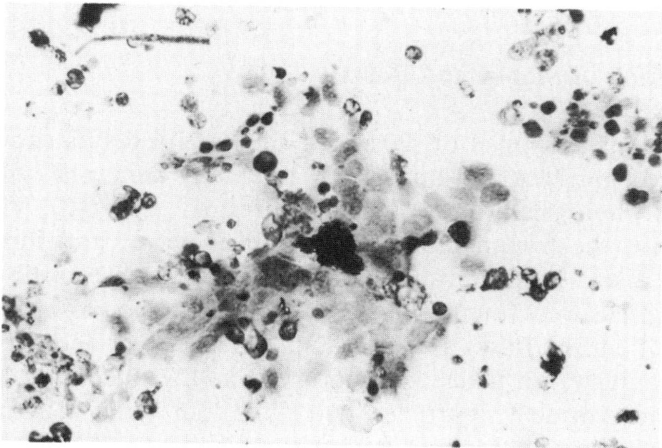

Figure 6-2 Smear of debris suspension. Transitions from carbonized particles into morphologically more intact cells (May-Grünwald-Giemsa, × 350).

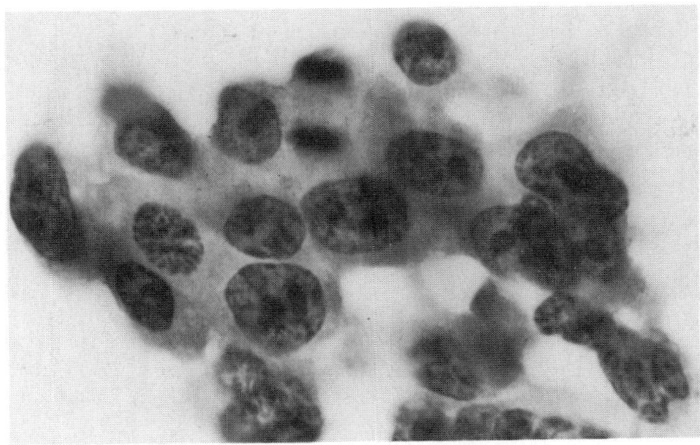

Figure 6-3 Smear of smoke suspension. Morphologically intact tumor cells. Note the mitotic figures (May-Grünwald-Giemsa, × 1400).

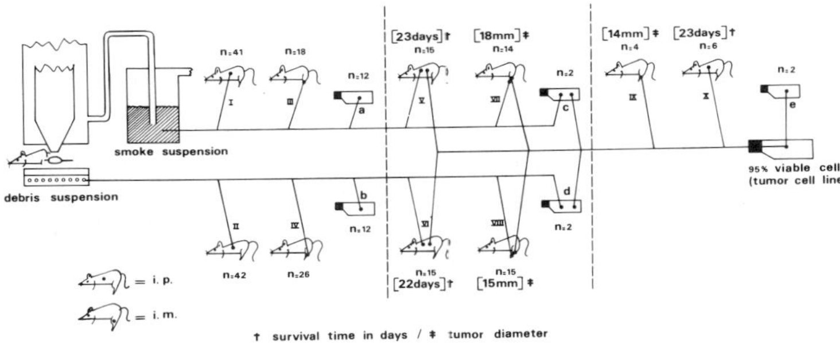

Figure 6-4 Results of in vitro culture and inoculation intramuscularly and intraperitoneally in syngeneic mice of suspensions of smoke and debris, resulting from CO_2 laser evaporation of Cloudman melanomas. Suspensions of smoke and debris alone never gave rise to growth in vitro (a and b) or tumor takes in mice (I, II, III, IV) (left side of figure). A suspension of viable tumor cells alone never failed to grow in vitro (e) or in vivo (IX and X) (right side of figure). Smoke and debris suspensions with added viable tumor cells gave rise to growth in all culture flasks (c and d) and showed only two take failures in group VII. Tumor growth was observed in all mice in groups, V, VI and VIII (center of figure).

CO_2 LASER VS CONVENTIONAL SURGERY

Radical Surgery

CO_2 laser and conventional surgery were compared in performing radical surgery on tumors in mice inoculated intramuscularly in the right hind leg. The mice were randomized before treatment.

The operations were performed in two experimental series. In the first series of experiments, the mean tumor size was 4 mm, and in the second, 9 mm (Figure 6-5). When the statistics for both series were added, it was found that the tumor was vaporized by the laser in a total of 112 mice

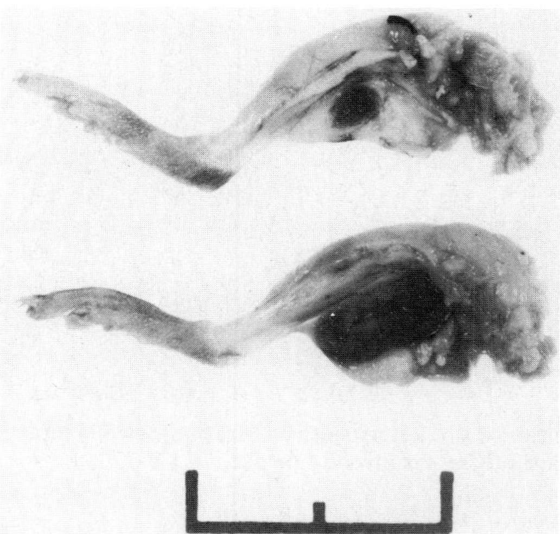

Figure 6-5 Amputated legs of mice from series I and series II showing medium-sized tumors.

and conventionally excised in 115 mice. All mice were killed and autopsied three weeks after treatment. The percentage of mice with local recurrences was the same in the laser and the conventionally treated mice, about 25% in series I and 5% in series II, proving that the CO_2 laser did not promote local tumor spread more than conventional surgery. Even more weight can be attached to this conclusion in view of the fact that the results were obtained by removal and damage of the same amount of tissue with both modalities. The statistics of mice with devitalized legs (Figures 6-6, 6-7) due to the treatment were equal for both treatment modalities, about 4% in series I and about 25% in series II. The differences between series I and series II (significantly less local recurrences and significantly more devitalized legs in series II) can be explained by the more uniform and superficial localization of the tumors in series II and by a more aggressive surgical approach.

The number of gross and microscopic metastases was uniformly low. They were the same in the laser and in the conventionally treated mice, as well as in a group of control mice, which had their tumor-bearing limb amputated after ligation of the femoral vessels, thus preventing iatrogenic metastases. It can be concluded that neither CO_2 laser nor conventional surgery increased the number of metastases. A superior role of the CO_2 laser, however, could not be demonstrated in this system. Virtually no blood loss occurred when operating with the CO_2 laser.

Incisional Biopsy

CO_2 laser and conventional surgery were compared in performing incisional biopsies from tumors with a mean size of about 15 mm. Mice in which the skin was incised after intraperitoneal pentobarbital anesthesia, and mice anesthetized with no skin incision acted as controls. In an additional group of mice, the tumor was massaged under intraperitoneal anesthesia. The total number of mice in these five groups was 66. The animals were randomized before treatment. The mice were killed with ether four hours after manipulation. The lungs and the right parailiac lymph nodes were investigated microscopically. Tumor emboli, consisting of at least two tumor cells, were used as the criterion for distant tumor spread (Figure 6-8). Tumor emboli in the lungs were found only in those mice which had established microscopic lung metastases as well. The incidence of microscopic tumor (metastases + tumor emboli) was the same in the five treatment groups, about 58%. Apparently, tumor emboli were related to the stage of evolution of the tumor and not influenced by manipulation. No tumor emboli were found in the lymph nodes. Neither a detrimental nor a beneficial influence of the CO_2 laser on distant tumor spread was, therefore, demonstrated.

Incision of Radioactively Labeled Tumor

We compared lymphatic and hematogenous migration of radioactively labeled tumor cells from ^{3}H-thymidine-labeled Cloudman S_{91} melanomas in DBA/2 female mice after CO_2 laser incision and convention scalpel incision. Melanoma cells growing exponentially in vitro were labeled by adding ^{3}H-thymidine (specific activity 2 Ci/mmole) to the culture medium overnight at a concentration of 13.3 μCi/ml. The cells were then harvested by trypsinization, washed, and resuspended to a concentration of 2×10^7 cells/ml. The radioactivity of the cells was 3×10^7 d.p.m./10^6 cells. The viability of the suspension was over 95%.

Forty-three mice were inoculated in their right calf muscles with 10 μl

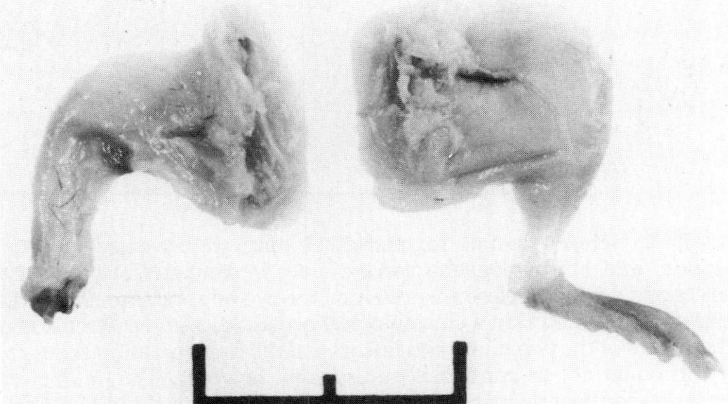

Figure 6-6 Devitalized leg of a laser-treated mouse from series II. The normal left leg is shown for comparison.

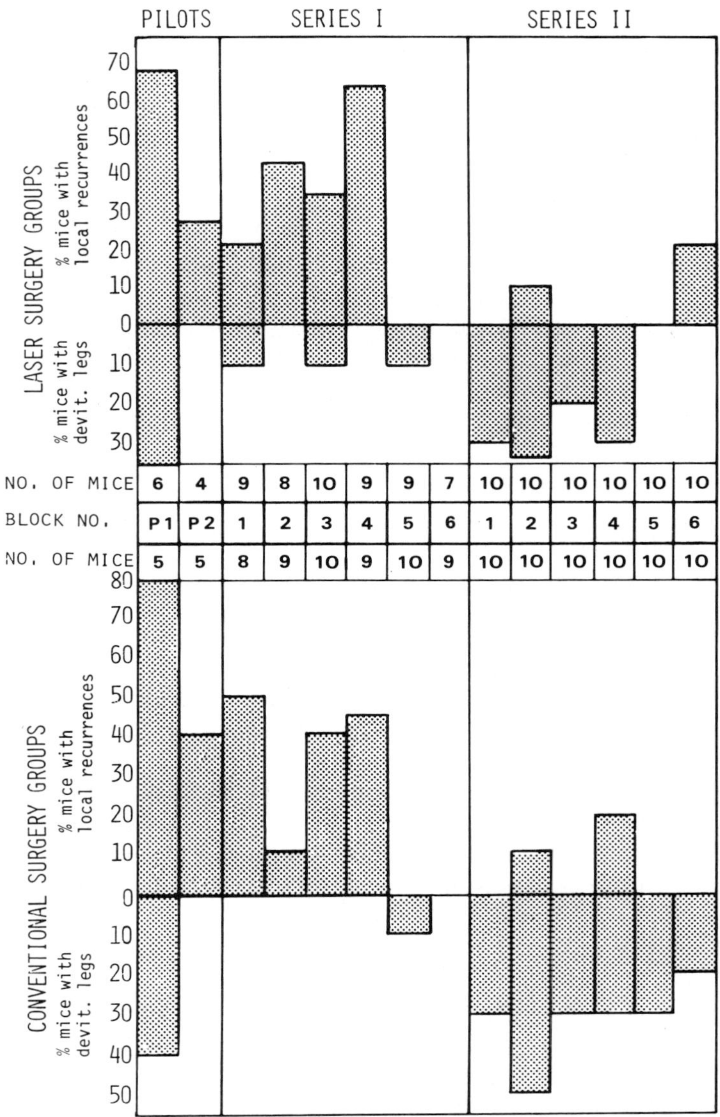

Figure 6-7 In series I and II together, 112 mice were treated by CO_2 laser vaporization, and 115 by conventional excision. Percentages of mice with local recurrences and devitalized legs are presented for two pilot experiments and for the 12 blocks of series I and II in a chronological order. A learning effect is suggested when the results of the two pilot experiments and the first operation series are compared. This could not be confirmed statistically, however. The number of local recurrences is significantly higher in the first series (χ^2-test, $p < 0.001$). The number of devitalized legs is significantly higher in the second series (χ^2-test, $p < 0.001$).

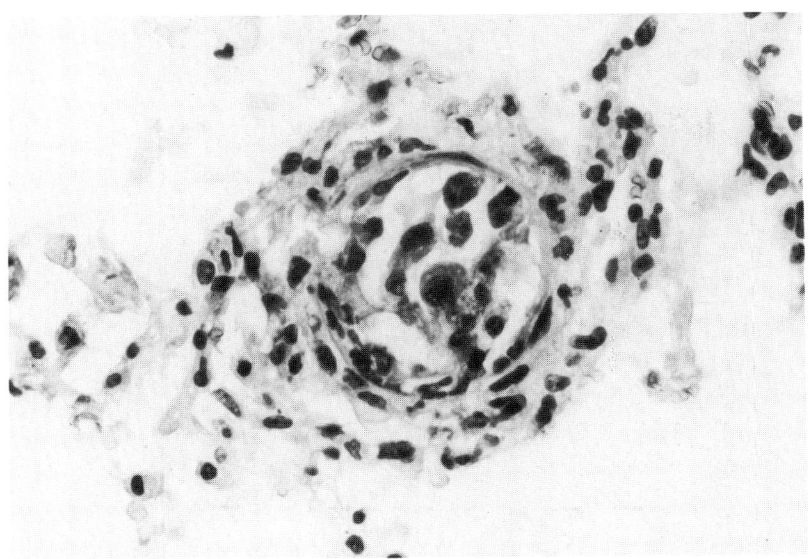

Figure 6-8 Tumor embolus in a pulmonary arteriole (H and E, × 560).

of this suspension containing 2×10^5 cells with a total activity of 6×10^6 d.p.m. The mice were randomized into three groups: laser incision (17), scalpel incision (17), and no incision (9). After eight days the cells had "taken," the size of the tumors being about 3 mm, and the animals were operated upon. Laser incisions were made with the 165-mm focal length handpiece of the Americal Optical CO_2 laser at an output of 10 to 20 watts. In all three groups the skin overlying the tumor was conventionally incised; in addition, the tumor and adjacent muscle were incised with the laser in the first group and with a conventional scalpel in the second group. The mice were killed 30 minutes after surgery. The tumor, the right parailiac lymph node, and a lung sample were removed and solubilized with "N.C.S." (Amersham) for liquid scintillation counting. One mouse of each group had to be discarded because of technical failures.

The results were reported in d.p.m. and tested by the Mann-Whitney U test (Figure 6-9). The radioactivity in the right parailiac lymph nodes was significantly higher in the scalpel-incision group than in either the laser-incision ($p < 0.01$) or no-incision ($p < 0.01$) groups. However, there was no significant difference in the radioactivity of the lymph nodes between the laser- and no-incision groups. Neither the tumors themselves nor the lung samples showed significant differences between the groups.

Conventional scalpel incision seemed to cause lymphatic migration of labeled cells, but laser incision did not. This favors the belief that the CO_2 laser might reduce dissemination of malignant cells via lymphatics,[3] possibly by sealing the cut ends of lymphatics.[10]

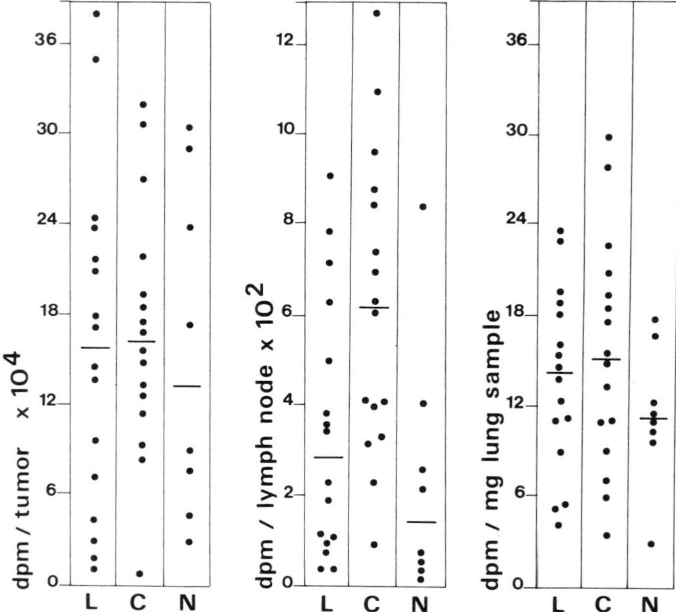

Figure 6-9 Lymphatic and hematogenous migration of label from ^{3}H-thymidine labeled Cloudman S_{91} melanoma in right calf of mice, 30 minutes after surgery. (L) laser incision; (C) conventional scalpel incision; (N) no incision. The median values are indicated by dashes. Significant differences between the groups were found only in lymph nodes. The radioactivity was higher after conventional scalpel incision than after laser incision ($p < 0.01$) or no incision ($p < 0.01$). The laser-incision group and no-incision group showed similar results.

SUMMARY

The results of these experiments demonstrated that the continuous wave CO_2 laser does not give rise to airborne and local tumor spread. This is in contradistinction to the pulsed laser. Promotion of iatrogenic distant tumor spread by the CO_2 laser as compared to conventional surgery could not be demonstrated. The reduction of iatrogenic spread of radioactive-labeled tumor cells, on the other hand, suggests that the CO_2 laser might reduce iatrogenic distant tumor spread. It is premature, however, to consider the clinical use of the CO_2 laser to reduce iatrogenic distant tumor spread.

It can be concluded, therefore, that use of the CO_2 laser is permissible but not specifically indicated on oncological grounds. The CO_2 laser should be used only when it clearly offers technical surgical advantages over existing methods.

ACKNOWLEDGMENTS

This work was supported by a grant from the Dutch Preventiefonds, and performed in close collaboration with Dr R.C.J. Verschueren in the Department of Pathology of the University of Groningen (head: Prof Dr Ph.J. Hoedemaeker).

REFERENCES

1. Polanyi TG, Bredemeier HC, Davis TW Jr: A CO_2 laser for surgical research. *Med Biol Engl* 8:541–548, 1970.

2. Verschueren RCJ: *The CO_2 Laser in Tumor Surgery.* Assen, Van Gorcum, 1976.

3. Hall RR, Hill DW, Beach AD: A carbon dioxide surgical laser. *Ann R Coll Surg Engl* 48:181–188, 1971.

4. Hall RR: Hemostatic incision of the liver: Carbon dioxide laser compared with surgical diathermy. *Br J Surg* 58:538–540, 1971.

5. Ketcham AS, Hoye RC, Riggle GC: A surgeon's appraisal of the laser. *Surg Clin North Am* 47:1249–1263, 1967.

6. Cloudman AM: The effect of an extra-chromosomal influence upon transplanted spontaneous tumors in mice. *Science* 93:380–381, 1941.

7. Staats J: Standardized nomenclature for inbred strains of mice: Fifth listing. *Cancer Res* 32:1609–1646, 1972.

8. Ketcham AS, Wexler H, Mantel N: The effect of removal of a "primary" tumor on the development of spontaneous metastases: I. Development of a standardized experimental technic. *Cancer Res* 19:940–944, 1959.

9. Oosterhuis JW, Verschueren RCJ, Oldhoff J: Experimental surgery on the Cloudman S_{91} melanoma with the carbon dioxide laser. *Acta Chiv Belg* 74:422–429, 1975.

10. Oosterhuis JW: *Tumor surgery with the CO_2 laser. Studies with the Cloudman S_{91} mouse melanoma.* Thesis, Rijksuniversiteit Groningen, 1977.

11. Oosterhuis JW: Lymphatic migration after laser surgery. *Lancet* 1:446–447, 1978.

12. Oosterhuis JW, Verschueren RCJ, Eibergen R, et al: The viability of cells in the waste products of CO_2 laser evaporation of Cloudman mouse melanomas. *Cancer* (in press).

13. Kaplan I, Ger R, Sharon U: The carbon dioxide laser in plastic surgery. *Br J Plast Surg* 26:359–362, 1973.

7 Anesthesia for Surgery with the CO_2 Laser

Martin L. Norton, MD, JD

The CO_2 laser is being used predominantly in the fields of otolaryngology, neurosurgery, plastic surgery, and gynecology.[1,2] The greatest problems for the anesthesiologist are presented in the area of otolaryngology because of competitive and concurrent interests in the airway. Basically, we are faced with the requisite of a noncombustible agent approach, coupled with the need for almost absolute surgical field quietude.

Protection of personnel is not an insignificant factor, but can be achieved relatively simply by the use of eyeglasses or shields, by attention to the distance from the emitted or reflected beam, and, above all, by education.

REGIONALIZATION OF USAGE

The fields of medicine that first found earliest practical use of this therapeutic modality are otolaryngology and gynecology. Neurosurgery, plastic surgery, dermatology, and urology have more recently been included in this listing.

The prime divisions are intracavitary vs surface surgery. The simplest anesthetic management for CO_2 laser surgery is in its use for surface surgery (dermatology and plastic surgery, eg, rhinophyma). However, this is also the area of highest risk to operating room personnel of laser-beam reflection or scatter radiation due to instrumentation.

Intracavitary laser surgery (laryngotracheobronchial and urologic) became possible and controllable by transmitting the beam via reflective mirrors guided by microscopic instrumentation. This controls the diffusion of the beam.

ANESTHETIC MANAGEMENT

The patient is evaluated according to standard methods.[3,4] For surgery involving the airway,[5] respiratory depressants are markedly limited or entirely omitted as premedicating agents. This is particularly true in pediatrics and in obstructive lesions of the upper and lower respiratory tracts. Ketamine should rarely be used due to the significant incidence of excitement with hyperventilation and the resultant hypercarbia and tissue oxygen demand, as well as the risk of ball-valve obstruction of bulky lesions. Diazepam is irregular in its pharmacologic pattern, and hydroxyzine may be painful. Narcotics should be used with great caution, and require the immediate availability of an antagonist, ie, naloxone.

Induction of anesthesia is done intravenously using thiopental (2.5%) until the patient can tolerate the mask. We usually continue with enflurane, although halothane is an acceptable substitute. The carrier is nitrous oxide and oxygen in a 1:1 ratio, followed by an intravenous drip of 0.2% succinyldiacetylcholine.

In any patient with obstructive symptomatology, and before use of muscle relaxants, inspection by rapid direct laryngoscopy is advisable to assure the intubationist of the practicability of endotracheal tube passage.

Endotracheal intubation is accomplished with succinylcholine, 80 mg to 100 mg intravenously. We do *not* use blocking agents such as pancuronium or curare since moment-to-moment control and rapid return of respiration are necessary. Additionally, antagonist agents have adverse side effects (see below). Almost all patients are initially intubated, even if it is intended to convert to venturi ventilation. This is to assure airway control and to allow the surgeon to place his instrumentation without undue urgency. The intubationist should inspect the upper laryngopharynx at the same time. Anesthesia is maintained with enflurane-nitrous oxide-oxygen plus an intravenous drip of succinylcholine, and has proven to be most efficacious.

Special comment must be made about the use of nondepolarizing relaxants in airway endoscopy and surgery. Concern is related not so much to the specific relaxant, but rather to the use of the antagonist combination of neostigmine and atropine. The muscarinic effect of neostigmine produces an increase in the volume and viscosity of secretions of the respiratory tract. Atropine tends to limit the volume of these secretions, but also may produce increased surface tension. Thus, there is a possibility of inducing patchy atelectases and, more particularly, capillary action, which may cause apposition at the anterior commissure of the larynx. The potential for webbing, if surgery occurred previously in this area, is self-evident.

The patient should be afforded ultrasonic nebulization for the first hour or two after surgery. All patients should be placed in a true Fowler's position (20° to 30° sitting), and carefully observed for signs of postsurgical edema. Some clinicians use corticoids during and after surgery to limit the degree of edema. Equipment for emergency reintubation should be available at the bedside for the first hour after surgery.

PROBLEMS AND HAZARDS

The primary problem with this modality of therapy is fire.[6] The laser is essentially an intensive beam of heat capable of raising the temperature of the substrate to a combustible level. Thus, strict avoidance of combustible substances such as plastic endotracheal tubes (possibly excepting the Milhaude tube[7]) and lubricants other than water or aqueous lidocaine, is indicated. Even aluminum-foil-wrapped, red rubber tubes have been implicated in this hazard.[8,9] The endotracheal tube cuff must be protected with wet Pattipads, and these *must be kept wet.*

Metal endotracheal tubes are now available, thus greatly reducing the fire potential.[10,11] However, there still is no absolute protection for the endotracheal tube cuff. Fortunately, the use of wet Pattipads, as noted above, is supplemented by the puff of air or fluid from the cuff when it is perforated. The latter has the effect of "lifting off" or quenching the flame. Unfortunately, continuing exposure of the pilot tube or deflated cuff to the laser beam may lead to combustion. However, there is a solution to this problem by using metalized or siliconized cuffs or protective collars.[7]

Surface burns of the eyes, lips, or other tissues can be avoided by strict attention to pre-focusing of the incident beam. Additionally, hand-held instruments should be utilized only with utmost caution. The common use of the foot-pedal switch is potentially fraught with danger. Development of an automatic on-off pressure switch on the handpiece is urgently needed. We have seen several instances of accidental beam emission when the foot pedal was inadvertently stepped on while the machine was in the emission mode.

Goldman and colleagues[12,13] have reported on the protection of operating personnel. Of particular note is the requisite protection of the eyes by special glasses. For the patient, we have routinely used porous Zona tape, saturated with water and *kept wet.* The moisture absorbs the heat energy; although the tape might visibly char, it will not burst into flame. However, this does not protect operating room personnel. They are somewhat protected by proper preoperative focusing of the instrument. Aside from this, their primary risk is related to reflection or scatter-beams from shiny retractors in the operative field. Here, we recommend use of protective glasses, although we have found no reason for specialized lenses specifically related to the wavelength of the CO_2 laser beam. Almost any plain glass appears satisfactory, although more study in this area is needed.

Another approach would be to ban all smooth reflective surfaces, and to require that all instruments used in the operative field be treated, eg, by "brush finishing," to disperse the incident beam into diffuse radiations so that the resultant emissions are below the energy level that might produce tissue trauma. This is the approach we have recommended in the manufacture of metal endotracheal tubes.[10,11]

SPECIALIZED TECHNIQUES

A technique employed when working in the airway is the use of venturi ventilation. The principle of the venturi, as we use it,[14] has proven most effective. The objective is to entrain room air, thereby increasing the volume of gas available for ventilation, while at the same time avoiding hyperoxygenation. This technique has been clinically available in endoscopy for some time[15] and more recently adopted for endolaryngeal application.[16] Basically, it involves placement of an "injection needle" within the lumen of the laryngoscope. Oxygen is then forced through the needle at relatively high pressures (8 to 16 psi for children, and 20 to 40 psi for adults), entraining (or sucking in) room air for volume and dilution. To accomplish this, the laryngoscope must be aligned in the same axis as the larynx. Additionally, the injection must be made at constant pressure/volume flows and *not* in graded or variable patterns.

The advantage of this system is that it provides a totally *unobstructed* view and free access to the surgical field (especially the vestibule and interarytenoid area) for the surgeon, while also permitting adequate ventilation of the patient.

Disadvantages include minimal tissue dehydration, tissue motion (vocal fold movements like a sail), and the blowing of free blood and particulate matter down the trachea. This is compensated for by repeated irrigation with a spray of aqueous lidocaine, synchronizing the surgery with the "rest phase" of ventilation, and meticulous attention to hemostasis. This technique must *not* be used if cold-knife surgery has opened tissue planes leading into the mediastinum, because of the danger of pneumomediastinum.

Another specialized technique is the use of the laser for endobronchial tumor extirpation.[17,18] In this approach we use a standard Holinger or Wolff ventilating bronchoscope, with the lower peripheral ports covered by aluminum sensor tape. An endotracheal tube cuff is placed on the bronchoscope to produce airway control, particularly when working in the lumen of the trachea or upper main-stem bronchi.

SPECIALIZED MONITORING

All patients should be monitored electrocardiographically and with a precordial stethoscope and the usual Riva-Rocci blood pressure cuff. Additionally, random arterial blood gas samples should be taken in both the operating room and recovery room. This is particularly important in patients with significant medical or operative problems.

MEDICOLEGAL CONSIDERATIONS

Medicolegal considerations in the use of venturi ventilation and the laser must be addressed. There are two factors to be considered: 1) the technique or procedure itself and 2) instrumentation.

Venturi ventilation has been clinically used since 1966. In various forms, often called jet ventilation, it has been used for laryngobronchoscopic procedures. By virtue of its duration of usage, it might be considered an accepted procedure. Similarly, the use of the CO_2 laser in endoscopy has been in clinical use since it was first applied by Strong and Jako.[19,20]

The question of when an innovative procedure becomes an accepted technique was addressed by this author in 1975.[21] It was concluded that each situation must be evaluated on its own merits, ie, on a case by case basis. The basic problem for both the anesthesiologist and the surgeon relates to its apparent ease of usage and application. As a result, the risk of exposing patients to these procedures without adequate training and experience may raise a major question of "informed consent." The patient is entitled to be aware of the physician's training and experience with these modalities. With the availability of semiannual training courses (eg, Boston University, Department of Otolaryngology), failure to obtain formal instruction places the burden on the physician to demonstrate his preparation for this relatively new therapeutic modality.

With respect to the instrumentation, physicians must be cognizant of regulations of the U.S. Food and Drug Administration, particularly as to categorization.

If the company manufacturing these instruments (laser units, venturi needles, etc), either unilaterally or by virtue of limitations of governmental regulations, imposes special requirements on the physician before purchase or use of the instrumentality, this must be considered as a potential medicolegal warning, even though the manufacturer's requirement is based on unwarranted fear of product liability and self-protectionist motivations. This information *is* available for submission in evidence should a negligence action or other legal recourse be resorted to by an injured party.

SUMMARY

The anesthetic management of microsurgery and endoscopic surgery with the CO_2 laser presents unique problems. It must be recognized that mismanagement can only serve to inhibit the justly deserved increased usage of this new modality of therapy. It is incumbent upon every anesthesiologist and surgeon to proceed with due respect for the technique and potential of this major advance in medical therapeutics.

REFERENCES

1. Strong MS, Jako GJ, Polanyi TG, et al: Laser surgery in the aerodigestive tract. *Am J Surg* 126:529–533, 1973.

2. Stellar S, Polanyi TG, Bredemeier HC: Lasers in surgery. *Laser Appl Med Biol* 2:241–293, 1973.

3. Birch AA: Anesthetic considerations during laser surgery. *Anesth Analg (Cleve)* 52:53–58, 1973.

4. Strong MS, Vaughan CW, Mahler DL, et al: Cardiac complications of microsurgery of the larynx: Etiology, incidence and prevention. *Laryngoscope* 84:908–920, 1974.

5. Snow JC, Kripke BJ, Strong MS, et al: Anesthesia for carbon dioxide laser microsurgery on the larynx and trachea. *Anesth Analg (Cleve)* 53:507–512, 1974.

6. Snow JC, Norton ML, Saluja TS, et al: Fire hazard during CO_2 laser microsurgery on the larynx and trachea. *Anesth Analg (Cleve)* 55:146–147, 1976.

7. Milhaude A, Vaquette C, Starobinsky E, et al: Sonde d'intubation en silicone pour l'anesthesia general en microchirurgie du larynx par le laser au CO_2. *Cah D'Anesth* 27:717–720, 1979.

8. Hirshman CA, Leon D: Ignition of an endotracheal tube during laser microsurgery, letter to editor. *Anesthesiology* 53:177, 1980.

9. Hirshman CA, Smith J: Indirect ignition of the endotracheal tube during CO_2 laser surgery. *Arch Otolaryngol,* in press.

10. Norton ML, de Vos P: A new endotracheal tube for laser surgery of the larynx. *Ann Otol Rhinol Laryngol* 87:554–558, 1978.

11. Porch D, Hirshman C, Leon D, et al: Improved metal endotracheal tube for laser surgery of the mouth, larynx and trachea. *Anesthesiology,* in press.

12. Goldman L, Rockwell RJ, Fidler JP, et al: Investigative laser surgery: Safety aspects. *Biomed Engin* 4:415–518, 1969.

13. Goldman L, Hornby P, Rockwell RJ: Laser laboratory design and personnel protection from high energy lasers, in *Handbook of Laboratory Safety.* New York, C.R.C. Publishing Co, 1967, pp 75, 294–301.

14. Norton ML, Strong MS: Anesthesia for endoscopic diagnosis and surgery. *Otolaryngol Clin North Am,* in press.

15. Sander RD: Two ventilating attachments for bronchoscopes. *Del Med J* 30:170–176, 1967.

16. Norton ML, Strong MS, Vaughan CW, et al: Endotracheal intubation and venturi (jet) ventilation for laser microsurgery of the larynx. *Ann Otol Rhinol Laryngol* 85:656, 1976.

17. Shapshay SM, Davis RK, Vaughan CW, et al: Endoscopic management of airway obstruction from tracheobronchial neoplasia: Use of the CO_2 laser. Presented at Scientific Session, American College of Chest Physicians, October 1980.

18. Strong MS, Vaughan CW, Polanyi TG, et al: Bronchoscopic carbon dioxide laser surgery. *Ann Otol Rhinol Laryngol* 83:769, 1974.

19. Strong MS, Jako GJ: Laser surgery in the larynx: Early clinical experience with CO_2 laser. *Ann Otol Rhinol Laryngol* 81:791, 1972.

20. Strong MS, Jako GJ, Vaughan CW, et al: The use of the CO_2 laser in otolaryngology: A progress report. Presented at Scientific Session, American Academy of Ophthalmology and Otorhinolaryngology, September 1975.

21. Norton ML: When does an experimental/innovative procedure become an accepted procedure? *Pharos* 34:161–165, 1975.

PART II
The CO_2 Laser in Otolaryngology

8 Accessory Instruments and Basic Laser Techniques in Laryngology

Albert H. Andrews, Jr., MS, MD
Howard M. Baim, MD

INSTRUMENTS

Surgery with the CO_2 laser demands specialized instruments for making full use of the accuracy and control of the infrared beam. In laryngologic endoscopy the instruments include laryngoscopes, laryngoscope holders, targets, tooth protectors, Cottonoids, steam and smoke evacuators, retractors, and mirrors.

Laryngoscopes

As in any type of surgery, exposure of the larynx in laser surgery is the key to precise and accurately controlled lasing. The larger the instrument, the better is the exposure of the larynx. Jako laryngoscopes are high and wide, and furnish the best exposure of the larynx. The wide opening at the proximal end enables easy adjustments for binocular vision with the Zeiss operating microscope. For those patients whose larynx cannot be adequately exposed with the Jako laryngoscope, the Dedo laryngoscope may be suitable. The lumen of this instrument is somewhat square in shape, and the distal portion slopes away from the long axis, giving improved exposure of the anterior commissure. The Dedo laryngoscope is narrower than the Jako laryngoscope, and more precise adjustment of the microscope is required to give binocular vision. When neither the Jako nor Dedo laryngoscope gives satisfactory exposure of the larynx, the standard hourglass laryngoscope is used. Although it provides good exposure in difficult situations, its narrowness prevents binocular vision with the operating microscope. If the right eye is used, vision is along the right side of the laryngoscope and, if the left eye is used, vision is along the left side of the laryngoscope (Figure 8-1). Saline-moistened gauze wrapped around the proximal end of the laryngoscope protects the lips. This is a wise precaution when using the hourglass laryngoscope.

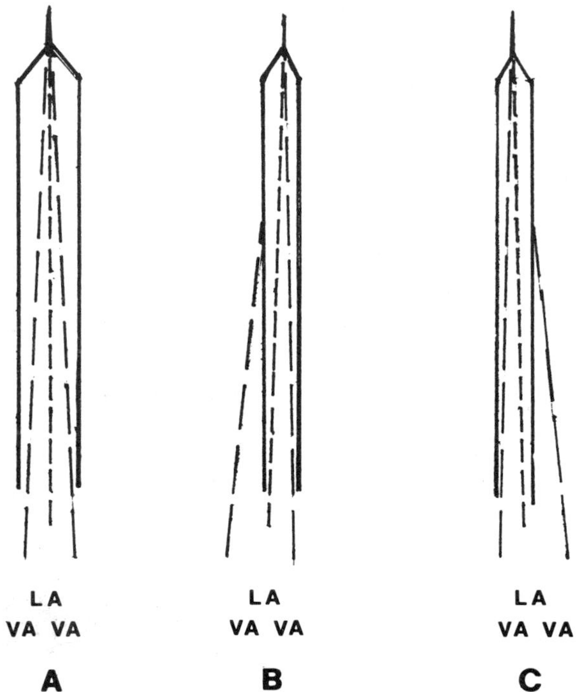

Figure 8-1 Diagrammatic representation of visual axes through laryngoscopes. (A) Binocular vision through a wide laryngoscope. (B) Right-eye monocular vision through narrow laryngoscope. (C) Left-eye monocular vision through narrow laryngoscope. LA = laser axis; VA = visual axis.

Laryngoscope Holders

The laryngoscope is held firmly in place so that the exposure of the larynx is maintained while lasing through the operating microscope. Both hands are free for lasing and to control the retractors, aspirators, and other instruments. Conventional chest supports resting on a surface, such as the chest, or a Mayo stand or bridge are generally unsatisfactory.

The Killian gallows gives stability to the laryngoscope. It can be attached to the laryngoscope using an extension piece* which screws into a threaded hole in the laryngoscope handle (Figure 8-2) or slips over the handle[1] (Figures 8-3, 8-4). The Boston University system† (Figure 8-5) allows force to be exerted in the proper direction without using the upper teeth or jaw as a fulcrum, as occurs in "lever" laryngoscopy or when holders are improperly used.[2] The "upper hand" retractor holder* (Figure 8-6) is fastened to each side rail of the operating table.[3] A special movable piece locks the Lewey chest support to the cross rod. This device, as well as the Killian gallows, requires that the larynx be first exposed manually; only then does the holder maintain exposure.

---

*American V. Mueller
†Narco Pilling

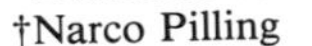

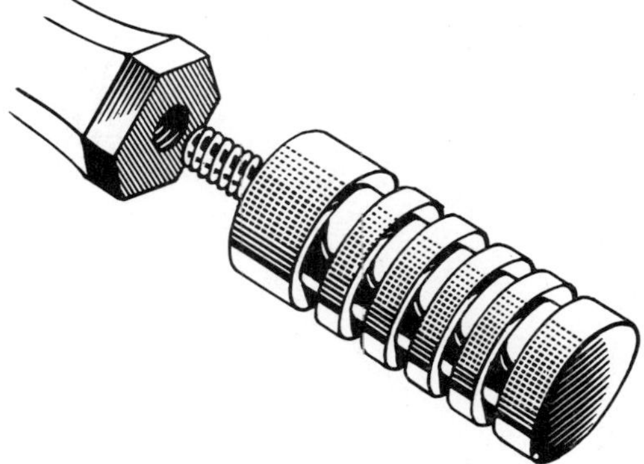

Figure 8-2 Laryngoscope extension handle that screws into the scope. Grooves facilitate attachment to Killian gallows of Boston University system.

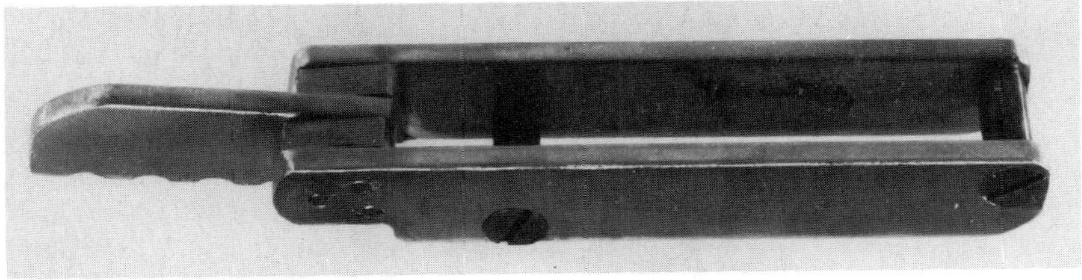

Figure 8-3 Andrews slip-on laryngoscope handle, viewed from above.

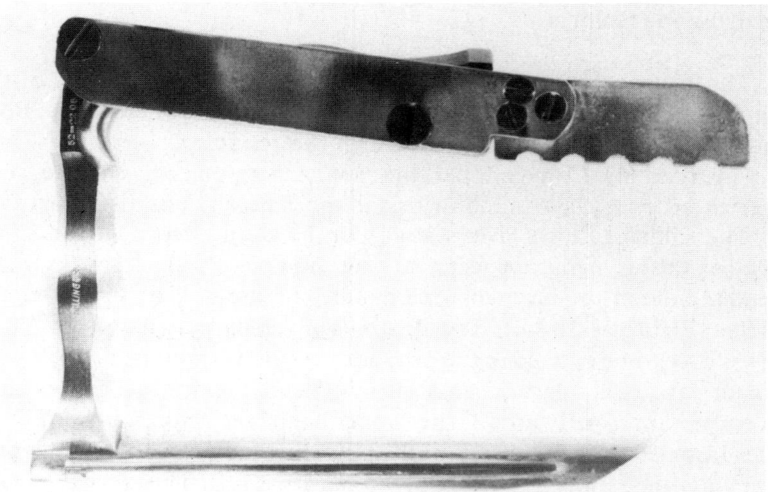

Figure 8-4 Andrews slip-on handle on laryngoscope.

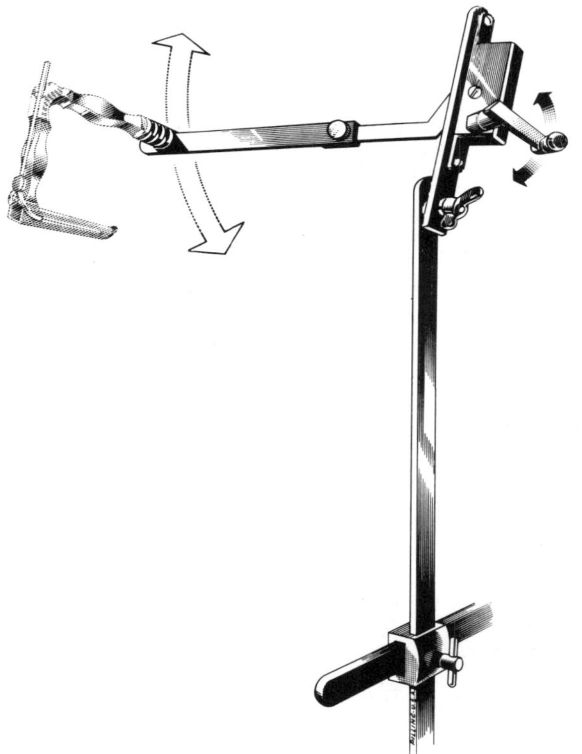

Figure 8-5 Boston University suspension system.

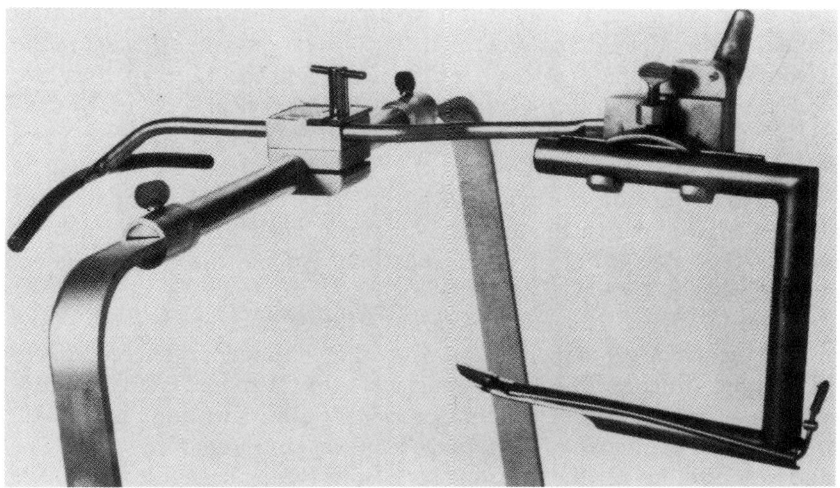

Figure 8-6 Upper hand rigid chest support holder.

Targets

The CO_2 laser is tested before each use for the relation of the aiming spot to the burn area. A rough check on the power output is also done. The target used for the test may be an asbestos block, wooden tongue depressor, or paper; the asbestos block is preferred. The test is usually done at a short exposure and low power (0.1 sec at 3 W). A holder is useful for placing the target at the right position and distance for the test.

Tooth Protectors

The teeth and gingivae are susceptible to injury from the pressure of the laryngoscope resting on them during the procedure. A teeth guard* is placed between the laryngoscope and the teeth or gingivae. This device is a better cushion than folded gauze, which might extend upward and partially block the proximal opening of the laryngoscope. If gauze is used, it must be positioned accurately because it might ignite when in contact with the laser beam unless it is thoroughly moistened and kept so during the lasing.

Neurosurgical Sponges

The laser is used to destroy pathologic tissue with accuracy and minimal injury to surrounding normal tissue. A stray beam from the

*Narco Pilling

laser, either misaimed or reflected from a shiny metal surface, can destroy tissue that was meant to be preserved. The lips or gingivae adjacent to the proximal end of a laryngoscope, or the mucosa in the upper trachea, are most susceptible to injury. Gauze pads or neurosurgical sponges, or Cottonoids saturated with normal saline are placed below the larynx and above the cuff of the endotracheal tube. The energy from the laser will be dissipated as the moisture evaporates from the Cottonoid. The pad is not allowed to dry because the laser may ignite it, with obviously disastrous results. These pads protect the tracheal mucosa and the cuff of the endotracheal tube from rupture.

Cottonoids are available in a variety of sizes, smaller ones being used in children and larger ones in adults. More than one pad is often required to fill the upper trachea. The thread attached to the Cottonoid is a definite advantage during removal. Even though the thread is moistened, it may still protrude into the lumen of the laryngoscope and interfere with vision. The laser may also destroy the thread in spite of its having been moistened. We have replaced the thread with a fine jewelry chain passed through a small hole in the end of the Cottonoid (Figure 8-7). Like the thread, it can be clamped to the head cover to prevent accidental loss. Unlike the thread, the chain is not damaged by the laser and lies posteriorly in the laryngoscope where it does not obscure vision. The chain reflects the laser beam with divergence so that accidental burns of the mucosa do not occur.[4]

Steam and Smoke Evacuators

The laser surgeon soon realizes that, despite the selection of the proper laryngoscope and holder and the optimal positioning of the microscope and Cottonoids, the view of the larynx is soon obscured by smoke and steam. The steam comes from the vaporization of water within the tissues and the smoke from vaporization of the solid material. With an airtight seal between the trachea and endotracheal tube cuff, there is little air flow in the larynx to remove the steam and smoke. Several solutions to this problem are available. A mouth aspirator with side holes, ie, "velvet

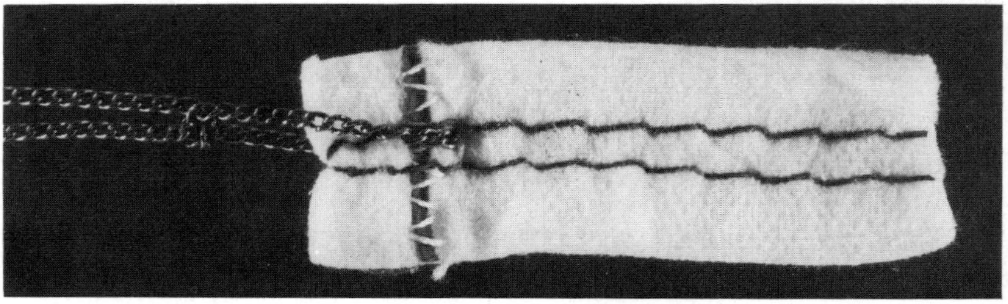

Figure 8-7 Cottonoid with fine jewelry chain.

eye," may be inserted along the side of the laryngoscope as far as the distal end of the posterior edge. This clears the smoke nicely. The aspirator may be passed through the laryngoscope and held to the side with a clip from a pen or pencil. This has limited use in small laryngoscopes, and the first method is generally preferred. Laryngoscopes are available with built-in evacuators.

Retractors and mirrors are made with hollow shafts so that when they are attached to the aspirator tubing, steam and smoke are eliminated. Compressed air can be passed through the shaft of the mirror and blown across its surface. This will eliminate steam and smoke as well as reduce the deposition of particulate matter on the reflecting surface.

Retractors

As more precise endolaryngeal surgery became possible, specialized instruments were designed to meet the needs of the laser surgeon. Laryngeal retractors were made to meet five needs: 1) to bring an area of the larynx into view; 2) to retract an area out of the way; 3) to shield an area from the laser beam; 4) to stroke or scrape an area to remove char or bring out abnormal tissue such as a papilloma; and 5) to remove smoke and steam. A number of different retractors have been developed,[5] but the only one still used is the anterior commissure retractor (Figure 8-8). It is made in right and left types, and large and small sizes.* The handle is

*American V. Mueller

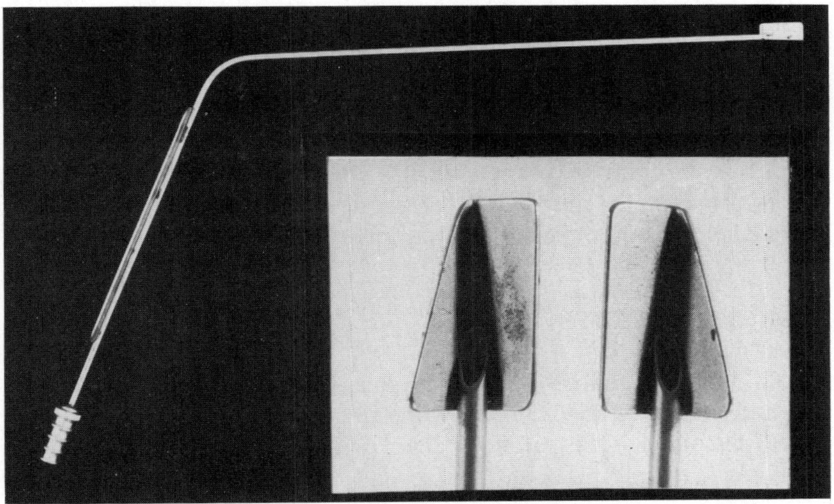

Figure 8-8 Andrews anterior commissure retractors, left and right.

designed to lie posteriorly at a 45° angle so that the fingers are well away from the path of the laser. The shaft of the handle is hollow so it can be used to aspirate steam and smoke. The blade is bent to a 90° angle. With the handle extending posteriorly, the horizontal portion of the blade is tapered toward the distal end. This allows the extent of separation of the vocal cords to be controlled by the depth of passage between the cords. The Tucker-Levine† retractor is not tapered. The free edge of the vertical portion of the blade is placed at the anterior commissure to protect the other vocal cord from the laser beam.

The retractor may also displace the endotracheal tube laterally and expose the posterior portion of a vocal cord, although a generally more satisfactory procedure is to displace the tube anteriorly with the tip of the laryngoscope.

Mirrors

Certain areas of the larynx are not directly accessible to the laser beam. The under surface of the vocal cords and the lateral portion of the laryngeal ventricle are two such areas. A mirror may be used to reflect the laser beam to these areas with good accuracy (Figure 8-9). The laser energy is absorbed by glass so that back-surfaced mirrors cannot be used. Front-surfaced glass mirrors are hazardous because a small bit of blood or secretion on the mirror can cause localized heating of the glass when struck by the laser beam. This can result in cracking and fragmenting of the glass and create foreign bodies in the larynx. Highly polished stainless steel mirrors reflect a reasonably good visual image as well as the laser beam. The mirrors may be round, oval, or rectangular with rounded corners.* The latter type mirror, when held at a 45° angle from the long axis of the laryngoscope, appears square. The size varies from 2 mm to 5 mm in width and is 1.7 times as long as it is wide. The handle is placed at a 45° angle to the hollow shaft. The tubular shaft allows clearing of smoke and steam by aspiration or compressed air, which also helps prevent deposition of debris on the mirror. Mirrors larger than those used in the larynx may be helpful in the mouth and nasopharynx.

BASIC TECHNIQUES

The primary goal of proper technique is to make full use of the precision and control of the CO_2 laser with safety to the patient and operating room personnel. This section deals with techniques applicable to

---

†Narco Pilling
*American V. Mueller

laryngology in a general fashion. Specific techniques are covered in the chapters dealing with specific diseases and surgical specialities.

Preparation

Microscope The Zeiss operating microscope is an integral part of the laser system. The laser components must be securely attached to the microscope to avoid possible injury to the patient if they become dislodged. Objective lenses of different focal lengths are available for the microscope. The 400-mm lens matches the focusing lens of the laser and permits the introduction of long-handled instruments into the laryngoscope. The oculars are adjusted to the vision of the surgeon, as is the interpupillary distance. The focusing rack is set in midposition prior to bringing the microscope into position. This allows adequate focusing on different portions of the larynx during the procedure.

Laser After the laser is attached to the microscope, it is adjusted so that the aiming spot is superimposed on the burn area or adjacent to it, as the surgeon may desire. For lasers without adjustment, the coincidence of the burn and aiming spot is confirmed. Using one of the test targets previously described, the surgeon can safely aim the laser and confirm the power output by judging the brightness and appearance of the burn on the target.

Endotracheal tubes Although always an obstacle for the laser surgeon, endotracheal tubes are necessary for a successful procedure. In spite of the high degree of accuracy of the laser, certain techniques place

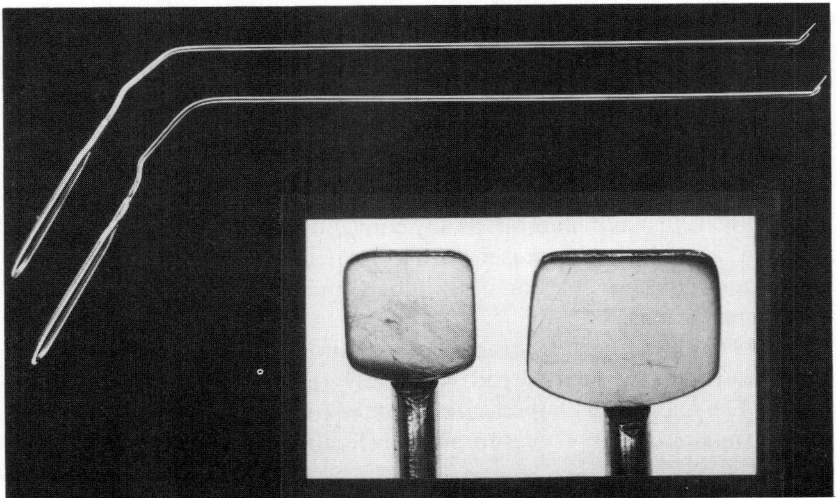

Figure 8-9 Andrews laser mirrors, small and large.

the endotracheal tube at risk of being damaged by the laser. Therefore, certain precautions must be taken to prevent damage to the endotracheal tube. If a red rubber tube is used, it is wrapped with adhesive aluminum tape* by overlapping one-third to one-half of the tape width. The wrapping starts at the cuff and continues until the portion potentially exposed to the laser is covered. The tube is then sterilized. A nonflammable tube such as the Norton tube can be used and left unwrapped. *Plastic tubes are dangerous and should never be used.* It must be remembered that the tube may be farther anterior in the trachea than in the larynx, and Cottonoids must provide protection.

Laryngoscopy and Preparation for Lasing

Prior to using the laser, a standard microlaryngoscopy is performed with the endotracheal tube in place. The larynx is exposed in standard fashion and the laryngoscope holder is attached to keep the laryngoscope stabilized. The microscope is positioned and a thorough inspection of the larynx is accomplished.

A biopsy of the abnormal area is then taken, using either the conventional method with cupped forceps, or with the laser as a knife. Histologic diagnosis is necessary prior to treating any lesion which may be malignant, and may give significant information on the pathologic process in nonmalignant disease. Cottonoids are then placed to protect the endotracheal tube and trachea. When the lesion is so large that it prevents placement of the Cottonoids, it is safe to lase, providing the surgeon recognizes the hazard. Lasing must be done to avoid having the beam go down the trachea. Cottonoids should be inserted as soon as there is adequate room.

Basic Lasing Technique

The CO_2 laser is a dangerous instrument in untrained or undisciplined hands, and is just as dangerous as any conventional cutting instrument. In addition, a fire hazard is present and the reflected laser beam can also be dangerous. The laser surgeon must understand the hazards and know the safety precautions.

Short exposure: The spread of heat to surrounding tissue is the cause of tissue reaction. This spread is directly related to time rather than power. The maximum temperature is limited to the vaporization temperature of water (100°C). Therefore, it is preferable to increase power rather than time.

---

*Radio Shack; 3M Co.

High power: Increasing the power does not increase the maximum temperature rise in adjacent tissue, but it does increase the depth or volume of tissue destroyed. Thus, it is a good technique. The power is adjusted as frequently as required to achieve the desired result.

Skip technique: By not repeating exposure at one area, the remaining tissue has time to cool and the reaction is low.

Repeated exposure: The desired depth of tissue destruction is obtained by repeatedly exposing the same area to the beam. Quickly repeated exposures should be avoided, since they usually indicate insufficient power and cause heating of the remaining tissue. It is better to use one exposure than two exposures at one-half the power.

Removal of char: The oxidation of the solid elements in the tissue or blood produces the char, which absorbs the energy and becomes hot. Because the char contains no water, its temperature can rise above 100°C and increase the degree of tissue reaction. The char is best removed by scraping it away with a retractor, blunt-end aspirator, or closed forceps. It can be removed by an open-end aspirator, but this procedure frequently causes bleeding and more charring as the lasing proceeds.

Palpation: The sense of touch and the response of tissue to pressure applied with an instrument are helpful clues to the progress of the lasing.

Shaving: At times it may be helpful to remove thin layers of tissue from a lesion. By using just the edge of the beam, extreme accuracy of destruction can be attained. Most of the beam passes the lesion and is absorbed by the moist Cottonoids.

REFERENCES

1. Andrews AH Jr: Suspension handle for laryngoscopes. *Ann Otol Rhinol Laryngol* 86:626, 1977.

2. Grundfast KM, Vaughan CW, Strong MS, et al: Suspension microlaryngoscopy in the Boyce position with a new suspension gallows. *Ann Otol Rhinol Laryngol* 87:560–566, 1978.

3. Andrews AH Jr: Rigid chest support holder. *Ann Otol Rhinol Laryngol* 87:567, 1978.

4. Andrews AH Jr: Jewelry chain on Cottonoids for CO_2 laser surgery. *Ann Otol Rhinol Laryngol* 88:827, 1979.

5. Andrews AJ Jr, Moss HW: Experience with the carbon dioxide laser in the larynx. *Ann Otol Rhinol Laryngol* 83:462–470, 1974.

9 Recurrent Respiratory Papillomas

M. Stuart Strong, MD

Recurrent respiratory papillomatosis (RRP) is a diffuse diathesis of the mucous membranes of the respiratory tract. It is encountered in all parts of the world. While the incidence of seven per million per year in the United States is relatively low, the effects of the disease on an individual or his family can be devastating.[1] Depending on the area of involvement and the pattern of recurrence, RRP can be a threat to the airway and even life itself. It can overwhelm the financial resources of the patient or the social services that may be responsible for the funding of his care, and frequently interferes with educational and vocational commitments. The disease affects all ages from infants to the aged, and all areas of the respiratory tract from the nostrils to the larynx, and to the tracheobronchial tree and pulmonary parenchyma.

At the present time there is no known treatment that can be relied upon to eradicate the disease consistently and permanently. Fortunately, spontaneous remission often occurs following treatment, so that patients are spared decades of recurrences and repeated treatments.

RATIONALE FOR THE USE OF THE CO_2 LASER

The relatively inaccessible location of the papillomas in the anterior nasal cavity, the subglottis, or the mainstem bronchi makes their removal difficult at best. The ability of the CO_2 laser to destroy the papillomas by vaporization without the introduction of an additional probe or instrument makes the laser almost an ideal instrument for removal of all visible papillomas.

The vascularity of the papillomas interferes with precise removal by cup forceps, for example, because of the "nuisance" bleeding that occurs. Occasionally, the bleeding can interfere with pulmonary ventilation and the orderly completion of the operation. The capacity of the CO_2 laser to obliterate all of the vessels in papillomas makes it possible to destroy all visible lesions under constant visual control. Hemostasis during laser destruction of papillomas is usually complete.

The diffuse distribution of the papillomas over wide areas of the respiratory mucosa makes their removal tedious when conventional instruments are employed. The CO_2 laser provides a method of speedy destruction while at the same time avoiding unnecessary injury to adjacent nasal perichondrium, vocal cord muscles, and tracheal cartilage.

TECHNIQUE OF USING THE CO_2 LASER

Nasal Vestibule

Generally, local anesthesia is adequate when removing papillomas from the mucosa of the anterior nasal cavity and the adjacent vestibular skin, if the latter is involved.

After suitable premedication, the eyes are covered with wet eye pads, which are completely covered with moistened, cloth adhesive tape. Care must be taken to insure that the tape is adherent to the skin of the infraorbital area and the bridge of the nose. In this way the eyes are protected from the laser beam if it is inadvertently misdirected outside the nasal vestibule. Thereafter, the skin of the nasal vestibule and adjacent skin of the face is cleansed with a suitable antiseptic. Topical anesthesia is induced by 250 mg cocaine hydrochloride in a 5% solution applied to the nasal mucosa of the involved nostril. Supplemental local anesthesia with 2 ml to 3 ml of 2% lidocaine should be infiltrated into the vestibular skin, which may be involved with papillomas or is close to an area of papillomas on the mucosa.

When it is certain that local anesthesia has been achieved, the CO_2 laser, fitted with a 300-mm lens, is brought into position so that the anterior nasal cavity can be viewed through the microscope, which is similarly fitted with 300-mm front lens (Figure 9-1). The use of 400-mm lenses on the microscope and the laser by tall surgeons is convenient.

The lesions are exposed by spreading the nostril with a self-retaining nasal speculum, or by vein retractors that are held by an assistant (Figure 9-2). A biopsy is taken for histological verification, and the lesions are systematically vaporized with the CO_2 laser beam. Smoke, steam, and secretions are removed by a right-angled suction tip. The base of the papilloma is removed, but the cartilage and perichondium are preserved. There is usually no bleeding and the wounds are lubricated with antibiotic ointment (eg, bacitracin ointment).

These procedures can almost always be done on an ambulatory basis but, because of anxiety, the patient will occasionally elect to have the operation performed under endotracheal general anesthesia.

Pharynx

General anesthesia is required for use of the CO_2 laser when removing multiple papillomas from the oropharynx and nasopharynx in order to achieve wide exposure with a gag and prevent motion of the target area. The eyes are protected by wet eye pads and cloth adhesive tape. Routine premedication and induction are followed by intubation with a minimally

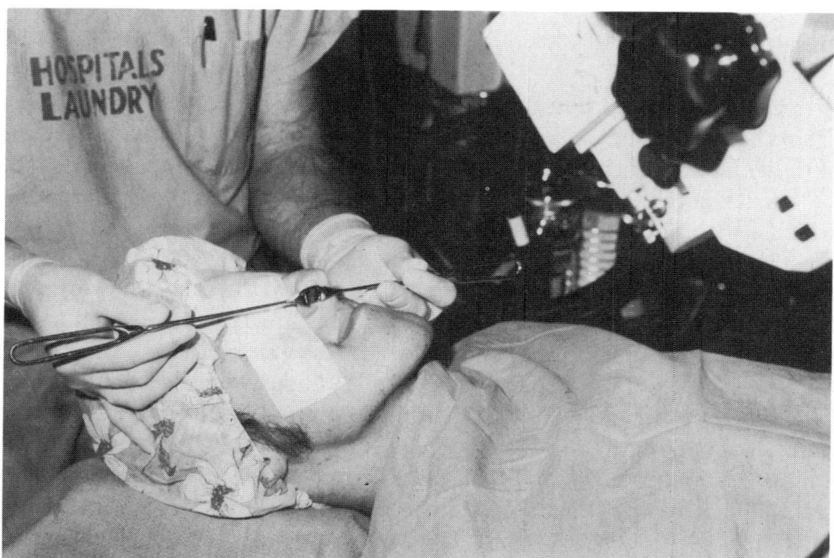

Figure 9-1 The nostrils are being spread with vein retractors and the anterior nasal cavity is being inspected through the microscope with the laser attachment in place. Note the protection of the eyes.

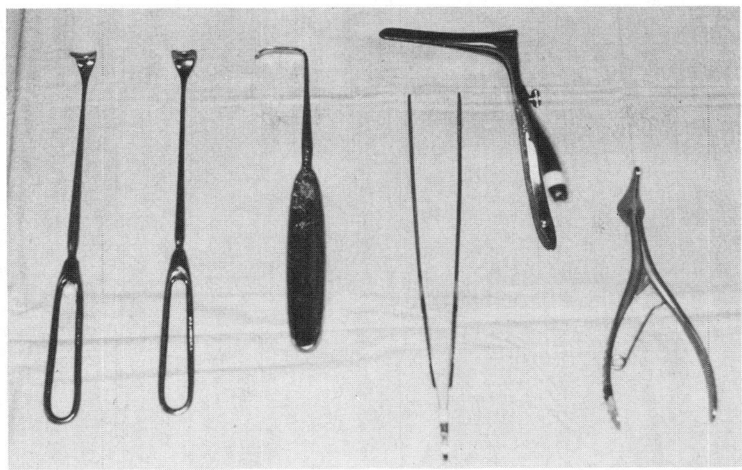

Figure 9-2 Instruments used during laser destruction of intranasal papillomas.

combustible endotracheal tube (eg, a tube made of red rubber or stainless steel). Although the tube is likely to be retracted out of the target area by the tongue blade of the gag, highly combustible tubes, such as those made of polyvinyl chloride, should not be used.

The patient is placed in the Boyce endoscopic position to facilitate the best view of the nasopharynx.

The most suitable gag is the Dingman cleft palate gag fitted with an appropriate tongue blade to accommodate the anatomy of the patient's oral cavity and pharynx. With cheek retractors in place, the Dingman gag gives excellent exposure of the entire oropharynx. The nasopharynx can be exposed by retracting the soft palate forward with transnasal catheters. An excellent view of the entire nasopharynx can be obtained in a 2-cm, front-face steel mirror.

The microscope and the laser should be fitted with a 300-mm front lens, although 400-mm lenses can be used by tall surgeons without inconvenience. The apparatus is positioned over the patient's open mouth so that the operator can stand above the patient's head (Figure 9-3).

Multiple papillomas of the pharynx are most often encountered on the soft palate, tonsillary pillars, posterior wall of the nasopharynx, and occasionally on the dorsum of the soft palate. A biopsy is taken for histological verification of the diagnosis. The papillomas are viewed directly through the microscope set at 6 or 10 power on the turret and are ablated along with their base. Smoke and steam are evacuated with a metal Yankauer suction tube. Papillomas in the nasopharynx are viewed with a steel, front-faced mirror, and the laser beam is reflected by the mirror onto the target papillomas. Steam and smoke are removed by a red rubber catheter placed in the choana through the nostril.

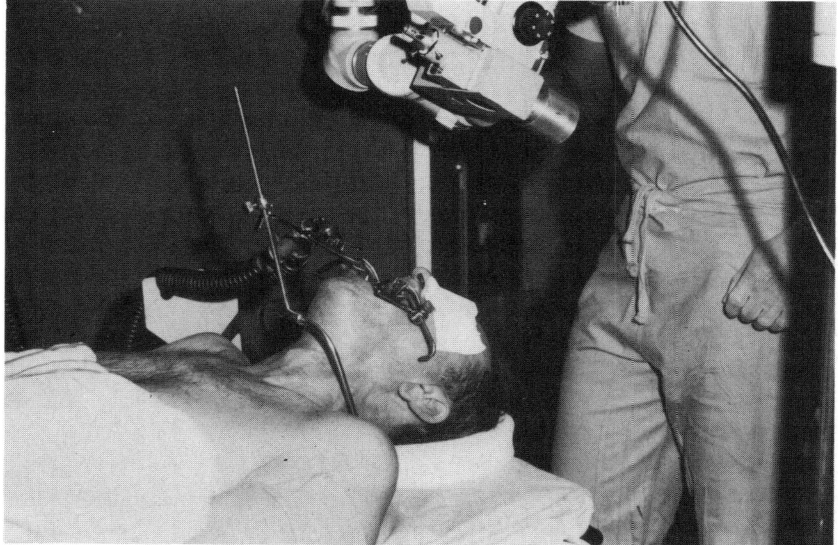

Figure 9-3 The oropharynx has been exposed with a Dingman gag and is being viewed through the microscope.

Larynx

In the presence of recurrent respiratory papillomatosis of the larynx, general anesthesia is employed for their removal. After induction of anesthesia, the patient is intubated with a metal tube or a red rubber tube which has been protected with self-adhesive aluminum.[2] If the patient presents with a tracheostomy in place, ventilation is maintained through the metal tracheostomy tube or through a metal- or aluminum-coated red rubber tube. This is necessary because the tube may be exposed to the laser beam as it passes through the trachea. Care must be taken to protect the patient's eyes.

The larynx is exposed with an appropriate large bore laryngoscope and placed on suspension. The larynx is brought into view with the microscope and attached laser, both fitted with 400-mm front lenses (Figure 9-4). A biopsy is taken and moistened Cottonoids are placed beyond the papilloma to protect the mucosa and the cuff of the endotracheal tube. The papillomas are then systematically destroyed down to and including their bases. If inspection of the interarytenoid space reveals the presence of papillomas, the endotracheal tube should be withdrawn and ventilation maintained with a venturi injection technique.[3] This allows complete eradication of all visible papillomas.

It is usually preferable to begin the dissection superiorly in the supraglottis and then proceed inferiorly toward the glottis and subglottis, depending on the distribution of the papillomas. As the dissection is completed in the anterior commissure, it is important to leave undisturbed 2 mm of mucosa covered with papillomas at the anterior end of one cord. The angled-suction, anterior-commissure retractor is useful for this purpose. If this precaution is not taken, anterior webbing will result.

This approach makes it necessary to remove the remaining fragment of papilloma during a second procedure six weeks later when the anterior end of the opposite cord will have become epithelialized. It is important, when dissecting the papillomas with the laser, to keep the tip of the suction tube, which is used for removing the steam and smoke, close to the side of dissection. Otherwise, the steam at 100°C will denude the adjacent mucosa of epithelium by causing a second-degree burn.

Except in the presence of a minimum number of papillomas, it is usually wise to administer a bolus of soluble steroid intravenously prior to induction of anesthesia (eg, 0.1 mg/k of dexamethasone). Because prolonged manipulation of the larynx during laser destruction of the papillomas may cause some degree of postoperative mucosal edema, short-term postoperative intubation may be required. This problem can be minimized by the elective use of intravenous steroids preoperatively.

Tracheobronchial Tree

Recurrent respiratory papillomas in the trachea and main-stem bronchi can be expeditiously removed with the laser bronchoscope.[4] General

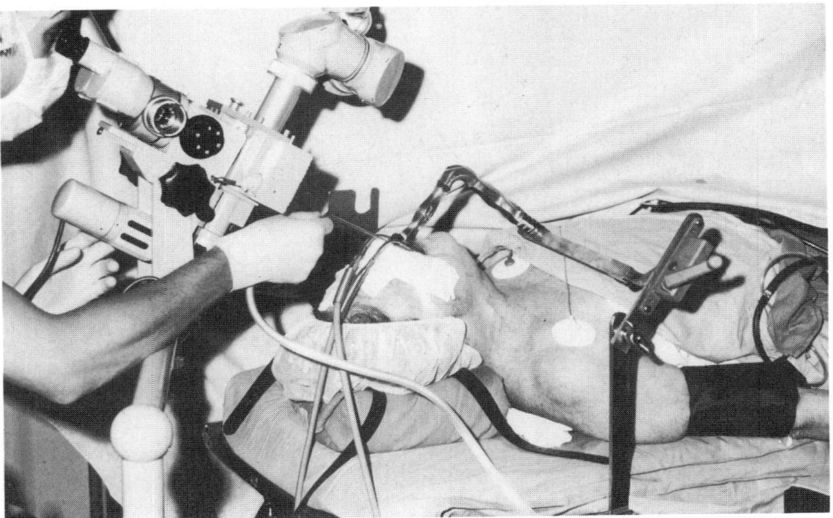

Figure 9-4 With the patient in the Boyce position and the laryngoscope suspended on the gallows, the larynx is being viewed through the microscope.

anesthesia is induced in the usual fashion and the patient is intubated with an ordinary endotracheal tube. This allows the orderly introduction of the ventilating bronchoscope through the larynx at the same time that the endotracheal tube is withdrawn. Ventilation of the patient is then maintained through the side arm of the bronchoscope. If a tracheostomy is present, the patient is first ventilated through the tracheostomy. The tracheostomy tube is removed as the bronchoscope is advanced through the larynx and upper trachea toward the lower trachea. In this way, complete control of the airway is maintained at all times. The patient's eyes must be carefully protected.

The tracheobronchial tree is inspected, the distribution of the papillomas is determined, and a biopsy is taken. The laser coupler is attached to the bronchoscope, and destruction is usually begun distally in the main-stem bronchi and lower trachea. Smoke and steam are removed as the patient is ventilated (Figure 9-5).

Occasionally, the tip of the bronchoscope may cause slight bleeding or a fragment of papilloma may become detached. These should be removed by the intermittent use of the suction tip. All visible papillomas are vaporized down to their bases, but neither the cartilage on the anterior and laterial walls nor the muscle on the posterior wall should be exposed.

Papillomas occurring on the wall of the tracheostomy stoma itself can be removed from the outside using the microscope and micromanipulator, while the patient continues to be ventilated through the

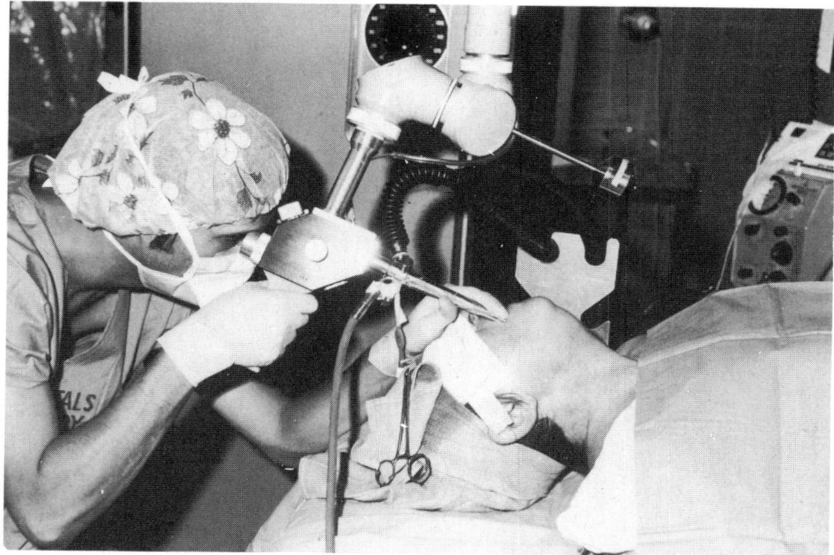

Figure 9-5 The ventilating bronchoscope has been attached to the laser coupler so that destruction of the papillomas in the tracheobronchial tree can proceed.

bronchoscope. An unprotected, combustible endotracheal tube should *not* be used in place of the metal bronchoscope at this stage.

Postoperative edema is not a problem unless there has been excessive manipulation in the larynx and subglottis; in this event preoperative intravenous steroids should be used.

RESULTS

The CO_2 laser has made it possible to remove all visible papillomas from the respiratory tract, except in those rare instances in which the tumors have extended into the secondary bronchi and the lung parenchyma itself. Removal is accompanied by minimal damage to the underlying tissue. We were able to maintain the airway so that tracheostomy could be avoided in all but two instances of a total of 210 patients. In these two cases the disease was so rampant and recurred so rapidly that the operation had to be carried out every ten days in order to keep the airway patent.

Recurrences were encountered in every case, but 42% of the patients went into remission for one year or more after two or more excisions with the CO_2 laser.

COMPLICATIONS

Early in our series, anterior glottic webbs were created on nine occasions by the injudicious dissection of both vocal cords simultaneously at the anterior commissure. Two patients developed slight contractures in the interarytenoid space because of repeated *deep* dissection in this area.

Before the use of aluminum-protected tubes or metal endotracheal tubes, there were three episodes of momentary combustion of the latex covering of the red rubber tube, but this resulted in no injury to the patients.

Prolonged suspension of the laryngoscope on the suspension gallows produced postoperative edema of the sublingual, submandibular, and soft palate areas in two patients due to prolonged cyanosis of the tongue. This required a nasopharyngeal airway for three hours postoperatively until the edema dissipated.

DISCUSSION

While CO_2 laser destruction of recurrent respiratory papillomas is not in itself curative, it does provide the most expeditious method of removal and the best method of preserving the airway and avoiding tracheostomy. The prognosis is always guarded because it is impossible to anticipate when spontaneous remission will occur. It is advisable in new patients to reduce the papilloma population to zero on three occasions in the hope of inducing remission. If the tumors recur despite three total removals, the operation should be repeated thereafter only as necessary to preserve the airway.

It is important, when removing papillomas from the larynx, to avoid *repeated* exposure of the underlying muscle on the vocal cord. Exposure on one or two occasions is not harmful, but if it is repeated, scar formation and contracture will ensue. Treatment should not be heroic if a pattern of relentless recurrence has been established!

Although CO_2 laser destruction is the best method of patient management in recurrent respiratory papillomas available at this time, an effective form of adjuvant therapy is urgently needed. Whether the clinical trials presently being conducted with adjuvant topical chemotherapy will prove to be successful, remains to be seen.

SUMMARY

Recurrent respiratory papillomatosis is an old problem that continues to defy complete solution. The CO_2 laser is a safe and effective method of management, provided that proper precautions are taken. Its use reduces the need for tracheostomy to a minimum and gives the patient the best chance of going into spontaneous remission.

The technique of using the CO_2 laser for this purpose is one which can easily be acquired by any surgeon experienced in suspension laryngoscopy and rigid-tube bronchoscopy.

The use of the CO_2 laser is to be recommended at this time, but the availability of an effective adjuvant therapy is urgently needed if a higher proportion of prolonged remissions is to be achieved.

REFERENCES

1. Strong MS, Vaughan CW, Healy GB: Recurrent respiratory papillomatosis in laryngotracheal problems in pediatric patients, in Healy GB, McGill T (eds): *Textbook of Ear, Nose, Throat.* Springfield, Ill, Charles C Thomas, 1979, pp 88-98.

2. Norton ML, DeVos P: New endotracheal tube for laser surgery of the larynx. *Ann Otol Rhinol Laryngol* 84:554-557, 1978.

3. Norton ML, Strong MS, Vaughan CW, et al: Endotracheal intubation and venturi ventilation for laser microsurgery of the larynx. *Ann Otol Rhinol Laryngol* 85:656-663, 1976.

4. Strong MS, Vaughan CW, Polanyi TG, et al: Bronchoscopic CO_2 laser surgery. *Ann Otol Rhinol Laryngol* 83:769-776, 1974.

10 Benign Laryngeal Diseases

Geza J. Jako, MD

The foundation of microsurgery started in otologic surgery with the use of magnification. In the 1950s, binocular Galilean magnifying telescopes (surgical microscopes) revolutionized ear surgery.[1] In the next decade, Jako,[2,3] and then Kleinsasser[4] developed the instrumentation and techniques for endoscopic microsurgery of the larynx. This new technique greatly improved the surgical precision in laryngoscopic surgery. Further improvement in precision was achieved by application of the carbon dioxide laser. The removal of a vocal cord nodule in a dog marked the beginning of the practical clinical application of carbon dioxide laser microsurgery[5] (Figures 10-1A, B). Initially, it was applied in the surgical management of papillomatosis and the major breakthrough appeared to be the hemostatic effect.[6] After this, the precision and clean cutting with the CO_2 beam and the excellent healing was realized as equally or more advantageous in surgical treatment of benign laryngeal diseases.[7,8]

Since most endolaryngeal microsurgical procedures are carried out using the Jako-Pilling fiberoptic laryngoscopes or similar instrumentation, familiarity with these instruments and the techniques of using them are essential.[9,10] Adequate aspiration of vapor and smoke created by the

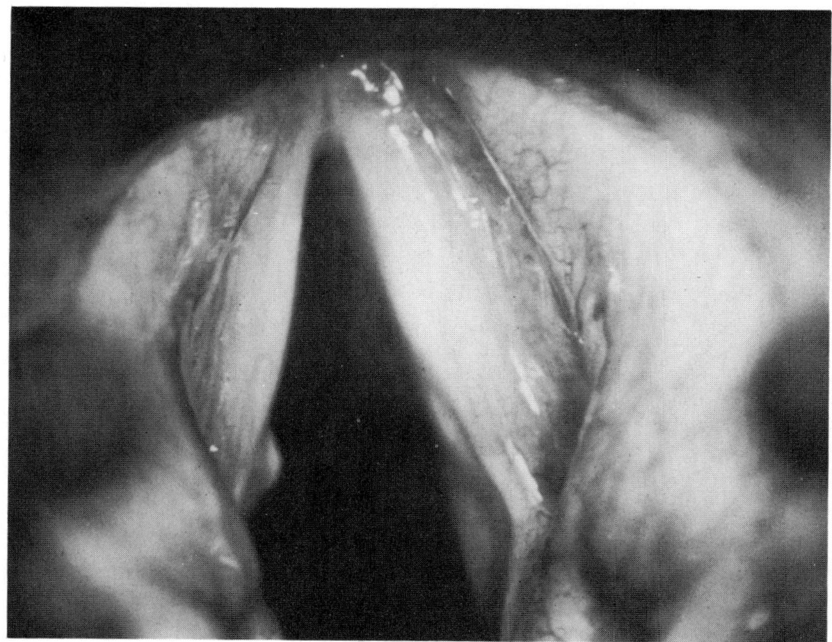

Figure 10-1A Vocal cord nodule of a dog.

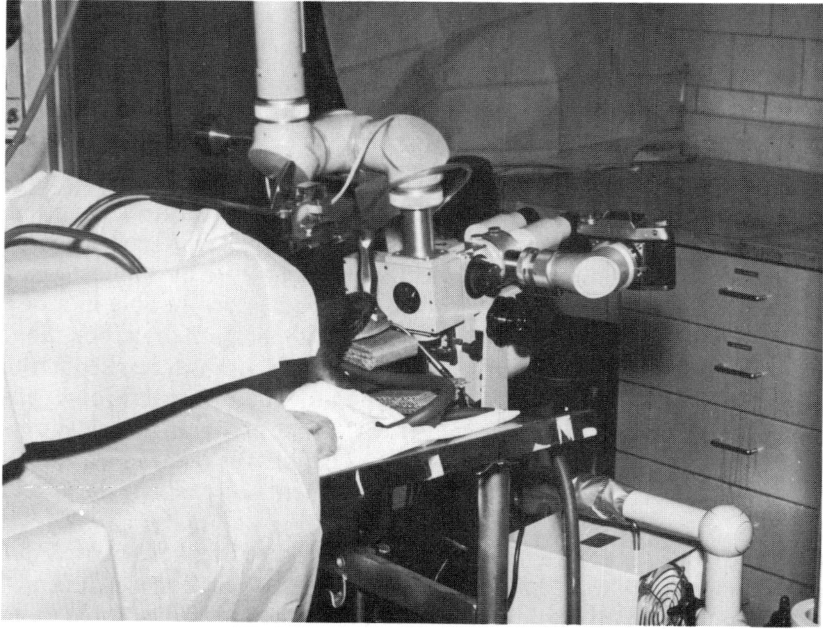

Figure 10-1B CO_2 laser microsurgical set-up for removal (1968).

laser is important to avoid heat damage to the surrounding tissue. This is accomplished by inserted aspirator tubes or suction retractors (Andrews).[11] The new Jako-Pilling laser laryngoscope has a built-in aspirator (Figure 10-2). Adequate visualization of the lesion to be removed is important. Larger lesions are held by a cup forceps and put under tension by pulling (Figure 10-3). This way, the tissue is stretched and the width of the cutting is diminished. Since most benign lesions contain small blood vessels, most procedures on the true and false vocal cords are almost bloodless. Small bleeding can be controlled with the laser by slightly defocusing the beam or turning the power down to increase coagulation. If the bleeding cannot be stopped easily with the laser, a suction tip designed for electrocoagulation connected to the diathermy equipment provides good coagulation for practically all blood vessels in the endolarynx.

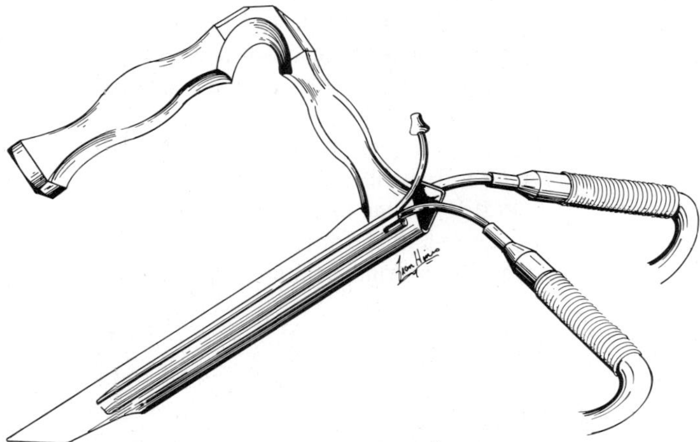

Figure 10-2 Jako-Pilling laser laryngoscope.

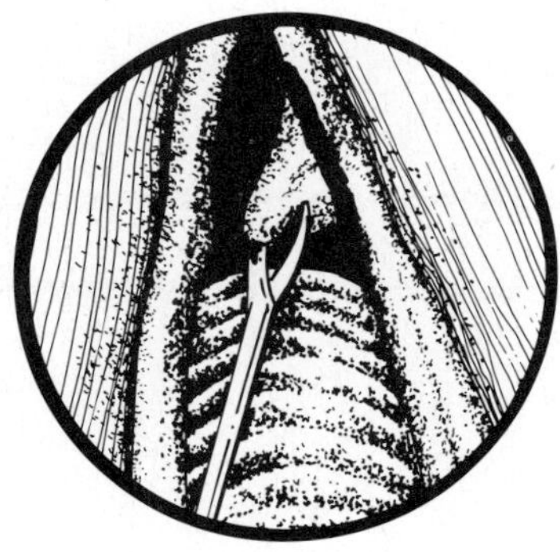

Figure 10-3 Holding vocal cord lesion with cup forceps and cutting around with the laser beam.

Removal of a larger benign growth always should provide a satisfactory amount of material for histological examination. The removed material can be measured and marked for orientation (Figures 10-4, 10-5). The specimen can also be marked with a suture using the Jako biopsy forceps for oriented biopsies[10] (Figure 10-6). A specimen cannot always be obtained on removal of small nodules. In these cases, photographic documentation preoperatively and postoperatively is especially important. Colored photography in these instances gives good documentation for the patient and the surgeon. Toluidine blue staining[12] is an excellent diagnostic tool to differentiate hyperkeratosis from more advanced lesions.

Generally, for benign lesions, 3 to 10 watts laser output power is used on the tissue target. The spot size of the laser beam in most present conventional instruments is 1.5 to 2 mm. The laser beam itself should be in a Gaussian mode to avoid unnecessary thermal injury to the surrounding tissues that might not be obvious at the time of surgery. If the beam is not a "good one," due to mirror deterioration or misalignment, the unnecessary heat damage could manifest in prolonged postoperative edema.[13-15]

Endoscopic laser microsurgery of the larynx almost exclusively can be carried out with general anesthesia.[16-19] Since most of the procedures are performed using endotracheal intubation, adequate safety and experience of both the surgeon and the anesthetist is of extreme importance to avoid potentially tragic consequences (see Chapter 7).

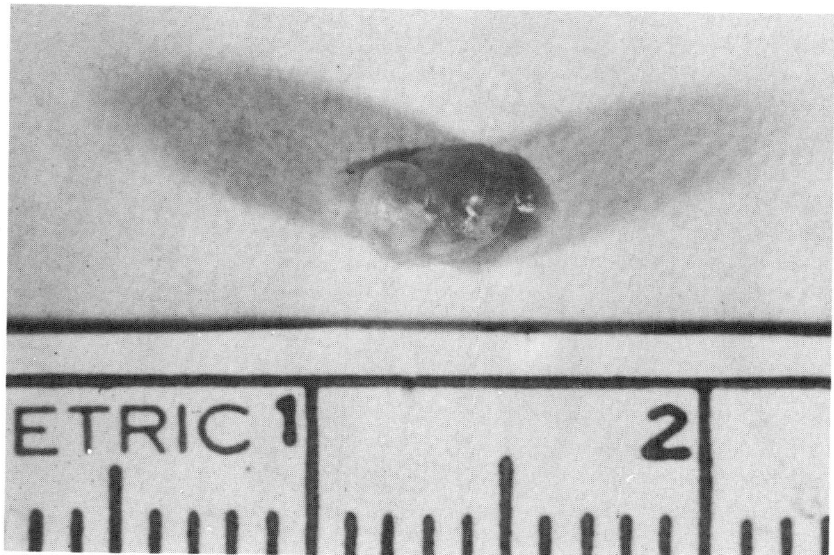

Figure 10-4 Measurement of removed vocal cord tissue.

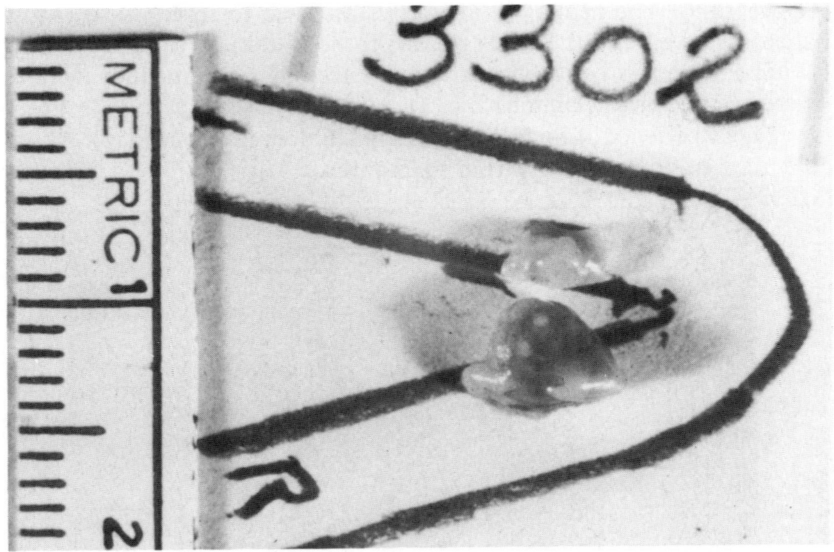

Figure 10-5 Marking removed tissue for orientation.

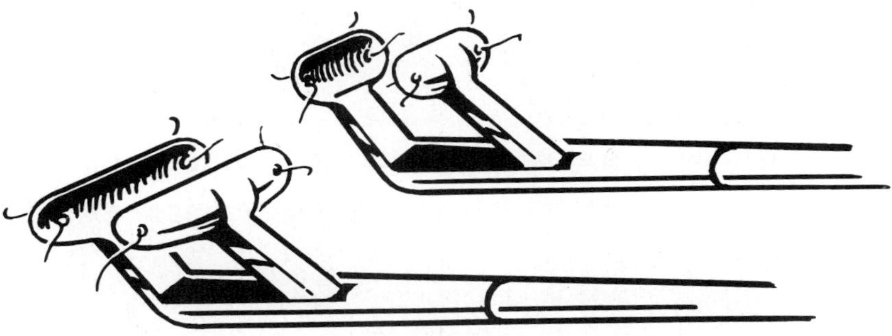

Figure 10-6 Biopsy forceps for "oriented biopsy."

SURGICAL APPLICATIONS

Vocal Cord Nodules

In cases where conservative treatment is not applicable, the removal of nodules with the CO_2 laser is a practical and precise one. In cases of soft nodules, laser surgical removal offers the advantage of quick removal and good healing postoperatively. Hard nodules will not respond to voice therapy; therefore, the choice of treatment is surgical removal. In the cases of small nodules, usually no specimen is obtained and the nodule is evaporated with the edge of the laser beam (Figure 10-7A, B). The part of the beam passing into the trachea is absorbed by a wet surgical pad

(Figure 10-8). The healing is relatively fast, two to three weeks. Most patients do well and the voice returns to normal in three to six weeks. Documentation by color photography is strongly recommended in cases where no specimen is obtained.

The experience of nodule removal in children is inconclusive. About 50% of the nodules recur within six months.

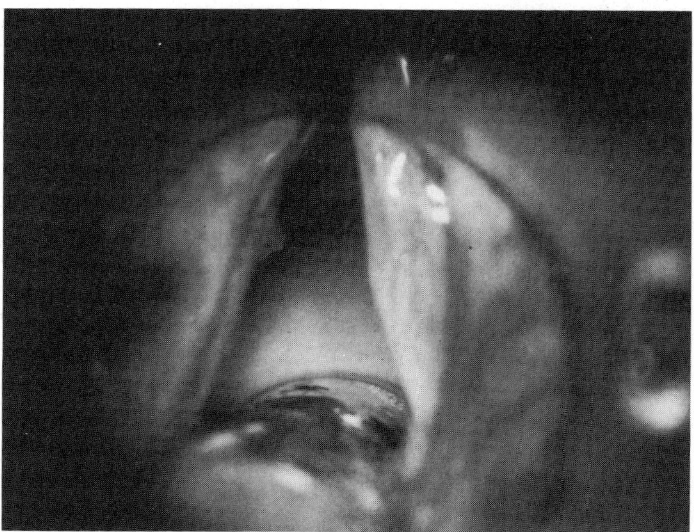

Figure 10-7A Small vocal cord nodule left, and polyp on right.

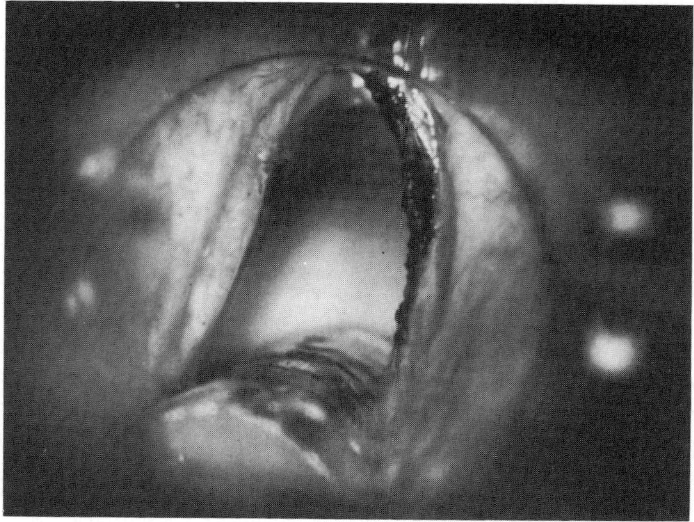

Figure 10-7B After removal.

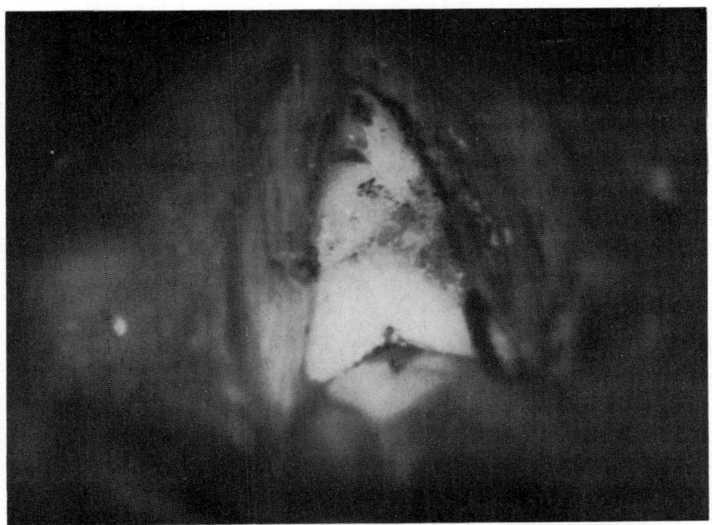

Figure 10-8 Protection of the trachea and the cuff with soaked pad.

Polyps

Sessile or pedunculated polyps are removed using an upcurved round cup forceps or larger oval-shaped cup forceps. By pulling the cup forceps toward the opposite side, the tissue is stretched, and the polyp is separated from its base. The specimen obtained is marked and sent for histological examination. The remaining epithelial edges are cleaned with the laser beam until a reasonably smooth surface is achieved. In most cases, there is no bleeding and an occasional minor bleeding vessel easily can be coagulated by turning the beam intensity to approximately three watts.

Occasionally, there is slightly more bleeding during the removal of teleangectatic polyps. Hyperkeratotic polyps are removed similarly with a cup forceps. In cases of hyperkeratotic polyps, hyperkeratotic patches involving the epithelial cover of the vocal cord are frequently seen. These epithelial patches including the underlying epithelium are then evaporated with the laser.

When polyps or small benign lesions are removed from the vocal cord edges, it is practical to remove some extra epithelium at the lower edge of the excision. This usually diminishes postoperative edema (Figure 10-9A, B).

In cases of bilateral lesions, similar principles as used in instrumental surgery are applied. At least 3 mm to 4 mm of normal epithelium should be left in the anterior commissure on one vocal cord. If the lesion is large in the anterior commissure, it is safer to do surgery on one vocal cord only and to do the other about two months later.

Caution should be exercised during laser surgical procedures inside the larynx to avoid overheating areas surrounding the lesion. This is accomplished using special suction retractors (Andrews), wet pads, and adequate aspiration. Unnecessary damage is created sometimes if the laser beam is not in a good mode, which creates more postoperative swelling and prolongs healing.

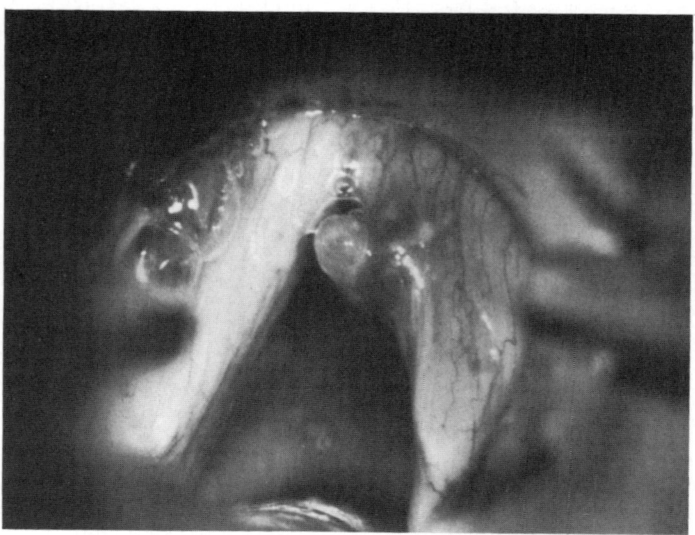

Figure 10-9A Circumscribed polyp right anterior vocal cord.

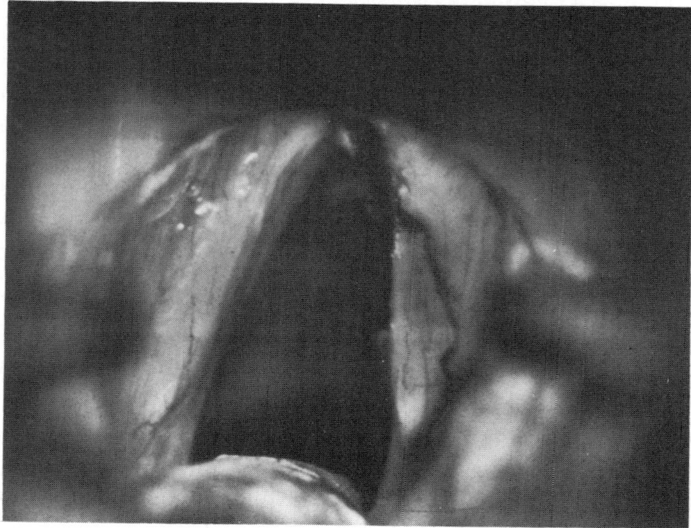

Figure 10-9B After removal.

Reincke's Edema

In cases of frequently occurring Reincke's edema and where the voice is affected to a degree that the patient desires improvement, selected excisions of the epithelium and some of the loose edematous subepithelial tissue is usually curative. Examination of the nose and sinuses is important in these patients because, frequently, marked postnasal discharge is found. The irritation and coughing caused by the postnasal discharge as well as allergy are factors in the development of Reincke's edema.

A strip of epithelium at the edge, including the lower edge of the cord, is excised. If the edema involves the upper surface of the cord, small holes can be drilled into the cord until the vocal muscle is reached (Figure 10-10A, B). Through these openings, the edema fluid can leak out and secondary scarring will adhere the epithelium firmer to the underlining structures.

Vascular Lesions

Vascular corditis has been described by Freche (personal communication). In these cases, slightly enlarged blood vessels can be seen under the vocal cord epithelium. According to Freche, this condition can

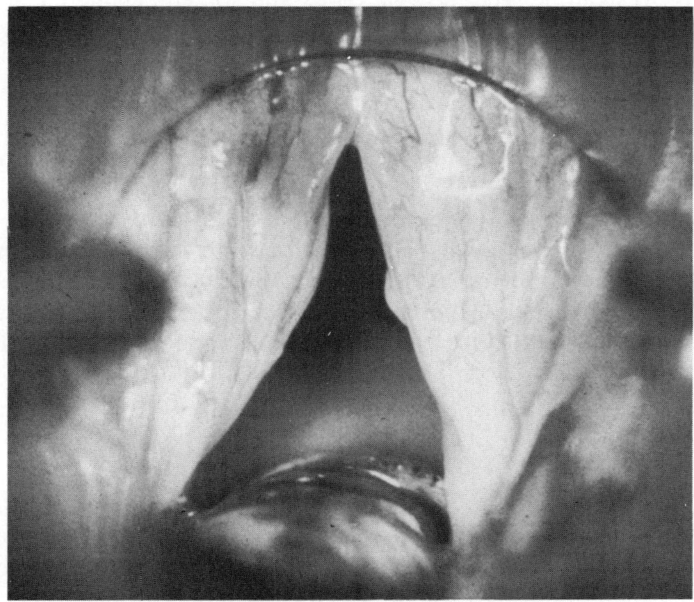

Figure 10-10A Reincke's edema.

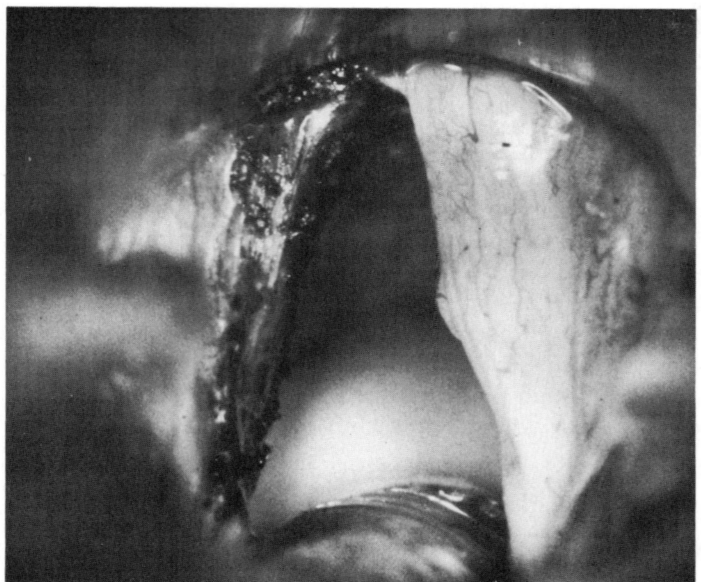

Figure 10-10B After removal one side only.

cause slight hoarseness or minor voice changes. He describes surgical excision of these vessels with the laser as a curative method. Occasionally, small varices can be seen in vocal cords and sometimes these can cause minor voice changes. These varices sometimes follow a hemorrhage into the vocal cord. Laser excision of these varices could be beneficial.

Cysts

Retention cysts involving one or both vocal cords manifest themselves usually as large polyps. Usually, these interfere with the vibration of the cords and cause marked hoarseness. The cysts can be removed best with laser excision since all parts of the cyst can be eliminated precisely. In cases of large bilateral cysts, it is advisable to do one side at a time (Figure 10-11A, B).

Cystic Polyps

These are polypoid-looking formations except, during removal, fluid escapes from the polyp (Figure 10-12,A,B). Occasionally, after the removal of cystic polyps, during healing, a small granulomatous polyp is formed. This manifests itself in severe hoarseness, which necessitates another surgical excision of the small lesion.

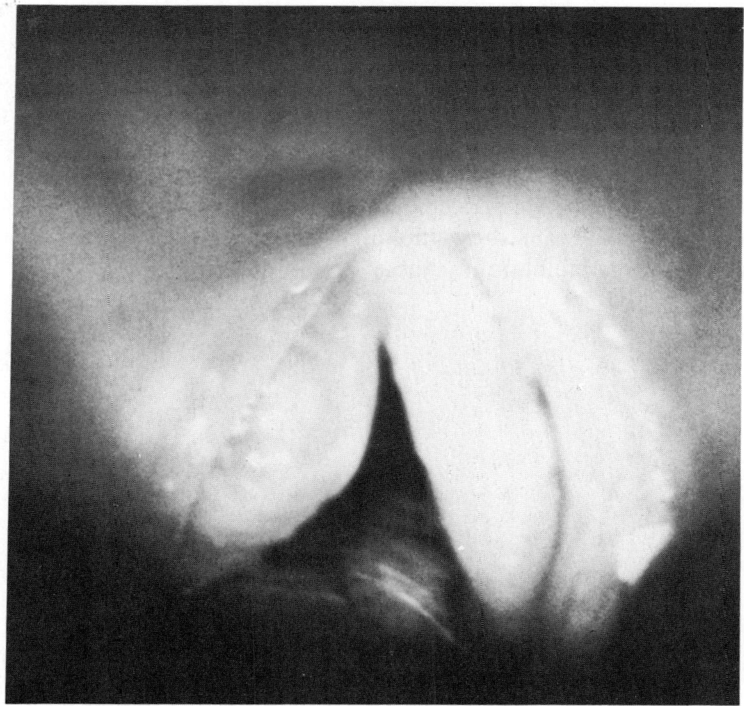

Figure 10-11A Bilateral vocal cord cyst.

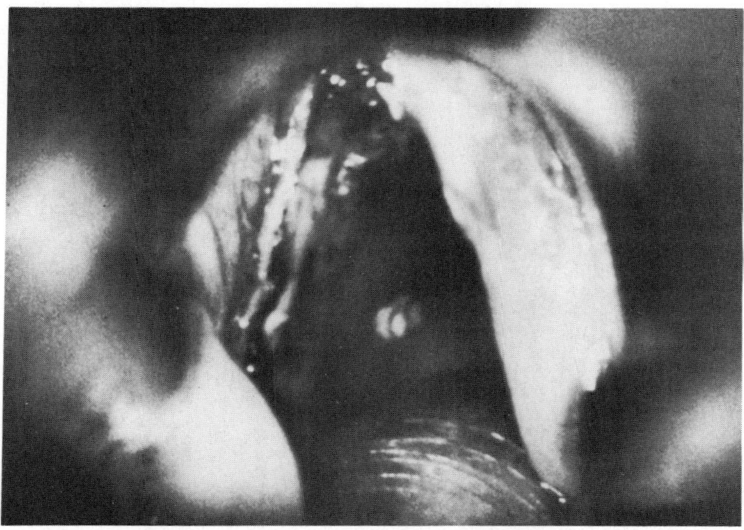

Figure 10-11B After removal, one side only.

Hyperkeratosis of the Vocal Cords

Under magnification, whitish unevenness and thickening of the vocal cord epithelium is observed. This is sometimes diffused, but more often seen as whitish patches. The upper and medial edges of the cords are involved more often but occasionally it can involve the undersurface. The whitish hyperkeratotic patches are also called leukoplakia. These are almost invariably caused by smoking, consuming hard liquor, poor oral hygiene, or a combination of these.

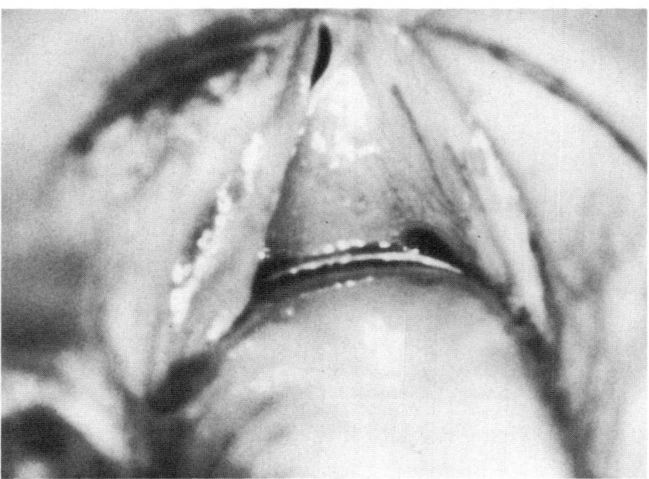

Figure 10-12A Large cystic polyp.

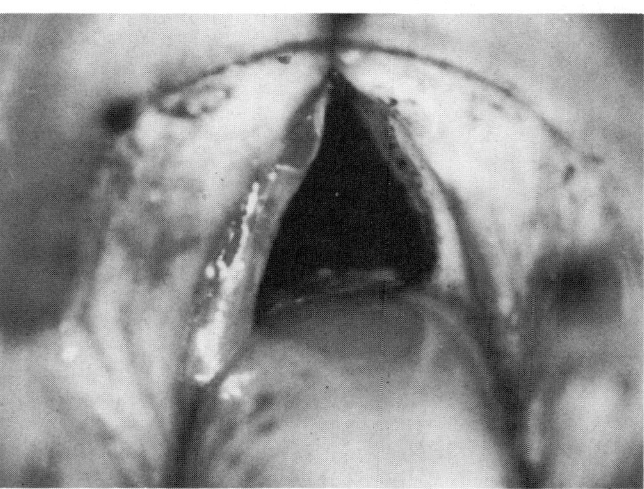

Figure 10-12B After removal.

Laser excision of the patches or, if the hyperkeratosis is generalized, shaving of the entire epithelium with laser evaporation is useful (Figures 10-13A, B, 10-14A, B). The newly grown epithelium, if it is not irritated, frequently shows a more normal appearance.

Future long-term control studies will provide information as to the usefulness of this epithelial shaving. If both cords are involved, the one showing more severe hyperkeratotic changes is shaved off first.

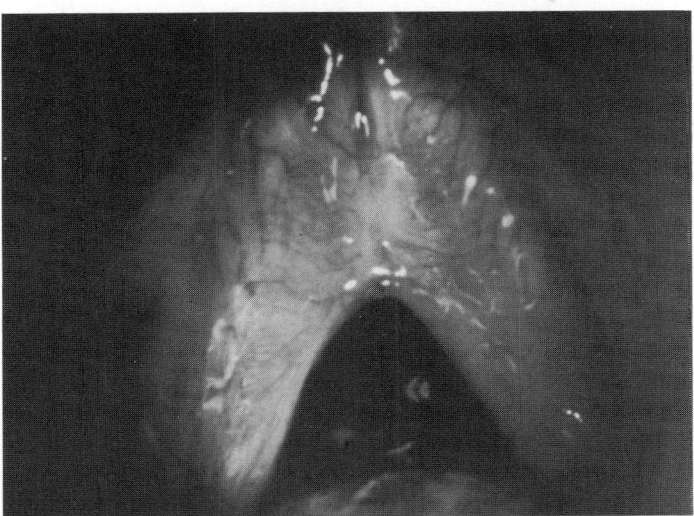

Figure 10-13A Hyperkeratotic polyp.

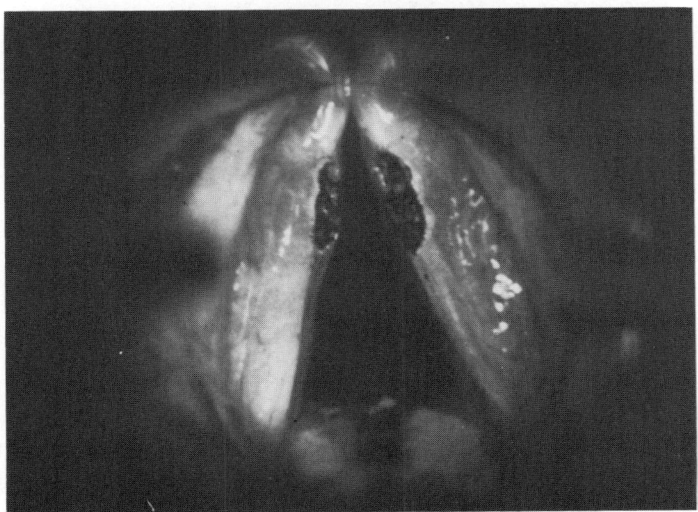

Figure 10-13B After shaving.

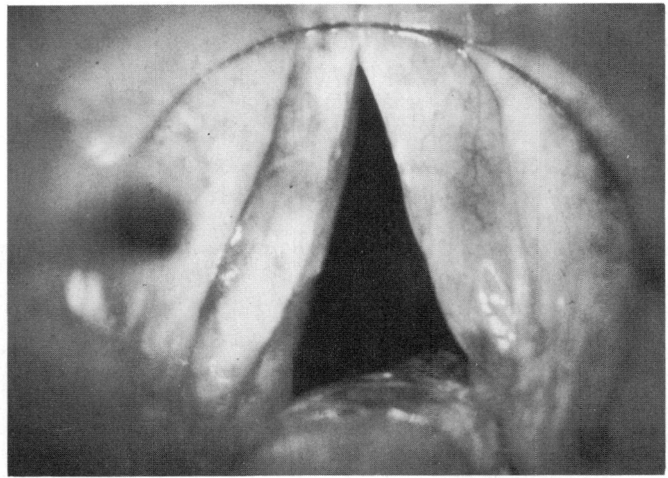

Figure 10-14A Hyperkeratosis and leukoplakia.

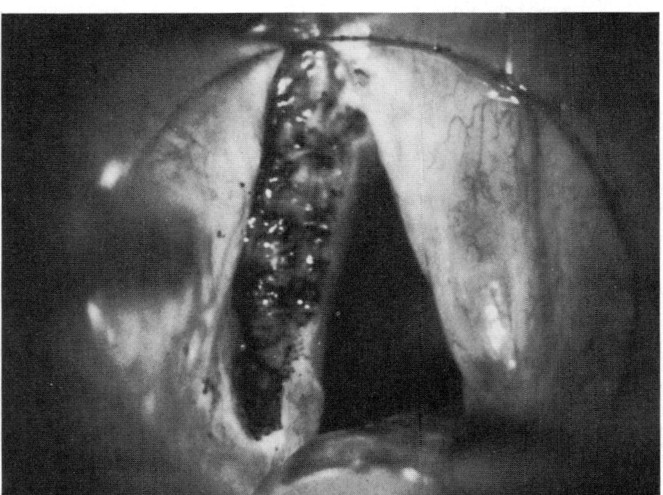

Figure 10-14B After shaving.

Webs and Synechias

Congenital lesions are addressed in Chapter 11. Acquired webs and synechias are traumatic, most frequently caused by surgical trauma. They occur most commonly in the anterior commissure when the epithelium of both cords is removed or injured. This removal or injury also applies to laser surgery. Therefore, one has to be careful of leaving at least 3 mm to 4 mm of intact epithelium in the anterior commissure.

The epithelial cover of one vocal cord can be preserved better with microsurgery of the larynx than with previous techniques. With laser surgery, similar criteria should be applied, protecting the epithelium on the opposite side from removal or burning. For this, Andrews special retractors or soaked wet pads are useful. The opposite vocal cord can be burned with the laser without removal of the epithelium. Secondary swelling can occur. This swelling might not be so obvious at the time of surgery and can be observed only with daily follow-up with mirror, telescopic, or fiberoptic laryngoscopy. Prolonged, total voice rest could contribute to the development of synechia or web. In a patient who did not use her voice for four weeks, against medical advice, a partial web, 3 mm posterior to the anterior commissure developed (Figure 10-15A) with severe hoarseness. At the patient's request, this area was opened with the laser, which resulted in prompt healing and excellent voice (Figure 10-15B).

Anterior webs are frequently created in surgery for papillomatosis when both anterior cords are denuded. In surgical management of papillomatosis, it is safer to remove the anterior commissure lesion from one cord and only partially from the other (see Chapter 9). Webs and synechias are also seen in surgery of vocal cord cancers. In these cases, it is an acceptable consequence of surgery. These usually improve by themselves over the years. In cases of massive laser surgery, special attention has to be paid to aspirate the hot smoke and vapor from the larynx to avoid diffuse burning. Posterior commissure webs occur more often from prolonged intubation and in children.

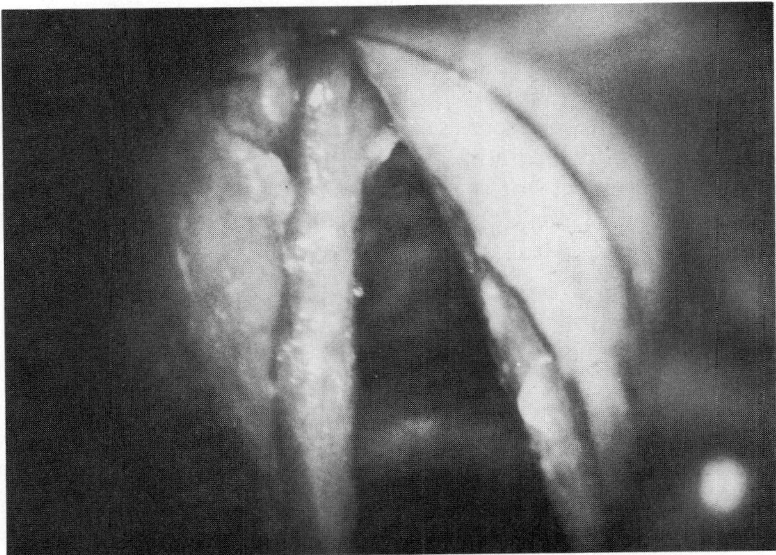

Figure 10-15A Partial web.

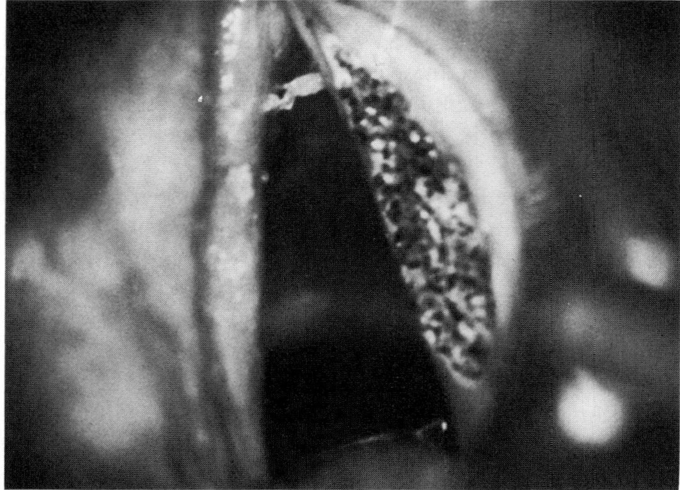

Figure 10-15B After excision.

Contact Granulomas

Large contact granulomas usually are removed for histological examination and possible treatment. In our experience, after laser surgical excision, about one half of these granulomas recur. They usually heal spontaneously in about a year.

Laryngocele and Prolapse of the Mucosa of the Ventricle

Small internal laryngoceles can be excised easily by holding the tissue under tension and separating it with the laser. Prolapsed, thickened, hypertrophied mucosa of the Morgagni's ventricle also can be excised similarly with the laser. Care should be taken to protect the surrounding area with wet pads. Healing usually is prompt and satisfactory.

Ventricular Folds

The ventricular folds easily can be cut with the laser since they contain small caliber blood vessels and any cutting procedure is relatively bloodless. In the past, cutting procedures involving the ventricle folds usually were avoided due to the profuse bleeding. Laser surgery is a definite advantage. Tissue excision of the ventricular folds often heals with more scarring than the true cords. Therefore, indications for surgical procedures involving the false cords should be limited.

Spastic Dysphonia

In spastic dysphonia, the patient phonates with his ventricular bands and has a deep, husky, unpleasant voice. The false cords are hypertrophied. In these cases, a wedge resection of the false cords with the laser is a useful and practical procedure. Partial removal of the false cords had been tried before, but due to the usually severe and profuse bleeding, it was not a popular procedure.

Technique of wedge resection The ventricular bands are exposed with a large size Jako-Pilling laryngoscope and wedges cut into the ventricular folds. The wedges could by symmetrical, or one can be cut more anteriorly and the other more posteriorly (Figures 10-16A, B, 10-17).

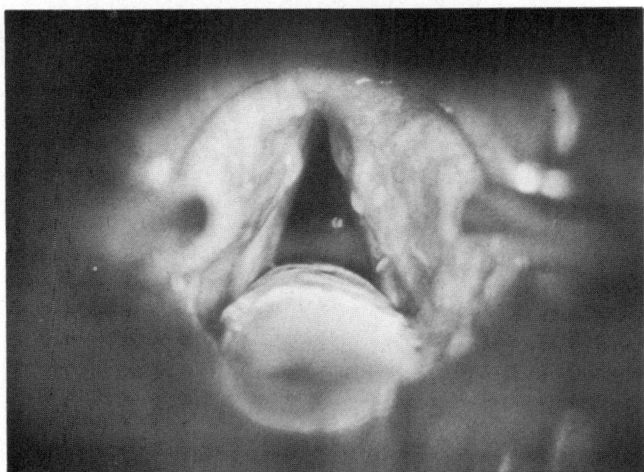

Figure 10-16A Hypertrophied false vocal cords.

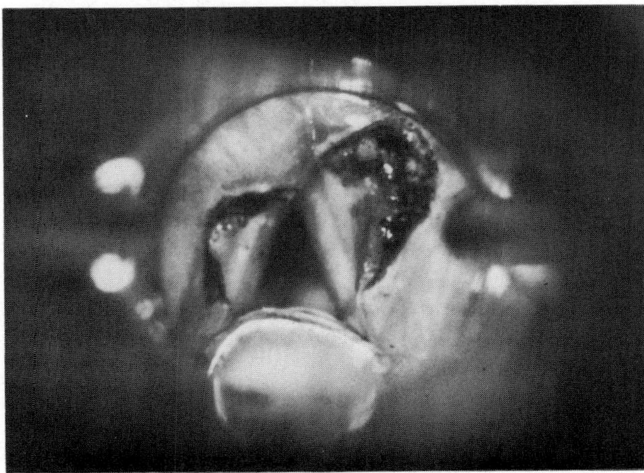

Figure 10-16B After wedge resection.

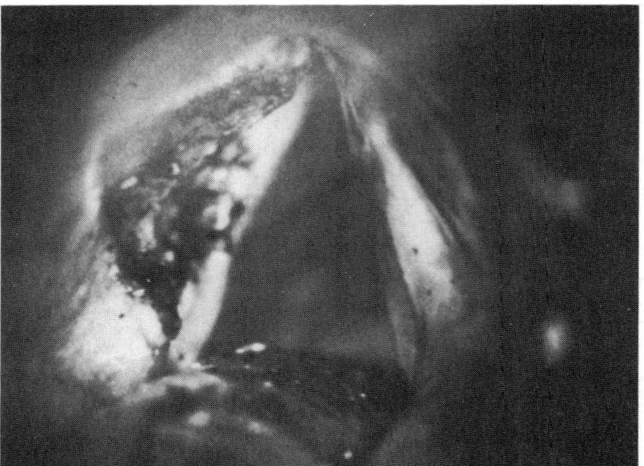

Figure 10-17 Wedge resection of left false cord (the right wedge resection is not shown.)

Postoperatively, the patient cannot phonate with his ventricular bands and he is forced to use his true cords. The healing false cords usually contract from scarring and are not able to approximate again.[10]

Amyloid Tumor

Isolated amyloidosis of the upper respiratory tract usually involves the subglottic trachea, distal trachea, but rarely the vocal cords and the false cords.[20,21] These tumors are whitish-pink in color and slightly hard. In a patient where both false cords were involved, wedge resection was carried out first on one side, then three months later on the second side (Figure 10-18A, B). The removal of the amyloid tumor of the false vocal cord was bloodless and the postoperative healing was excellent.

Cysts of the Epiglottis

These cysts originate from the free edge of the epiglottis or from the vallecula, in which case they are called glossoepiglottic cysts (Figure 10-19A, B). They can be small and symptomless or so large that they can create partial airway obstruction. For removal, a large size laryngoscope is inserted into the vallecula and the cyst is excised at the base with the laser. This is a relatively simple procedure.

Traumatic Laryngeal Stenosis

This is more often seen in children, and is dealt with in more detail in Chapter 11. Frequently, it is associated with granuloma formation. The removal of the granulomas with the laser is an elegant procedure because it is practically bloodless. The removal of scarred rings also can be accomplished easily with laser excision. Special care is taken here to interrupt the laser beam frequently so unnecessary heat flow into the surrounding tissues is diminished. These cases usually require postoperative stenting with the tracheostomy. A plastic chimney cannula with silicone tubular stent was developed for this purpose (Figure 10-20).

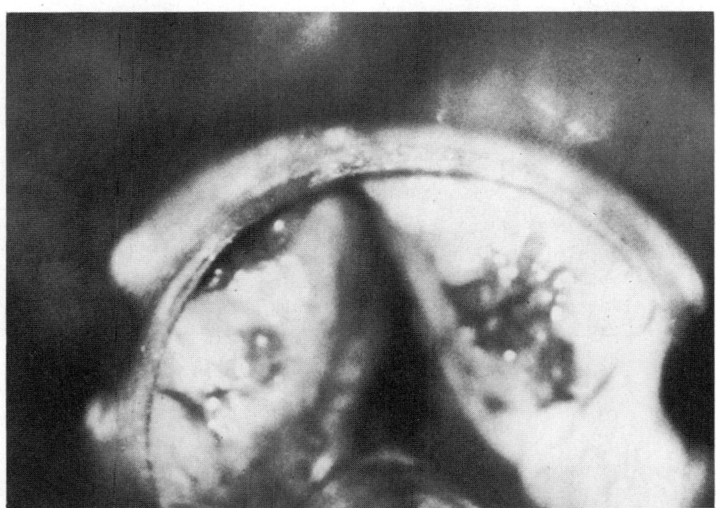

Figure 10-18A Amyloidosis of the ventricular bands.

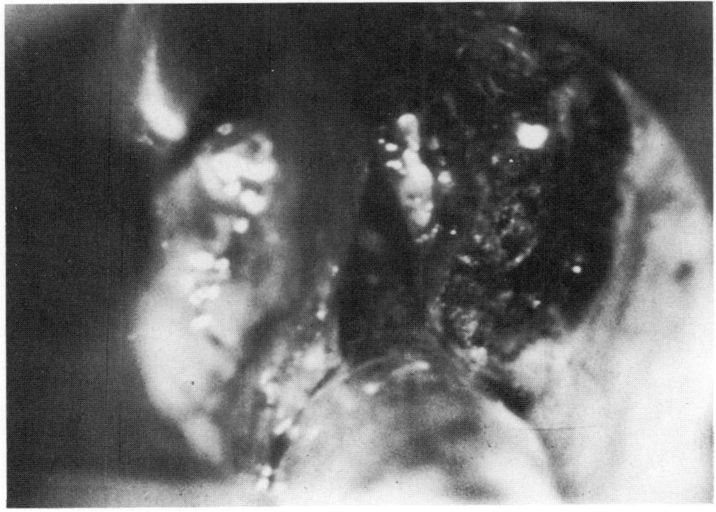

Figure 10-18B After excision (wedge resection)—right side.

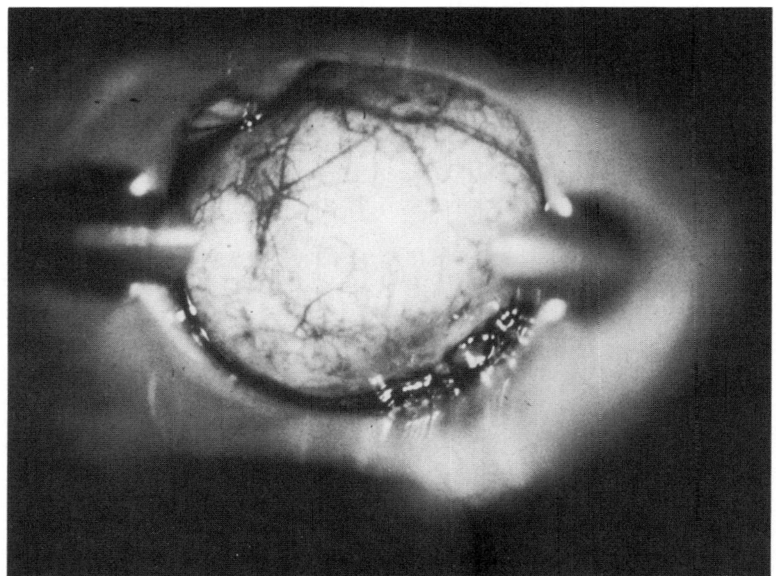

Figure 10-19A Glossoepiglottic cyst.

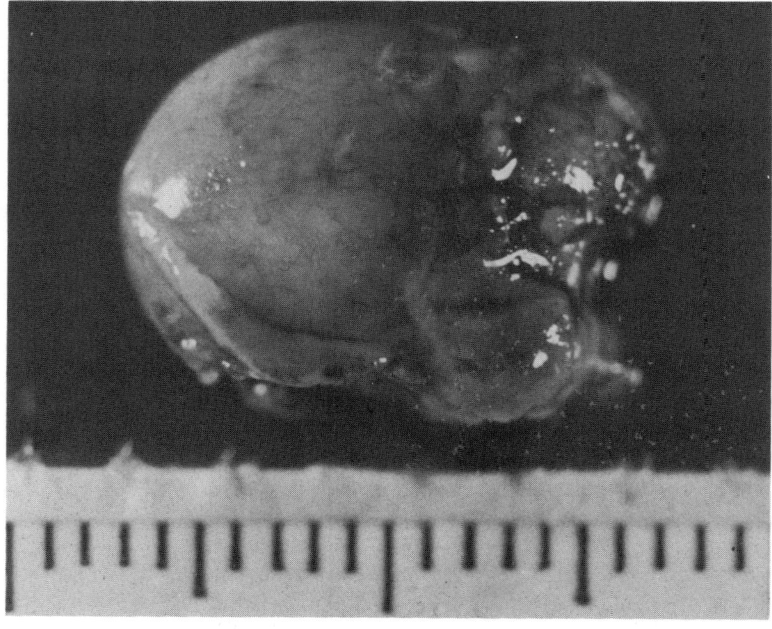

Figure 10-19B After excision.

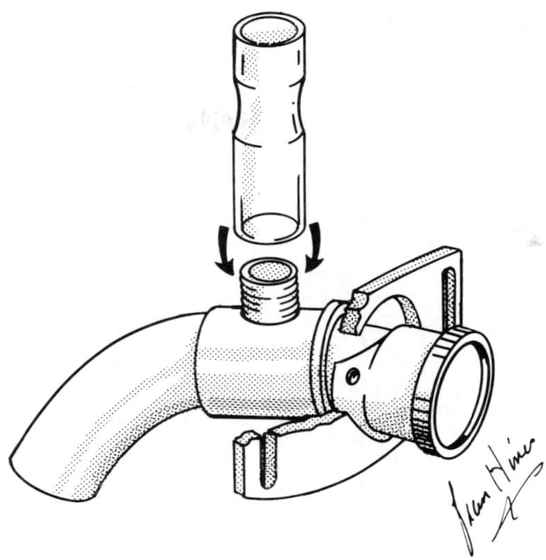

Figure 10-20 Plastic chimney cannula with tubular silicone stent.

REFERENCES

1. Wullstein H: The restoration of the middle ear in chronic otitis media. *Ann Otol Rhinol Laryngol* 65:1020–1041, 1956.

2. Jako GJ: Laryngoscope for microscopic observation, surgery and photography. *Arch Otolaryngol* 91:196–199, 1970.

3. Jako GJ: Laryngeal endoscopy and microlaryngoscopy, in Paparella MM, Shumrick DA (eds): *Otolaryngology,* vol 3, ed 2. Philadelphia, WB Saunders Co, 1980, pp 2410–2430.

4. Kleinsasser O: *Microlaryngoscopy and Endolaryngeal Microsurgery.* Philadelphia, WB Saunders Co, 1968.

5. Jako GJ: Laser surgery of the vocal cords. *Laryngoscope* 82:2204–2216, 1972.

6. Strong MS, Jako GJ: Laser surgery in the larynx. *Ann Otol Rhinol Laryngol* 81:791–798, 1972.

7. Jako GJ, Polanyi TG: Carbon dioxide laser surgery in otolaryngology, in Kaplan I (ed): *Laser Surgery.* Israel Academic Press, 1976.

8. Jako, GJ, Wallace RA: Carbon dioxide laser microsurgery and its applications in laryngology, in Waidelich W (ed): *Laser 77: Opto-Electronics, Conference Proceedings.* Schenectady, NY, Science and Technology Press, 1977.

9. Jako GJ, Vaughan CW, Polanyi TG: Surgical management of tumors of the upper aerodigestive tract with carbon dioxide laser microsurgery. *Int Adv Surg Oncol* 1:265–284, 1978.

10. Jako GJ: Microsurgery of the larynx with the CO_2 laser in Paparella MM, Shumrick DA (eds): *Otolaryngology,* vol 3, ed 2. Philadelphia, WB Saunders Co, 1980, pp 1–20.

11. Andrews AH Jr, Moss HW: Experience with the carbon dioxide laser in the larynx. *Ann Otol Rhinol Laryngol* 83:462–470, 1974.

12. Strong MS, Vaughan CW, Incze J: Toluidine blue in the diagnosis of cancer of the larynx. *Arch Otolaryngol* 91:515–519, 1970.

13. Abramson AL, Stern LS, Grimes GW: Qualitative and morphometric evaluation of vocal cord lesions produced by the carbon dioxide laser. *Laryngoscope* 90:792–808, 1980.

14. Jako GJ: Laser biomedical engineering: Clinical applications in otolaryngology in Goldman L (ed): *The biomedical laser: Technology and Clinical Applications.* New York, Springer Verlag, 1981.

15. Mihashi S, Jako GJ, Incze J, et al: Laser surgery in otolaryngology: Interaction of CO_2 laser and soft tissues. *Ann NY Acad Sci* 267:263–294, 1975.

16. Abrahamson AL, Raphael N, Ruder C, et al: Jet ventilation system for carbon dioxide laser microsurgery of the larynx, abstracted. Scientific exhibit SE-14, American Academy of Otolaryngology Annual Meeting, Anaheim, Calif, September 1980. *Otolaryngol Head Neck Surg* 88(5):212, 1980.

17. Norton ML, Strong MS, Vaughan CW, et al: Endotracheal intubation and venturi (jet) ventilation for laser microsurgery of the larynx. *Ann Otol Rhinol Laryngol* 85:656–663, 1976.

18. Rontal M, Rontal E, Wenokur M: Jet insufflation anesthesia for endolaryngeal surgery. *Laryngoscope* 90:1152–1168, 1980.

19. Snow JC, et al: Anesthesia for carbon dioxide laser microsurgery on the larynx and trachea. *Anesth Analg (Cleve)* 53–507, 1974.

20. Cohen AS: Amyloidosis. *N Engl J Med* 277:522–530, 1967.

21. Lenart Z: Amyloid tumors of the upper respiratory airway. *Weekly Med J* (Hungarian) 56:1–13, 1912

11 Treatment of the Pediatric Airway

Gerald B. Healy, MD
George T. Simpson, MD

The therapy of congenital and acquired lesions of the pediatric airway has always presented a challenge. Management of airway problems in children requires a thorough assessment, an accurate diagnosis, and selection of a therapeutic modality with minimal morbidity.

Since its introduction in 1968, the CO_2 surgical laser has proven to be a remarkably effective tool in the treatment of lesions of the upper airway. Its unique features demonstrated that this instrument would be an ideal tool for treating infants and children. Such features as excellent visibility, hemostasis, lack of postoperative edema, and minimal scarring are all extremely attractive features in treating pediatric patients.[1]

METHODS OF DELIVERY

The basic delivery system includes a 25 to 50 watt CO_2 surgical laser coupled to a Zeiss operating microscope. The accessory equipment required for laser surgery in children has been outlined in previous chapters.

In addition, a fiberoptic bronchoscope with an appropriate laser coupler is required for performing laser bronchoscopy.

Before laser surgery is undertaken, correct positioning of the patient is vital. A slight alteration in position may transform an extremely difficult procedure into a fairly easy one. As an initial step, the patient's head should always be placed at the "foot" of the operating table.

For procedures involving the nasal cavity, oral cavity, or oropharynx, it is usually convenient to lower the head of the operating table approximately 15° to 20° below the horizontal. This allows the surgeon to direct the laser from directly over the head of the patient (Figure 11-1). In procedures involving the hypopharynx, larynx, and tracheobronchial tree, the patient is placed in a horizontal position with the shoulders elevated and the head hyperextended. The entire operating table is then angled in the reverse Trendelenberg position by approximately 20°. This allows for proper angulation of the operating microscope and, thus, more comfort for the surgeon (Figure 11-2).

Protection of the patient and operating room personnel is vital. Eye protection is particularly important. The patient's eyes should be protected by the use of moistened eye pads, while the operating room personnel should be protected by eyeglasses or protective lenses. Safety must always be kept in mind when employing this or any other surgical modality.

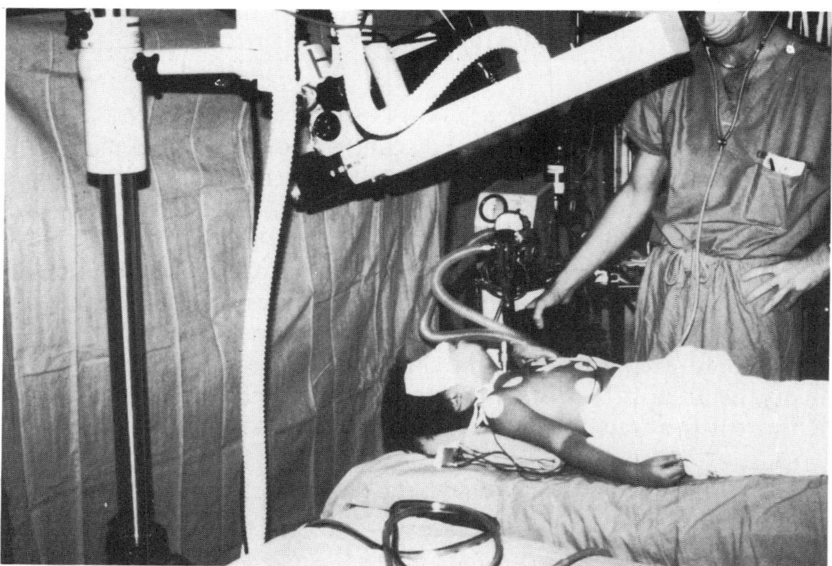

Figure 11-1 Position of patient and laser attachment for oral cavity and nasal procedures.

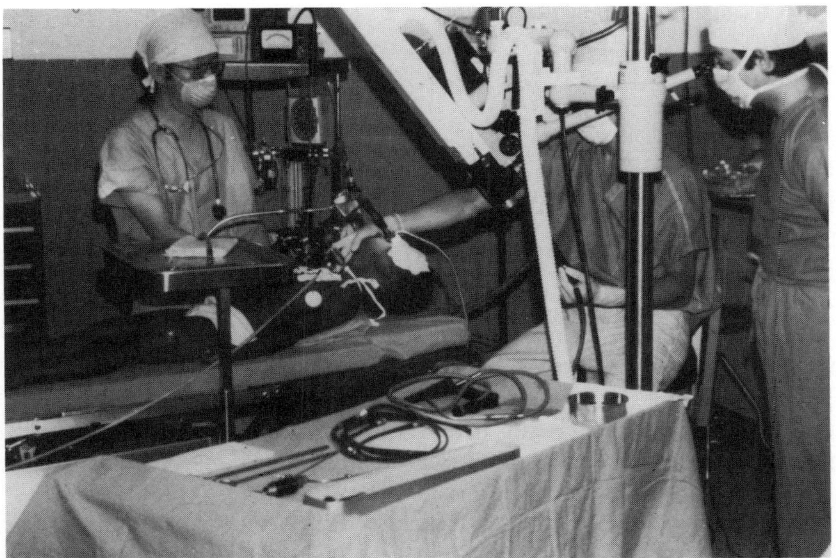

Figure 11-2 Position of patient and laser attachment for laryngeal and tracheobronchial procedures.

General anesthesia is employed in all patients as there is no place for local anesthesia in laser procedures in the pediatric population. Patients generally undergo induction via mask technique. Patients with a tracheotomy already in place are induced by direct connection to the tracheotomy tube. Tracheotomy tubes composed of combustible material must always be changed to a metal tube. This avoids any chance of fire when "blindly" lasing above the level of the tube.

If endotracheal intubation is employed, the surgeon should supervise the wrapping of the endotracheal tube with noncombustible aluminum tape. Inspection of this tube should be carried out by the surgeon and the anesthesiologist. It is particularly important to bend the tube before insertion into the patient to be sure there are no breaks in the overlapping layers of tape. The tube should always be wrapped completely to include the tip area as this is the most likely spot to ignite. Other combustible materials such as gauze sponges must be used cautiously if they are required in the field of surgery. Fires should not and must not occur!

The use of an endotracheal tube wrapped with aluminum tape may obscure some lesions of the larynx in very small children. The venturi device has proven to be exceptionally useful in pediatric patients. If laryngeal laser surgery is contemplated, the patient is prepared via endotracheal intubation. After the lesion has been adequately visualized by the conventional microscopic technique, the endotracheal tube is removed and the patient is ventilated with the venturi system.

AREAS OF APPLICATION

Nose

The most significant advance in the use of the laser in nasal lesions has been the repair of choanal atresia.[2] It has also been used to treat isolated cases of nasal papillomas and intranasal telangiectasia.

Nasopharynx

Small angiofibromas have been successfully treated with this modality.[3]

By utilizing appropriate reflecting mirrors, adenoid tissue may be precisely removed. This may be particularly important in patients with palatal incompetence, where a total adenoidectomy may be harmful to future speech production.

A few isolated cases of nasopharyngeal papilloma have also been treated.

Oropharynx

The most frequently performed procedure in this region has been tonsillectomy. It is particularly useful in patients with coagulopathies in whom precise hemostasis is important. (The laser is quite useful in coagulating vessels less than 0.5 mm in diameter.) As dissection of the tonsil is undertaken with the laser, the larger vessels are accurately visualized through the microscope and then cauterized with conventional diathermy. Due to the lack of significant postoperative scarring in laser wounds, laser tonsillectomy is also helpful in patients with palatal incompetence. Conventional tonsillectomy in such patients frequently causes scarring which further impairs palatal function.

The laser has also proven useful in resection of lingual thyroid (Figure 11-3), lingual tonsil (Figure 11-4), and cystic hygroma with oropharyngeal involvement.

Oral Cavity

Oral papillomas are usually the most frequently treated lesions. These are often isolated lesions that are not associated with any involvement in the remainder of the aerodigestive tract.

Gingival hyperplasia secondary to phenytoin therapy, as well as benign tumors of the tongue such as granular cell myoblastoma, have also been successfully treated.

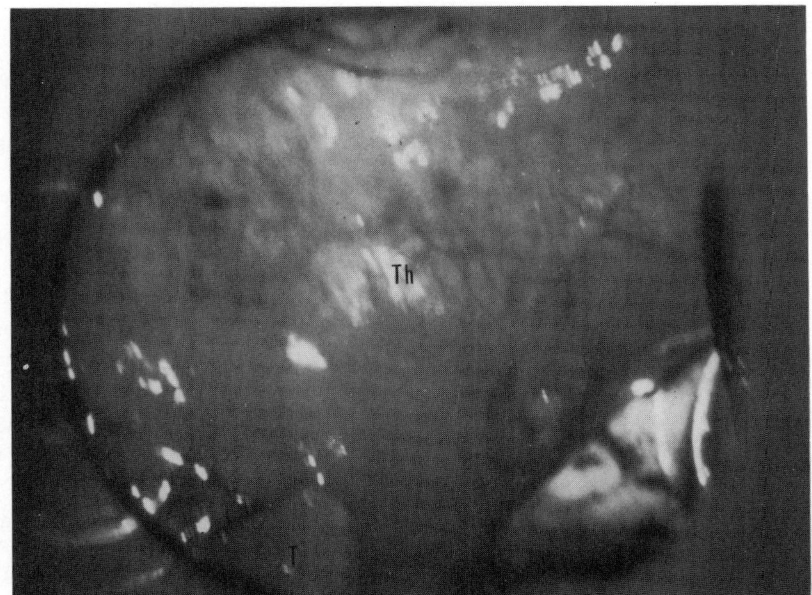

Figure 11-3 Large lingual thyroid before laser resection. (Th = thyroid; T = tongue)

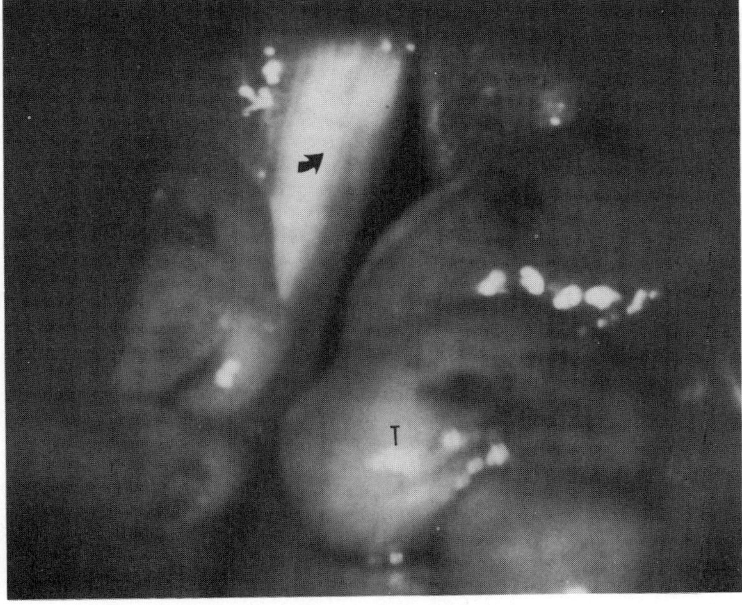

Figure 11-4 Lingual tonsil tissue obstructing the glottis. (arrow = vocal cord; T = tonsil tissue)

Larynx

The laser has its greatest utilization in pediatric laryngology. The commonest area of application has been in the difficult problem of recurrent respiratory papillomas where it has proven very useful in controlling this difficult disease process.

The laser has also been extremely helpful in treating two other difficult lesions: acquired subglottic stenosis and congenital subglottic hemangioma.

Twenty-four cases of acquired subglottic stenosis have been treated. Seventeen patients have been successfully decannulated without need for an external approach procedure. In treating these patients, it has become obvious that not all cases of subglottic stenosis are alike and, therefore, a uniform approach cannot be applied to every case. In patients presenting with total scarring of the subglottic space, all acquired scar tissue is removed (Figure 11-5), and the newly created lumen is maintained for approximately four weeks with a soft Silastic stent held in place with a through-and-through laryngeal wire.[4] These patients are maintained on prophylactic antibiotics, but no corticosteroid therapy is employed in order to avoid any delay in reepithelialization.

In cases where the lumen is narrowed but present, scar tissue is removed first on one side, and then on the other. In this instance, oppos-

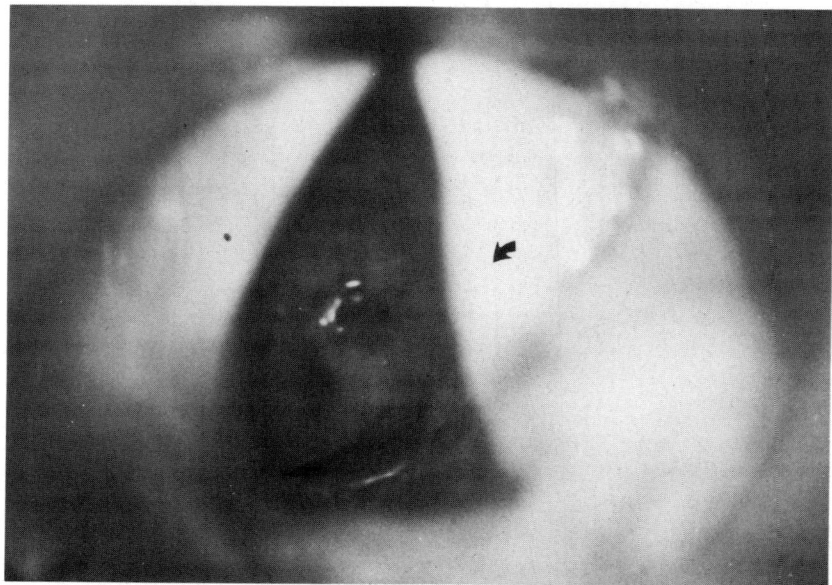

Figure 11-5A Subglottic stenosis with almost total occlusion. (arrow = vocal cord)

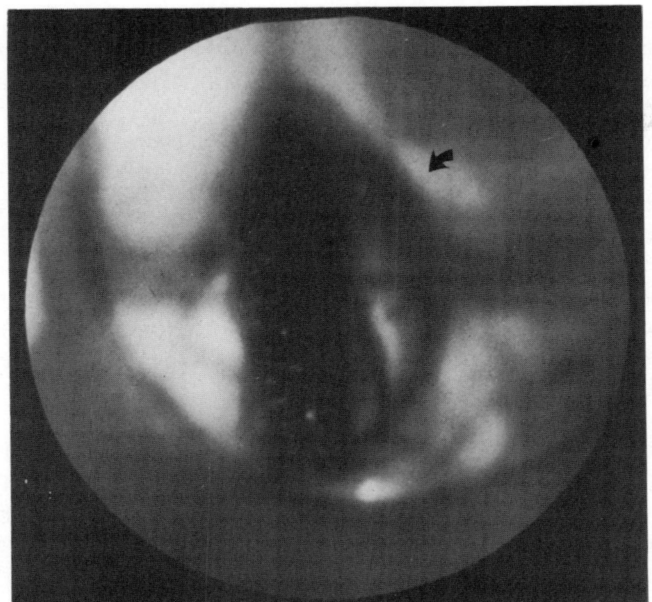

Figure 11-5B Appearance of subglottic space immediately after lasing. (arrow = vocal cord)

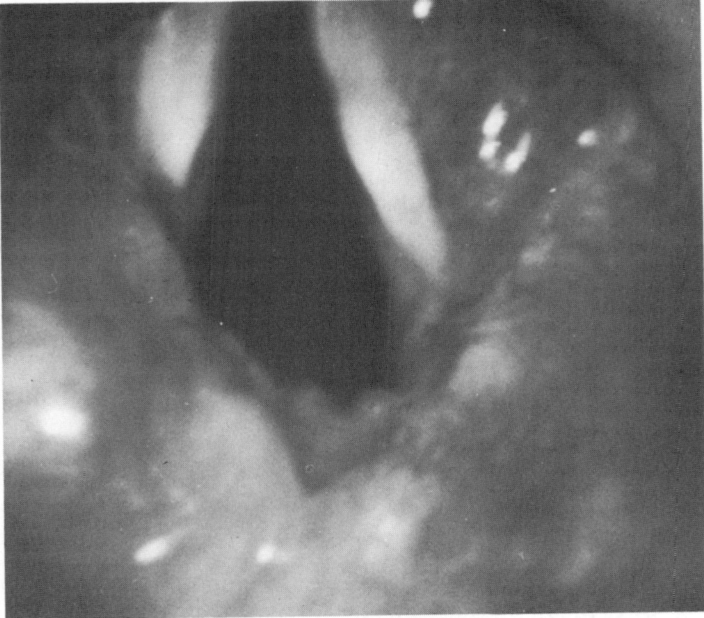

Figure 11-5C Appearance of subglottic space after healing has taken place.

ing denuded surfaces are not created, which appears to improve chances for a successful result. No stents are placed in these patients inasmuch as a lumen is already present. Prophylactic antibiotics are also employed in these cases as well.

Over the years, many types of therapy have been advocated for congenital subglottic hemangioma. Most of these patients have required tracheotomy, and their clinical course has been prolonged and tedious. Laser removal of this troublesome lesion has now been accomplished in 14 patients without complication. In these cases, a small amount of tissue is obtained for histological confirmation and the remaining lesion is vaporized, thus creating a patent airway. Tracheotomy is not required and complete removal can usually be accomplished in one procedure.[5]

Table 11-1 outlines the laryngeal lesions, both congenital and acquired, that have been successfully treated.

The CO_2 laser has proven to be a dramatically effective tool in pediatric laryngology because of its unique properties. The ability to resect lesions without inducing significant scarring, edema, or excessive bleeding is not found in any other type of conventional therapy.

Table 11-1
Pediatric Laryngeal Lesions Treated by CO_2 Laser

Lesions	No.
Papilloma	140
Subglottic hemangioma	14
Acquired subglottic stenosis	24
Subglottic cyst	2
Chondroma	1
Neurofibroma	3
Web	5
Cystic hygroma	2
Lymphedema	1
Nodule	1
Granuloma	6
Supraglottic cyst	1
Polypoid fibroma	1
Total	201

Tracheobronchial Region

The ability to connect the fiberoptically illuminated bronchoscope to the CO_2 surgical laser has been a great advance. The largest group of patients treated has been those with recurrent respiratory papillomas. A limited number of other lesions, such as small tracheal hemangiomas and posttracheotomy granulomas, have been successfully resected. The laser does not seem to be effective in treating significant tracheal stenosis.

POSTOPERATIVE TREATMENT

Pediatric patients require little in the way of postoperative therapy. Humidification must be vigorously employed in order to stimulate the resumption of mucosal ciliary activity. Frequently, crusts will accumulate on the eschar created by laser resection. This may lead to some degree of obstruction in the small airway. Vigorous use of mist will help alleviate this troublesome problem (Figure 11-6).

The use of corticosteroids as a prophylactic measure against postoperative edema may be employed if the surgeon desires. Edema from laser injury itself is almost nonexistent. However, iatrogenic trauma caused by instruments, suction tips, and the like may necessitate the use of steroids. Dexamethasone (1 mg/kg to a maximum dose of 20 mg) may be employed even in neonates in a single bolus dose.

Antibiotics are usually not necessary unless a stent is required for maintenance of a newly created lumen. Thus, their use is recommended in choanal atresia repair and the correction of acquired subglottic stenosis where stents are usually placed. It is apparent that antibiotics dramatically reduce the amount of granulation tissue present when the stent is removed.

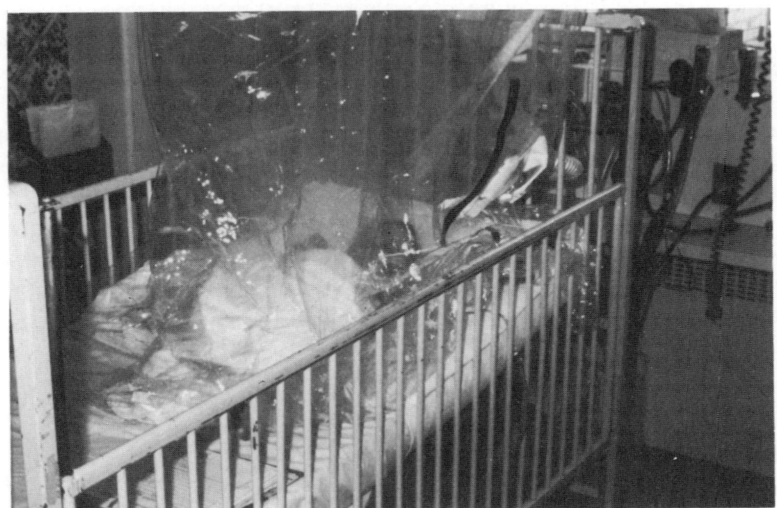

Figure 11-6 Patient in mist tent postoperatively.

COMPLICATIONS

Complications are usually directly related to the inappropriate application of the laser. For example, a large amount of energy delivered over a prolonged period to an infant's larynx will generate an unacceptable amount of heat. This may well lead to unwanted tissue destruction with resulting edema and scarring.

If a patient should develop any postoperative edema from excessive manipulation or instrumentation, reintubation may be required. Many of these patients, however, may respond to racemic epinephrine therapy delivered by positive pressure ventilation, thereby avoiding the need for intubation.

The danger of fire must again be emphasized. Meticulous attention should be paid to all phases of laser surgery so that this unfortunate outcome does not occur. In the event of fire, the endotracheal tube should be removed immediately and the patient ventilated by positive-pressure mask technique. An appropriate dose of muscle relaxant should be administered so that the glottis does not close and, therefore, adequate access to the airway for ventilation can be assured.

SUMMARY

The CO_2 surgical laser has proven to be a safe, effective, and unique way of dealing with lesions of the pediatric airway. It markedly reduces the need for an external surgical approach in many lesions which were formerly treated in this manner. Very few recurrences have been observed in any lesions treated except patients with recurrent respiratory papillomas.

The laser has also proven to be remarkably cost-effective, in that most pediatric patients can be discharged from the hospital on the morning following surgical intervention. Some patients with prior tracheotomy may be discharged on the evening of surgery.

The spectrum of treatment with the laser will probably widen over the years with the advent of flexible instrumentation and an appropriate delivery system. Greater avenues may be achieved when the CT scanner and the CO_2 laser can be joined to provide a unique means of managing even microscopic lesions.

REFERENCES

1. Healy GB, McGill T, Strong MS: Surgical advances in the treatment of lesions of the pediatric airway. *Pediatrics* 61:380–383, 1978.

2. Healy GB, McGill T, Jako G, et al: Management of choanal atresia with the CO_2 laser. *Ann Otol Rhinol Laryngol* 87:658–662, 1978.

3. Fearon B: Personal communication.

4. Strong MS, Healy GB, Vaughan CW, et al: Endoscopic management of laryngeal stenosis. *Otolaryngol Clin North Am* 12:797–805, 1979.

5. Healy GB, Fearon B, French R, et al: Treatment of subglottic hemangioma with the carbon dioxide laser. *Laryngoscope* 90:809–813, 1980.

12 Management of Oral Lesions

Charles W. Vaughan, MD

The use of the CO_2 laser has made easier the revival of an old idea, that transoral resection of accessible lesions of the tongue, floor of the mouth, buccal mucosa, retromolar area, and palatine arch may be performed with relative ease, with minimal morbidity, and with success. This straightforward, and often simple, approach has been used since medical history was first recorded. The ancient Hindus mention destroying a lesion in the throat by the application of a hot iron passed through a metal tube.[1] Surgical techniques grew bolder, however, and when the composite operation was developed in the 1940s,[2] interest in the transoral management of many lesions waned. Many surgeons felt such an approach was likely to be inadequate and therefore not sound. The pendulum undoubtedly swung too far; many mandibles were sacrificed unnecessarily when a discontinuous approach would have been adequate.

Interest in transoral resection was rekindled when it was discovered that resection in continuity was not essential.[3,4,5] Advances in anesthesia, airway control and surgical instrumentation including the CO_2 laser made the technique easier.

A variety of surgical instruments have been utilized to destroy or remove the tumors. This suggests that none of them have been ideal. Sharp dissection with the cold knife or scissors is complicated by nuisance bleeding, which often interferes with visual control of the resection, so that while it is adequate for accessible lesions of the anterior tongue, it is often quite difficult elsewhere in the oral cavity.

Cryosurgery has been used occasionally as the primary modality in the treatment of early tumors. It has been used more often for palliation of advanced or recurrent tumors. If the entire tumor can be twice frozen to at least $-20°C$, as measured by thermocouples, cryosurgery is a predictable method of destroying localized tumors. Unfortunately, it is impossible at the time of surgery to determine if, in fact, the entire tumor has been frozen since there is no specimen for histologic examination. Significant edema, unpredictable in its extent, follows the cryotherapy. It is not controlled by the use of steroids and a tracheotomy is usually necessary. Healing begins only after the destroyed tissue has sloughed some two to three weeks postoperatively.

Hot knife electrosurgery utilizing the cutting current is rapid and fairly easy to carry out since nuisance bleeding is kept to a minimum. However, the extent of adjacent tissue damage is unpredictable. Again, postoperative swelling is often enough to require a tracheotomy, and wound healing is delayed until the destroyed tissue sloughs, allowing the wound to granulate and heal by secondary intention. The resultant scar contracture is often considerable and if resection has been in the area of the retromolar trigone, trismus is expected. Pain is often severe in the immediate postoperative period. The excised specimen is distorted because of heat coagulation, and evaluation of the resection margin becomes difficult.

The CO_2 laser overcomes many of the difficulties associated with these instruments. The excision is essentially bloodless and when the laser is combined with the operating microscope, visual control of the resection is excellent. The lesion may be excised adequately with a minimal amount of normal tissue. The specimen is in good condition; the margin can then be evaluated histologically.[6] The excision usually requires minimal manipulation and there is little or no accompanying edema, thus the need for tracheotomy is avoided. Since there is a minimum of adjacent tissue destruction secondary to heat transfer, no slough occurs. Healing is undelayed and is associated with minimal scar formation.[7]

All soft tissues of the oral cavity, including mucous membrane, salivary glands, muscles, fat, etc, react similarly to the laser impact. Cutting or incising of these tissues may then be done in a predictable and reliable fashion.[8] Ducts of major salivary glands may be transected without concern and no effort need be made to maintain their patency with sutures or stenting. The surrounding area is allowed to granulate and to heal by secondary covering from the residual mucous membrane.

Teeth will be injured if impacted with the energy from the CO_2 laser. This energy absorption will be rapidly transformed into heat which cannot be dissipated as steam as occurs in soft tissue. Thermal damage may be extensive. On occasion, thermal shock has caused some teeth to chip and break in the manner of a glass goblet suddenly exposed to hot water. Therefore, laser energy should not be allowed to impact accidentally on the teeth.

Mandibular and maxillary bone may be treated with the laser. The cellular material is dissipated as steam and smoke, leaving behind a dry, crumbly white calcium material which may be scraped or wiped away to expose the residual bone. Lasers powerful enough to cut bone are not generally available, and therefore if a specimen of bone is necessary, reciprocating saws or dental drills should then be utilized for this purpose. If the tumor has invaded the periosteum or has entered into the bone, it is possible to destroy this tumor while progressively cooking the surface with the laser, wiping away the calcium residue, recooking the surface, etc, until the desired level of destruction has been reached. Bone treated in such a way heals by granulation and secondary covering from adjacent epithelium.

For reasons unknown, the postoperative wound is relatively painless unless it later becomes secondarily infected; therefore, morbidity is minimal and most patients can be discharged from the hospital on the first postoperative day, eating a normal diet, and with minimum analgesic requirement.

The laser, however, is not a perfect instrument for surgery in the oral cavity. Its use requires the lesion be visible in a direct line of sight or visualized with the use of mirrors. These mirrors must be front surfaced, fully reflective, and not subject to thermal damage. Lesions behind large teeth or towards the posterior floor of the mouth may be technically difficult or impossible to treat with the laser.

The technique is tedious when large amounts of tissue must be excised or vaporized. In such instances, the hand-held delivery system is more rapid and more maneuverable than the unit attached to the operating microscope. It is still clumsy to use, however, and its bulk tends to obscure visualization. The electrosurgical instrument (Bovie) will allow for rapid removal of the tumor bulk. The wound may then be examined with the microscope and further tissue excised with the laser as necessary. If it appears that the lesion has been completely removed with the Bovie knife, the laser will still be useful to remove the tissue injured by the electrocautery. This will hasten the healing process and reduce the amount of postoperative pain.

GENERAL CONSIDERATIONS IN SURGERY IN THE ORAL CAVITY

Anesthesia is necessary since the application of the laser is painful. When general anesthesia is used, it must be of a nonflammable type and the endotracheal tube must be the least inflammable type available. Polyvinyl chloride, portex and latex rubber tubes are highly inflammable and must not be used. Commonly available red rubber tubes are relatively resistant to inadvertent laser impact but should be covered with a reflective, self-adhesive aluminum foil. It should be remembered that uncovered areas such as the cuff and the tip of the tube remain at risk. Norton metal tubes are the only nonflammable tubes available and should be used whenever possible.[9] Nasotracheal intubation is preferred for lesions in the anterior portion of the mouth. An oral tracheal tube is satisfactory when the Dingman gag is used.

Water-soaked gauze should be used to further protect any area likely to be harmed by the laser. The eyes, especially, risk injury and should be taped shut and further protected by covering them with moist eye pads. A strict aseptic technique is unnecessary. Surgeons and assistants should wear gloves. Instruments placed within the mouth should be sterilized and kept on a surgically clean table.

A bite block is used for exposure of lesions in the anterior oral cavity. The lips and cheeks are retracted with McBurney retractors and traction sutures may be placed on the tip of the tongue if necessary. The Dingman gag is excellent for exposure of lesions of the buccal mucosa, of the retromolar area or the palatine arch. Extra cheek retractor holders may be utilized to hold and guide light cables, suction tubes, etc.

In treating lesions in the oral cavity, the laser should be attached to the Zeiss microscope whenever possible so that the beam may be precisely controlled by the micromanipulator. The microscope light provides fair illumination of the operative field. This may be supplemented by fiberoptic light bundles attached to the Dingman gag assembly or held by assistants. The magnification allows close inspection of the lesion and of tissue planes as the dissection proceeds.

If the lesion is thought to be suitable for excision, the laser is first used to outline its surface limits and the incision is then carried through the mucous membrane. The lesion is put on traction to open wide the laser incision. With sufficient traction, the laser will cut more rapidly. Blood flow in all but the larger vessels is easily controlled. Bleeding from larger vessels may require electrocoagulation or suture ligation. If bone removal is necessary to provide a margin of safety, the desired area of destruction may be accomplished with the laser, or by excision with an air drill or oscillating saw. If the saw is used, the laser may be helpful in smoothing the rough bone edges and to provide hemostasis. Frozen section monitoring of the tumor bed should be performed as necessary.[10] The wounds are left open and allowed to granulate and heal by secondary intention. Postoperative oral hygiene includes the use of saline irrigations, or hydrogen peroxide mouth washes until healing occurs.

PRINCIPLES OF DISSECTION IN SPECIFIC LESIONS

All benign lesions suitable for excision are readily managed with the laser. Recurrent respiratory papilloma may occur on the lips, on the gingiva and on the palatine arch. These should be biopsied and then vaporized down to their bases. However, care should be taken to preserve the maximum amount of mucous membrane. It should be remembered that there is no known cure for these lesions and therefore removal is only palliative. Until they undergo spontaneous remission, they will recur repeatedly. Repeated mucous membrane destruction will produce scarring.

Ranula may be unroofed easily and left to fill in and become obliterated. Granular cell myoblastoma may be excised and/or vaporized and the bed left to granulate and heal by secondary intention. Capillary hemangioma that are relatively superficial may be completely excised and/or vaporized. In contradistinction, cavernous hemangioma should not be treated with the CO_2 laser since bleeding from the dilated veins will not be controlled by the laser.

Hyperkeratosis, which arises in response to chronic trauma such as the frequently noted *white line* on the buccal mucous membrane, resulting from its interdigitation with teeth, is completely benign and without atypia. It requires no treatment. Hyperkeratosis resulting from exposure to carcinogens, and with evidence of atypia, represents a continuum of pathology from premalignant to malignant lesions in a diseased mucous membrane. It does require treatment. Unfortunately all of the mucous membrane exposed to the carcinogen is diseased and subject to further development of atypia. At present, we have no method of preventing this epithelial deteriorization, nor do we have any method of restoring this damaged tissue. We cannot totally remove it or destroy it. Therefore, treatment of this specific area of atypia should not preclude any option for treatment of further cancers that may occur, nor should it make this unhealthy mucous membrane less healthy over the long term. Instead, the atypism should be removed with the CO_2 laser in its entirety while preserving the maximum of surrounding *normal* tissue.

A supravital dye, such as toluidine blue,[10,11] should be applied to the mucous membrane to demonstrate the areas of significant atypism, and then only these are excised and the specimen examined by the pathologist (and by the surgeon). The wound heals by secondary intention.

In an occasional patient with field cancerization, the atypism may even involve the spaces between the teeth. The laser should not be used in such areas. This mucous membrane must be removed by other modalities such as cold knife excision, or the teeth should be extracted to afford better exposure and observation of the entire area.

Superficial lesions of the lips are easily removed with the laser, but when the tumor invades deeply into the musculature, the lesion may be treated just as easily with a sharp knife. Primary closure is necessary to produce an acceptable cosmetic result.

Lesions of the anterior two-thirds of the tongue can be treated for cure by laser excision if there is normal mobility of the tongue and if all margins of the tumor are visible, or will become visible during the dissection. Lesions in the posterior lateral portion of the tongue are generally unsuitable for transoral resection since exposure in this area is limited.

Noninfiltrating lesions of the floor of the mouth are easily removed with the laser. The field is dry and the extent of the tumor may be followed. Tumors that overlie bone may require bone removal. When this is necessary, the use of the air drill is recommended since it is much faster. The cut surface of the bone then may be coagulated and smoothed with the laser.

Retromolar lesions that show no evidence of trismus or bone invasion may be suitable for excision with the laser. In the past, treatment of these lesions with the electrosurgical cautery has resulted in incapacitating trismus. With the CO_2 laser, however, the mandible and masseter and pterygoid muscles may be exposed during the resection without concern for postoperative disability.

Lesions of the palatine arch are often superficial and multicentric. Wide areas of mucosa need to be removed. However, when the tumor extends to the posterior pharyngeal wall or base of tongue, or toward the eustachian tube, it is usually impossible to obtain an adequate margin with healthy tissue around the specimen. Such lesions should not be treated for cure.

If full thickness of the palate is to be removed, the endotracheal tube should be protected from inadvertent laser impaction. Tumor removal at the junction of the posterior tonsillar pillar and the posterior pharyngeal wall carries risk of danger to the carotid artery. If the tonsillar artery or a main branch of the descending palatine artery is encountered, suture ligation will be required.

The laser may be used in the management of lesions of the oral cavity for purposes other than *cure*. Large lesions may be reduced in bulk in order to define the tumor limits. Such cyto-reduction is also theoretically appealing in that both radiotherapy and chemotherapy should be more effective with a reduced tumor burden. Conventional surgical procedures, radiation therapy or chemotherapy may be instituted in the immediate postoperative period without waiting for “healing.”

The laser has also been used for palliation in patients physically unable to undergo treatment by conventional surgery or radiotherapy. Bulky or painful tumors may be removed, with improvement in their alimentation and reduced requirements for analgesics.

REFERENCES

1. Wright J: *The Nose and Throat in Medical History.* St. Louis, LS Matthews, 1898, p 23.
2. Martin H: *Surgery of Head and Neck Tumors.* New York, Hoeber-Harper, 1958, p 13.
3. Spiro RH, Strong EW: Discontinuous partial glossectomy and radical neck dissection in selected patients with epidermoid carcinoma of the mobile tongue. *Am J Surg* 123:544–546, 1973.
4. King GD: Transoral resection for cancer of the oral cavity. *Otolaryngol Clin North Am* 5:321–325, 1972.
5. Healy GB, Strong MS, Uchmakii A, et al: Carcinoma of the palatine arch. *Am J Surg* 132:498–503, 1976.
6. Mihashi S, Jako GJ, Incze JS, et al: Laser surgery in otolaryngology: Interaction of CO_2 laser and soft tissues. *NY Acad Sci* 267:263–294, 1975.
7. Jako GJ: Laser of the vocal cords, an experimental study with the CO_2 laser on dogs. *Laryngoscope* 82:2204–2216, 1972.
8. Strong MS, et al: The role of the CO_2 laser in otolaryngology. *Trans Am Acad Ophthalmol Otolaryngol* 82:595–602, 1976.
9. Norton ML, deVos P: New endotracheal tube for laser surgery of the larynx. *Ann Otol Rhinol Laryngol* 87:4:554–558, 1978.
10. Byers RM, Bland KI, Bodase BS, et al: The prognostic and therapeutic value of frozen section determinations in the surgical treatment of squamous cell cancer of the head and neck. *Am J Surg* 136:525–528, 1978.
11. Strong MS, Vaughan CW, Incze JS: Toluidine blue in the management of carcinoma of the oral cavity. *Arch Otolaryngol* 87:527–531, 1968.

13 Nasal Applications

George T. Simpson, MD
Gerald B. Healy, MD
Stanley M. Shapshay, MD

Rhinologic laser surgery is in its infancy. Healy described the first use of the laser in correction of choanal atresia.[1] Other reports have mentioned nasal uses of the lasers.[2,3] Future uses of the laser in nasal surgery, however, may match the pattern of growth of the laser's other surgical applications. This pattern has been one of steady expansion to incorporate the use of laser surgical techniques throughout the upper aerodigestive tract. These applications have been described previously and are discussed in detail in other chapters.

A number of unique characteristics have been noted to be associated with CO_2 laser surgery. They make the laser most attractive for use in rhinologic surgery. These characteristics include the hemostatic properties of CO_2 laser energy, the absence of damage to surrounding tissues, minimal postoperative edema, and rapid wound healing with minimal scar tissue formation.[4]

Despite these attractive features, the use of the laser in nasal surgery has developed slowly since other satisfactory techniques are available for most surgical problems. When no good alternative technique has been readily available, or when other problems, such as blood dyscrasias, are present and render standard technique difficult, the laser has been used. The results to date have been most satisfying. While supporting a cautious approach to the use of the laser in rhinologic surgery, we believe this technique will continue to expand and, for many lesions, may replace other techniques.

METHODS OF DELIVERY AND GENERAL TECHNIQUES

All rhinological surgery has been performed with the 25 to 50 watt CO_2 surgical laser system coupled to the Zeiss operating microscope. Accessory equipment includes standard rhinologic surgical instruments and a variety of otologic microsurgical instruments. The nasal cavities and choanal areas can be readily seen with the microscope by using either self-retaining nasal specula or retractors, or by using standard surgical ear specula of the largest size which will fit through the nares. Ear specula have the added advantage of shielding the alar rim of the nares from the laser beam. The speculum can be manipulated by hand or secured by a speculum holder. Additional illumination for microscopic vision within the nasal cavity can be readily supplied by a fiberoptic light bundle from a laryngoscope. The tip of the bundle is passed along the sides of the specula. Small-diameter suction tips of either the Fraser, Barony, or laryngeal microsurgical types allow suctioning of the cavity without obstruction of vision. Suction is necessary to remove the smoke and steam from the laser vaporization, as well as blood and secretions.

The safety of the patient and the operating team is of paramount importance. The two significant hazards to both are injuries from laser radiation inadvertently striking unprotected tissue and from laser-ignited fires in combustible materials.

The first hazard is prevented by shielding the patient and operating team from undesirable exposure to direct or reflected laser energy. The patient's eyes are covered with saline-moistened gauze pads, secured with tape. The remainder of the face is then covered with several layers of moistened gauze (Figure 13-1). All surgery is performed under general anesthesia to avoid unanticipated patient movements. Operating room personnel must wear glasses or safety goggles to shield their eyes from reflected radiation. The surgeon's hands are kept outside the path of the laser beam.

Fire hazards can be prevented in several ways. All combustible materials are kept moistened. Cotton gauze is repeatedly moistened as necessary. If available, metal, Norton-type, flexible, endotracheal tubes are used in adults. For children, or adults if necessary, red rubber endotracheal tubes are completely wrapped with overlapping layers of aluminum tape. These must be inspected jointly by the surgeon and anesthesiologist to insure that no combustible material is exposed. Metal tube connectors are used.

Proper patient positioning is essential. The patient should be placed so that his head is at the "foot" of the table. A rolled sheet or thyroid cushion supports the shoulders. The neck is anteroflexed and the hyper-extended head is supported on a "doughnut." The patient and table are then lowered 15° to 20° in the Trendelenberg position. These details of positioning are of major importance as both the access of the laser

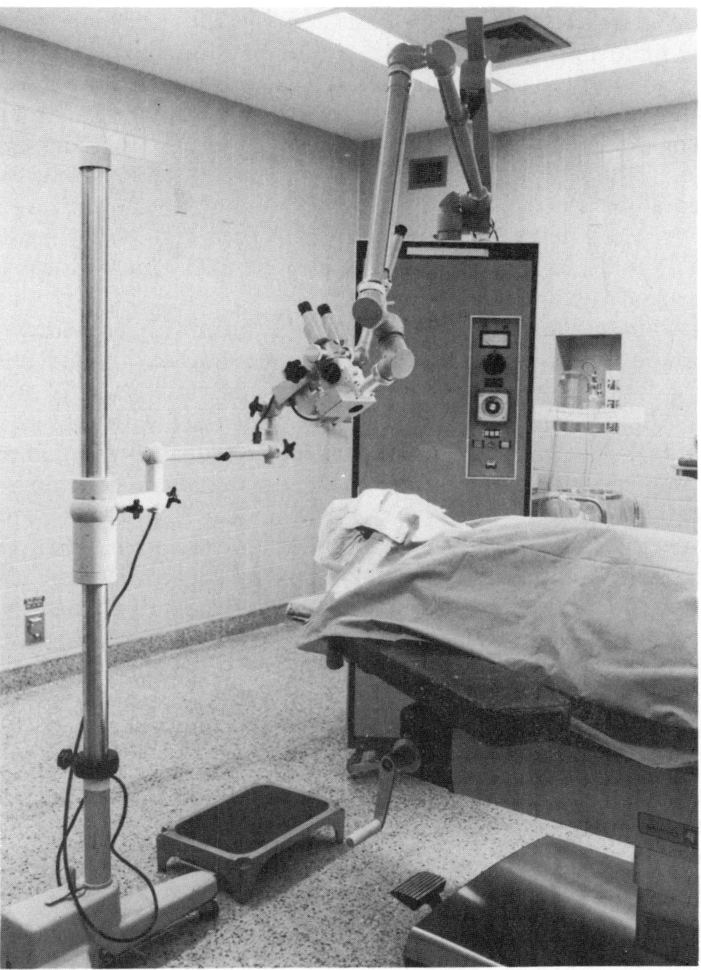

Figure 13-1 Patient positioned for external nasal laser surgery. Note face protection. For intranasal laser surgery the patient should be reversed with head at the foot of the table and the table in slight Trendelenberg position.

microsurgical system and the surgeon's physical comfort are dependent on them.

For intranasal surgery, mucous membranes are first vasoconstricted with 0.125% or 0.25% phenylephrine hydrochloride after clearing the nose of all secretions. A saline-soaked gauze sponge, or neurosurgical sponge, is placed in the nasopharynx to protect this region from laser radiation after removal of anterior tissue or opening of an atresia. The sponge also serves as an additional landmark to aid in determining the depth of surgery and the extent of tissue removal.

The nasal cavity is exposed with specula, as described above. The laser beam is directed within the nasal cavity by the micromanipulator and aiming light. For choanal atresia, the beam is directed along the nasal floor posteriorly to the atresic area. The nasal floor, the maxillary crest, and the turbinates provide excellent landmarks for the experienced rhinologic surgeon. Constant suction is important to remove steam, smoke, and secretions, and to allow continuous visualization of intranasal structures.

For laser surgery of the nasal dorsal skin, as in rhinophyma, infiltration with 0.5% or 1.0% lidocaine with 1:100,000 epinephrine is helpful for vasoconstriction and hemostasis.

Intranasal bleeding usually is not a problem with laser surgery. The hemostatic effect of the laser minimizes bleeding during and following surgery. If oozing persists, nasal packing can be employed. We prefer oxidized cellulose for small areas, or finger cots filled with packing gauze. Microfibrillar collagen can be helpful for persistent bleeding in patients with coagulopathies. If required, packing material can be removed in 24 hours.

When a lumen has been created, as in the correction of choanal atresia, stents of Silastic (preferably) or polyethylene tubing are placed to maintain the lumen. The posterior end should be cut on a bevel and the tube positioned with the bevel opening downward. The tubing is sutured to the septum with nylon sutures. Stents are usually left in position for four weeks. Humidification, including mist and saline drops, is important to reduce or prevent crusting. Suctioning of the tube lumen is necessary several times a day.

Stents usually are not necessary for other types of rhinologic laser surgery. If both the septum and lateral nasal wall mucosa have been extensively denuded, a Silastic sheet can be sutured to the septum with a nasal splint to prevent the possible formation of synechiae. This sheet can be removed in ten days.

When stenting is necessary, prophylactic antibiotics are given when the stents are in place. This appears to markedly decrease the amount of granulation tissue forming around the stents and, therefore, the likelihood of formation of stenosis.

SPECIFIC APPLICATIONS

The laser has proved useful in a number of rhinologic surgical problems (Table 13-1). Some of these will be discussed in detail.

Table 13-1
Nasal Surgery with the Carbon Dioxide Laser

Lesions	No of cases
Choanal atresia	17
Rhinophyma	4
Papilloma	7
Telangiectasia	4
Polyposis	2
Granuloma	2
Synechiae	2
Total	38

Choanal Atresia

The first and preeminent use of the CO_2 laser in rhinologic surgery has been in the correction of choanal atresia.[1] The laser provides a simple, rapid, and accurate means of performing this difficult operation.

This technique offers a number of advantages over other methods of treatment.[5,6] The transpalatal approach for surgical correction is a formidable procedure, especially in small children and infants. Many of the previously described transnasal approaches have been performed "blindly" and, therefore, pose considerable risks. Previously reported microsurgical techniques are time-consuming because "nuisance" bleeding may obscure the operative field. Laser correction is performed under direct vision; the hemostatic effect of the laser minimizes bleeding. Other structures are not endangered or violated.

In addition to the general surgical techniques described previously, a number of additional points should be emphasized. The laser beam is directed along the floor of the nose to the atresic area (Figure 13-2). This area is then vaporized until the neurosurgical sponge is seen in the nasopharynx (Figure 13-3). The choana is then slowly enlarged to a size appropriate to the patient's age and development. If the atresic area consists of a bony plate greater than 1 mm thick, the bone is removed with a small rongeur. This prevents excessive conduction of heat from the bone, which could injure adjacent tissue or produce necrosis or sequestration. An effort is made to remove as much of the posterior septum as possible.

Seventeen patients with choanal atresia have been treated to date. Eleven had bilateral atresia and six were unilateral. Patients ranged in age from 11 hours to 14 years. Twelve of the 17 patients required no further surgery. Three have required a second operation on one or both sides. One patient's unilateral atresia closed and has remained so. One patient has been lost to follow-up.

Following laser correction, some patients require periodic dilatation of the posterior choana in order to maintain the surgically-created lumen. The dilatation usually is readily accomplished in an outpatient setting without anesthesia. Rubber bougies are used. This additional technique has been quite effective in producing a final, acceptable result without necessitating further surgery.

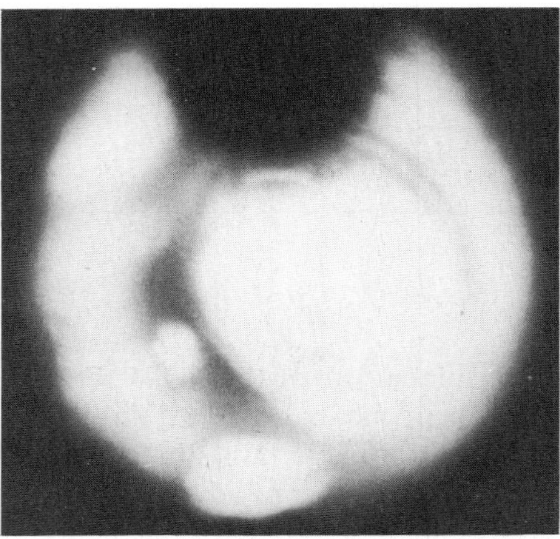

Figure 13-2 Choanal atresia, intranasal view of atresia plate.

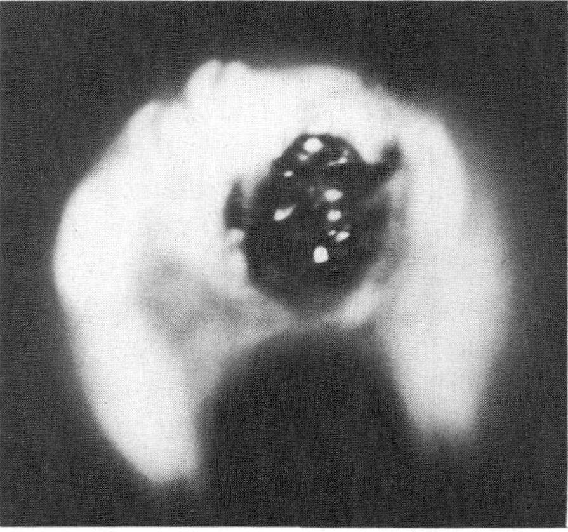

Figure 13-3 Choanal atresia, laser-created opening in the atresia plate. The saline-moistened gauze in the nasopharynx can be seen.

Rhinophyma

Rhinophyma is a condition of progressive enlargement of the nose resulting from hypertrophy of soft tissues, especially the sebaceous glands (Figure 13-4). The precise cause is unknown. A variety of surgical treatments have been described, including excision of tissues with full-thickness skin graft replacement, skin elevation with subcutaneous tissue excision, and subtotal excision (sculpturing with a scalpel or razor), followed by reepithelialization from remnants of glandular epithelium.[7-9] Each of these methods shares the common problems of moderately profuse hemorrhage impairing visualization and precise excision, and of creating a smooth transition to surrounding skin.

These problems may be largely overcome by using the operating microscope and CO_2 laser for microsurgical excision and sculpturing of the dorsal nasal tissues.[3] The hemostatic properties of the laser and excellent wound healing have been advantageous in the treatment of rhinophyma. Four patients have undergone laser excision of rhinophymas without complication and with excellent cosmetic and functional results.

The nasal skin is washed with a hexachlorophene solution and then dried. The eyes are protected with saline-moistened pads, and the remainder of the face, excluding the nose, is covered with several layers of moist gauze. Metal instruments are kept out of the operating field to pre-

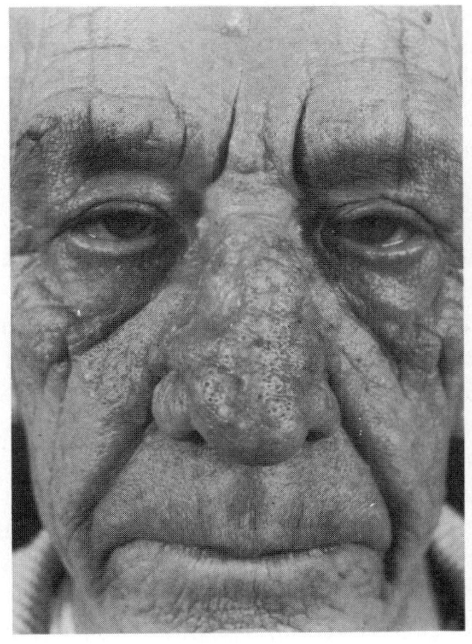

A

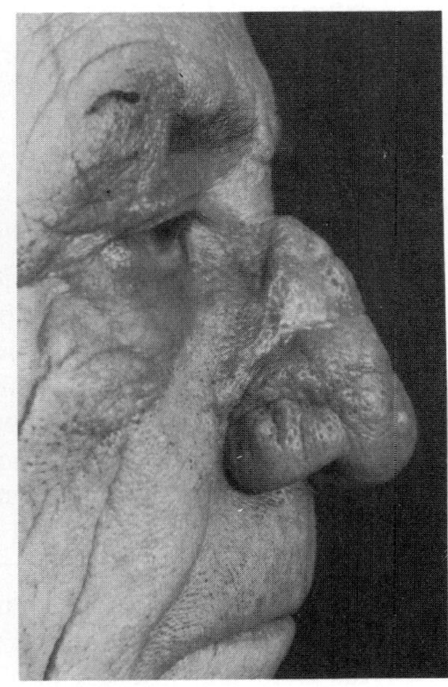

B

Figure 13-4 Rhinophyma, preoperative view. **A** Anterior **B** Lateral.

vent reflection of laser radiation. Other safety precautions are as previously described. A plastic suction evacuator is necessary to draw steam and smoke from the field.

The nasal skin is infiltrated with 1% lidocaine with 1:100,000 epinephrine. The laser is set on manual mode, with foot-pedal control. The power setting may be varied between 10 and 50 watts as necessary. A 400-mm lens is used on the operating microscope.

The bulk of the tissue is excised with the laser. The remainder is vaporized in incremental amounts under microscopic vision until the desired depth has been reached. A helpful guide in determining the desired depth of vaporization is the amount of sebum which can be expressed from the dilated sebaceous ducts. An assistant's finger is intermittently inserted into the nares to "milk out" sebum from the glands. When sebum is barely expressible, a satisfactory depth of tissue removal has been reached. Contouring of the tissue by "feathering" the edges with small amounts of laser vaporization creates a smooth transition to normal skin. Care must be taken, however, to leave a rim of uninterrupted skin around the nares to prevent secondary scar contracture.

Hemostasis is excellent. No measurable amount of blood loss has been noted during the procedures.

The nose is dressed only with a covering of bacitracin ointment. No prophylactic, systemic antibiotics are necessary.

Postoperatively, patients experience minimal discomfort which can be readily controlled with minor analgesics. A dark eschar forms within 24 to 48 hours and resolves in ten days. Complete epithelialization occurs in three to four weeks (Figure 13-5). Follow-up at six months has shown the cosmetic results to be good.

Intranasal Laser Surgery

A variety of intranasal lesions are readily excised with the laser (Table 13-1). Hemostasis is the primary advantage of the laser in intranasal surgery. Patients with blood dyscrasias or coagulopathies which make other techniques difficult may undergo laser excision with little or no blood loss. Vascular lesions such as telangiectasias or small angiomata can be discretely vaporized without significant bleeding or the necessity for skin grafts. Intranasal packs are generally not needed postoperatively.

Large masses of intranasal tissue from granulomatous disease or polyps can be vaporized in a relatively short period of time by using higher power settings. The septum, turbinates, and posterior choanae serve as landmarks and are preserved.

Adequate lighting is essential for proper vision. The microscope light must be supplemented with a fiberoptic light bundle as described above. This is especially important when working posteriorly within the nasal

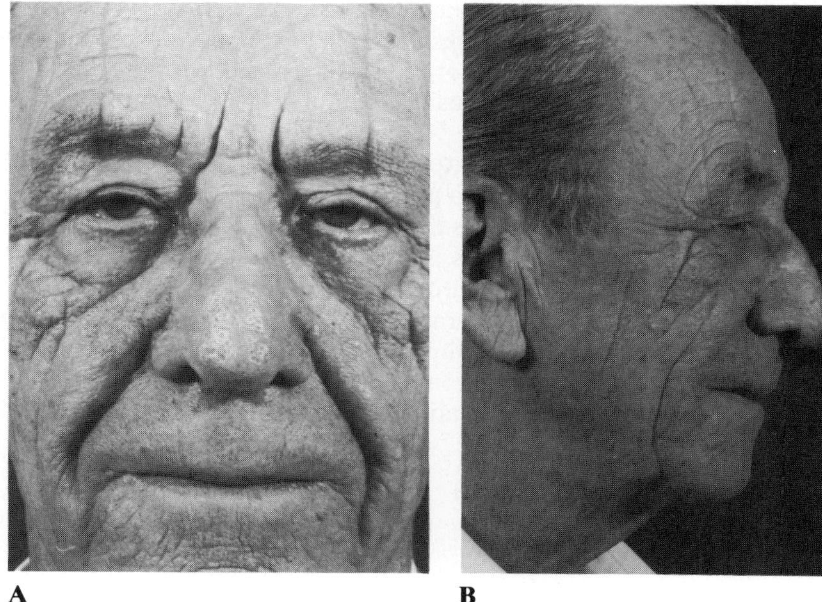
A B

Figure 13-5 Rhinophyma, postoperative view. **A** Anterior **B** Posterior.

cavity. Continuous suction removal of steam and smoke also aids visibility.

Occasionally, microlaryngeal cupped forceps are helpful to manipulate polypoid masses. This allows the stalk to be severed, and the polyp can be removed without vaporizing it, thus shortening operative time and preserving epithelial tissue.

Postoperatively, patients experience little or no discomfort. Bleeding is rarely a problem and can be controlled with the brief use of packs as previously described. Local swelling is mild, especially in comparison with that following other methods. Patients frequently note their ability to smell again, especially after obstructive lesions such as polyps have been removed. Crusts do form but can be minimized with saline or glycerol drops and saline douches. Pulsatile nasal irrigations with a Water-Pik are very helpful in removing crusts and improving patient comfort. Healing is rapid, occurring within a few days for small lesions and within two weeks following the removal of extensive lesions.

COMPLICATIONS

Complications have been virtually nonexistent. However, they can easily result from failure to follow the principles and techniques previously described. It should be pointed out that excessive applications of laser energy to a thick plate of atresic bone in the choana will produce an unacceptable level of heat absorption and subsequent necrosis and sequestration with resultant stenosis. Therefore, thicker bone should be removed with a rongeur.

Raw, unepithelialized surfaces and circumferential wounds may adhere or contract with healing to produce synechiae or strictures. These can be prevented by the judicious use of stents or Silastic splints, and by sparing the skin around the nares. Adequate humidification and the frequent use of suction and saline drops is important to minimize crusting and maintain patency of the stent tube.

Meticulous attention to detail is essential in maintaining safety precautions and preventing injury from laser-ignited fires or inadvertent injuries from misdirected laser radiation. These details have been described previously.

ADVANTAGES

The major advantages of nasal surgery include:

1. Marked hemostasis and decreased blood loss.
2. Minimal edema in surrounding tissues.
3. Excellent healing.
4. Minimal postoperative discomfort.
5. Applicability to all age groups.
6. Simplification of surgical technique.
7. Minimal hospitalization.
8. Maximal hospital utilization.
9. Capability of use despite coagulopathies or blood dyscrasias.

SUMMARY

CO_2 laser surgery offers distinct advantages in a variety of rhinological problems. It is especially useful in the early correction of choanal atresia and for intranasal surgery in patients with blood dyscrasia. It appears to offer a superior method of correcting rhinophyma.

Future applications for laser rhinologic surgery will be developed as greater numbers of surgeons become familiar with the laser's advantages and techniques of use.

REFERENCES

1. Healy GB, McGill T, Jako G, et al: Management of choanal atresia with the CO_2 laser. *Ann Otol Rhinol Laryngol* 87:658–662, 1978.

2. Healy GB, McGill T, Simpson GT, et al: The use of the carbon dioxide laser in the pediatric airway. *J Pediatr Surg* 14:735–740, 1979.

3. Shapshay SM, Strong MS, Anastasi GW, et al: Removal of rhinophyma with the carbon dioxide laser. *Arch Otolaryngol* 106:257–259, 1980.

4. Strong MS, Jako GJ, Polanyi TG, et al: Laser surgery in the aerodigestive tract. *Ann Surg* 126:529–533, 1973.

5. Flake CG, Ferguson CF: Congenital choanal atresia in infants and children. *Ann Otol Rhinol Laryngol* 73:458–472, 1964.

6. Caldarelli DD, Friedberg SA: Transnasal microsurgical correction of choanal atresia. *Laryngoscope* 87:2023–2030, 1977.

7. Smith AE: Correction of advanced rhinophyma by means of plastic reconstruction surgery: A new technique. *Ann Surg* 96:792–801, 1958.

8. Anderson R, Dykes ER: Surgical treatment of rhinophyma. *Plast Reconstr Surg* 30:403–414, 1962.

9. Matton G, Pickrell K, Hughes W, et al: The surgical treatment of rhinophyma: An analysis of 57 cases. *Plast Reconstr Surg* 30:403–414, 1962.

14 Diseases of the Pharynx

Ronald J. French, MD

The unique characteristics of the CO_2 laser are of particular advantage in the surgical treatment of lesions of the pharynx. Because of the anatomy and physiology of the tongue and pharynx, accessibility to lesions in this region may be difficult. Discomfort and gagging, as well as variations in anatomy, can make examination and treatment difficult in the unanesthetized patient. Substance abuse seems to enhance sensitivity, creating further difficulty of examination in those who may be at greatest risk. Under general anesthesia, redundancy of tissues often requires assistance in retraction to provide proper visualization, whether conventional surgical approaches or the CO_2 laser is used. The profuse blood supply of the pharyngeal structures further handicaps the surgeon. In such an operative field, extensive bleeding further compromises visibility.

Mucosal disease can often be subtle to clinical observation, despite the presence of histologically significant disease. Margins of malignant lesions are of crucial importance, and may be difficult to discern because of the reasons mentioned above. Therefore, the trauma sustained by these delicate mucosal structures because of retraction or instrumentation to obtain hemostasis may obscure important features.

The CO_2 laser is advantageous for the surgeon dealing with pharyngeal structures, because vascular coagulation is easily effected while tissue section visibility is enhanced. Mechanical trauma is minimized since less sponging, clamping, and suturing are required.

TECHNIQUES

One usually finds that vessels 0.5 mm in diameter or less will be coagulated when transected by the CO_2 laser. Bleeding from larger vessels may be controlled by conventional methods. We have found the energy of the CO_2 laser can be used to coagulate larger vessels held in the jaws of the hemostat, not unlike the technique used in electrocoagulation. Ebonization (blackening) of the hemostats to reduce reflection of the laser energy is desirable (Figures 14-1 and 14-2).

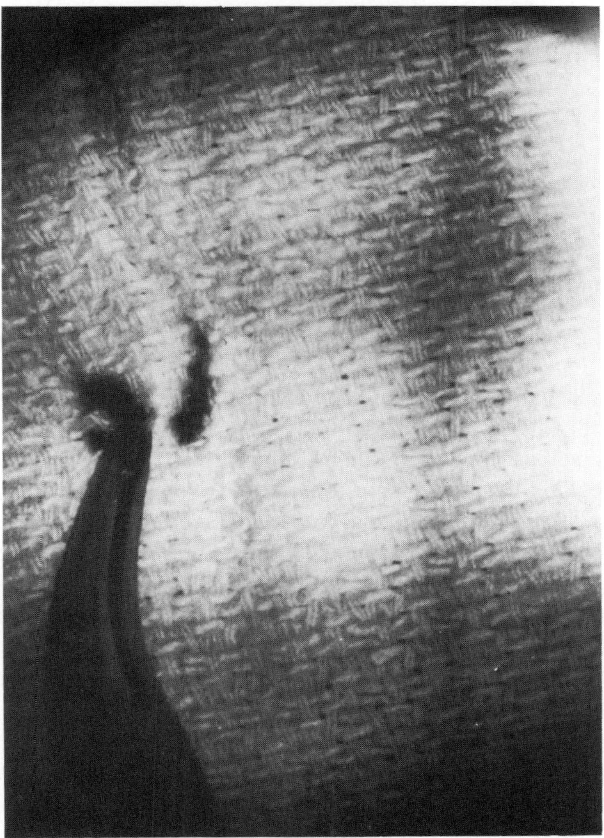

Figure 14-1 Laser energy deflected from standard hemostat.

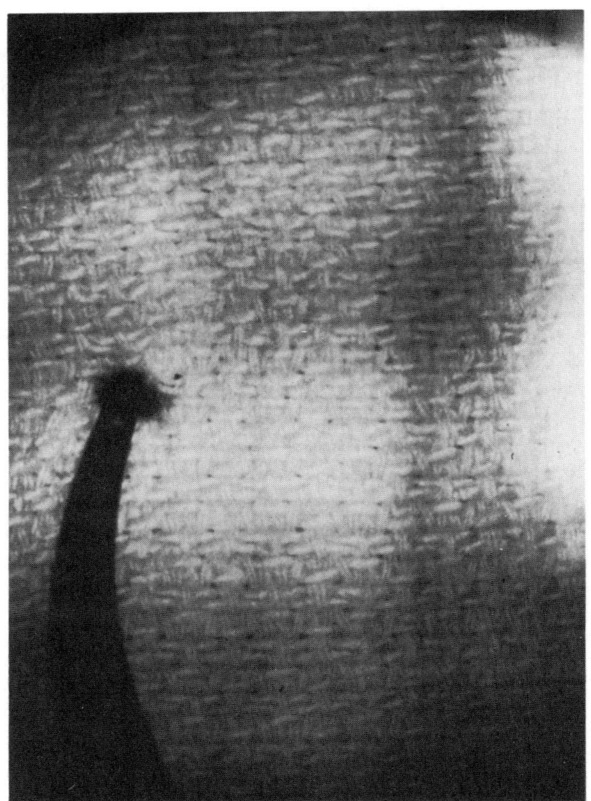

Figure 14-2 Laser energy not deflected from point of ebonized hemostat.

Although all bleeding cannot be controlled during larger pharyngeal surgical procedures, its reduction has great advantages. The visibility afforded, as well as lessened tissue trauma, allows the procedure to be done with more delicacy and discretion. Abraded and edematous operative fields can obscure lesion margins. Surface epithelium, particularly keratotic debris, may be so delicate that only dissection with the CO_2 laser can prevent fragmentation.

Because of the redundancy of mucosal structures, there is the likelihood of significant edema, both during a prolonged pharyngeal surgical procedure and, particularly, in the immediate postoperative period. Standard surgical removal of large oral lesions will certainly result in enormous postoperative edema. While tissue response to injury may be expected to result in pain and edema, it is particularly debilitating when it involves the pharynx. Edema prevents oral feeding and may require prolonged parenteral sustenance. Injured tongue musculature produces such pain that swallowing is often impossible, even when edema does not prevent it.

An even greater threat to the patient is concomitant airway obstruction because of edema, and the inability to handle secretions because of pain, edema, and decreased mobility.

A real asset is offered when a surgical procedure can be managed largely or entirely with the CO_2 laser. Coagulation of the blood and lymph vessels reduces postoperative edema. Swallowing, breathing, and the handling of secretions is much less compromised. Because pain is also reduced in the postoperative period, these benefits are enhanced. The wound progresses through the various stages of healing with noticeably less edema, pain, and infection. Necrosis and even slough resulting from edema and infection after conventional surgical excision of large oral lesions are rarely seen. Variations in healing rate occur depending on the amount of injury to the site, but the normal healing and rapid reepithelialization are to be expected.

MALIGNANT LESIONS OF THE PHARYNX

The use of the CO_2 laser does not allow the surgeon to compromise in any way in the removal of malignant disease. Rather, the laser may be helpful in performing the correct surgical procedure, and permit a less eventful recovery.

Determination of the correct surgical approach to a pharyngeal carcinoma depends on many factors. The size, location, histology, and localization (or spread of) the lesion are prime considerations. The patient's general medical condition and previous surgical procedures or irradiation must also be considered. The necessity of additional or combined lymphatic surgery is an important factor. If these factors suggest that an endoral resection is feasible, then the use of the CO_2 laser may be considered. In approaching the pharyngeal lesion, proper exposure must be obtained, usually by the use of self-retaining mouth gags, retraction sutures, and mechanical retraction by the surgeon and his assistant. Administration of anesthesia with a nasal endotracheal tube facilitates the procedure.

The CO_2 laser is generally used in conjunction with an operating microscope as described in previous chapters. This technique permits surgical resection without the introduction of additional instruments into the oral cavity. The hand pieces do offer the advantage of greater energy and may also be desirable if the surgeon must repeatedly turn from the microscope to effect hemostasis or visualize obscure areas.

Resection of lesions of the pharynx may be totally accomplished with the CO_2 laser, using the infrared beam as a hemostatic instrument. Unlike electrocauterization, the adjacent tissues do not suffer from the diffuse absorption of thermal energy. If larger vessels are sectioned, they will require electrocoagulation or suture ligature. In cases of a malignant lesion, one can examine, grossly and histologically, the wound edges for completion of resection. Defect closure, when this is desired, is made technically easier because of the lack of edema. Often, larger areas will granulate without epithelial or dermal grafting, as is the case after conventional excision. The lessened edema, necrosis, and infection, and the speed of reepithelialization follow the use of the CO_2 laser, and provide greater comfort during the accelerated healing period.

One will often be confronted by diffuse mucosal changes with multifocal areas of leukoplakia, carcinoma in situ, and frank invasive carcinoma. Frequently, there will be multicentric foci of carcinoma within a diffuse area of diseased membrane. These present a difficult problem to the surgeon, since complete eradication of the disease sometimes requires radical surgery. With the use of the CO_2 laser larger areas can be treated. Portions can be excised, while other areas are vaporized. Secondary wound healing can occur in huge areas which would not tolerate conventional surgery because of the morbidity so produced.

BENIGN LESIONS OF THE PHARYNX

While benign lesions requiring surgical removal from the pharynx are not common, they can be vaporized or excised with little morbidity and rapid healing as noted above.

TONSILLECTOMY

Discovery that surgical excision with speed and decreased bleeding, followed by rapid healing and decreased pain led us to use the CO_2 laser for tonsillectomy. This procedure can be done with the instrument in the microscopic laser configuration as described above.

The Davis-Crowe mouth gag with slotted tongue blade is used to provide visualization of the pharynx with the patient under general anesthesia. Since the endotracheal tube is retracted from the operative field it is usually not necessary to use special tubes or metallic wraps. The surgical assistant uses the Yankauer suction near the operative field to clear the resultant steam.

Dissection of the tonsils from their fossae is done as with sharp dissection. As the mucosa of the anterior pillar is incised, the muscle fibers can be easily identified and carefully dissected from the tonsillar capsule without injury to their depth. The entire procedure is usually bloodless in children. In adults, there are usually a few vessels in each fossa which will require coagulation with the CO_2 laser and ebonized hemostats or suture slipknots (or ligatures). Occasionally, the blood supply is so profuse that continuation of the procedure is fruitless. The blood itself absorbs laser energy and prevents further separation. Fortunately, this rarely occurs (Figures 14-3, 14-4, 14-5, 14-6).

The patients have little pain in the immediate postoperative period and are able to swallow and open their mouths with little distress on the evening of surgery. The recovery period is accompanied by some pain, but this seems less than that after a conventional tonsillectomy. Usually, the patient is pain-free after one week of recuperation. The eschar of the tonsillar fossa does not slough until two weeks after tonsillectomy, unlike the experience in conventional surgery. This is probably because the hemostasis and lymphatic coagulation at the time of the injury delays the acute inflammatory response and hence the other stages of wound healing. But it is interesting that, of several hundred tonsillectomies, only two have had late hemorrhage. In both cases it occurred one week after surgery. Delayed slough of the eschar is not accompanied by longer morbidity. There have been no acute hemorrhages or other complications following the procedure.

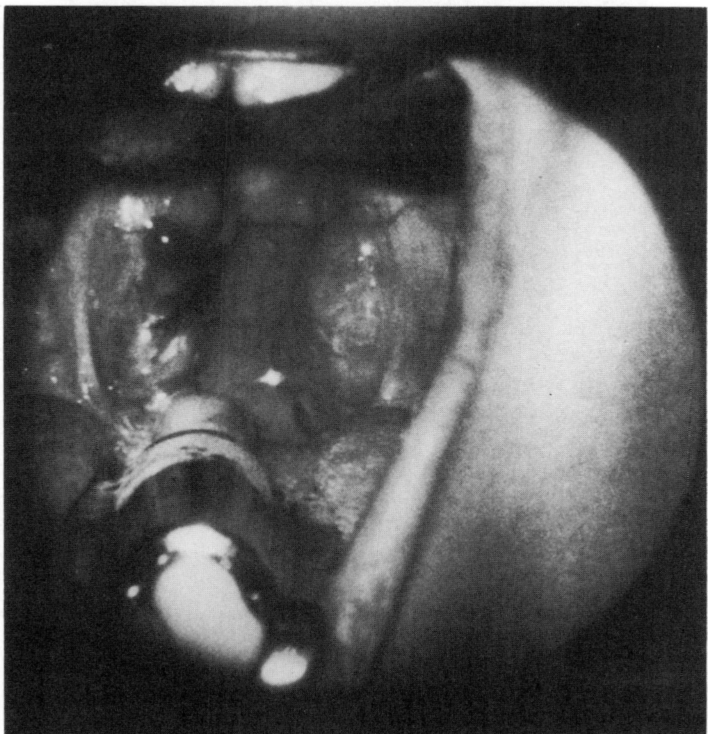

Figure 14-3 Laser tonsillectomy. View from cephalad.

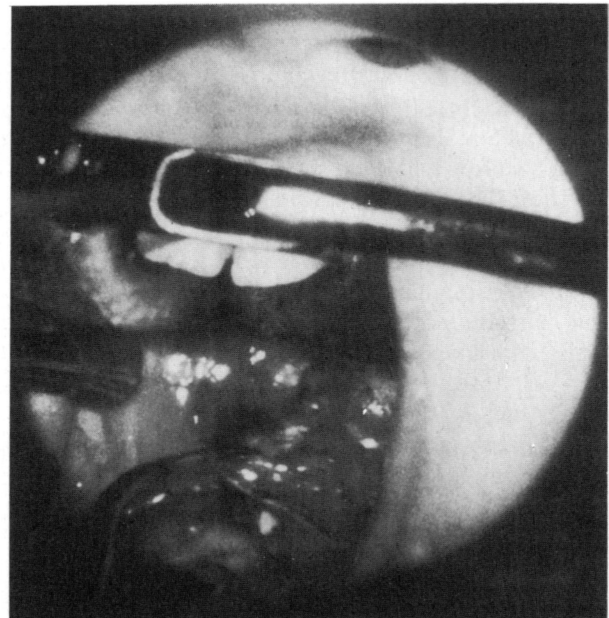

Figure 14-4 Laser tonsillectomy. View from cephalad.

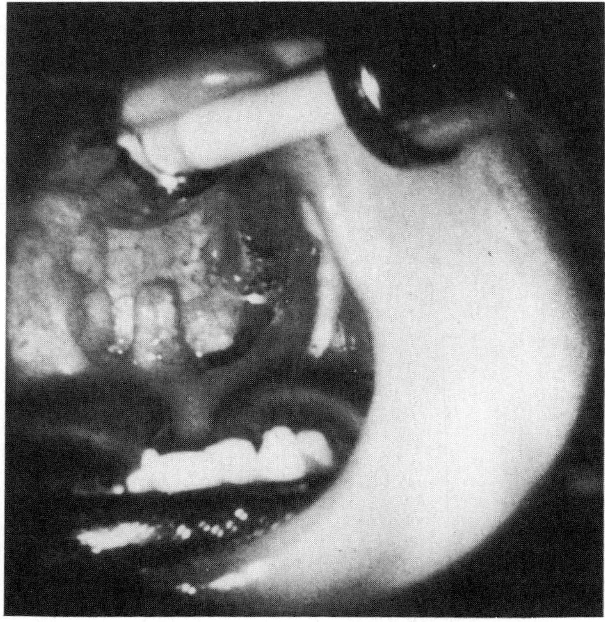

Figure 14-5 Laser tonsillectomy. View from cephalad.

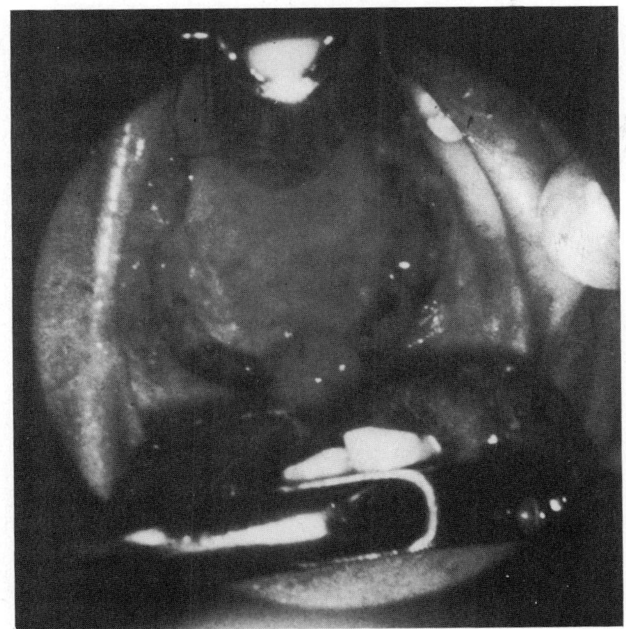

Figure 14-6 Laser tonsillectomy. View from cephalad.

15 Malignant Diseases

Charles W. Vaughan, MD

The laser has been used increasingly in the management of malignant disease in the area of the head and neck. Experience over the past ten years has proven it to be a very useful adjuvant.

Early studies with pulsed lasers did not suggest this would be true since their explosive power was difficult to control. However, continuous wave lasers are gentle in their action and are exquisitely controllable. The indications for their use in malignant disease have been slowly defined as laboratory and clinical experience has developed.

Of the three types of continuous wave lasers available for use in surgery, the CO_2 laser has been the clinical instrument of choice for theoretical and practical reasons in that its energy is effectively absorbed by tissue water, thus making it an accurately controlled instrument.[1] The neodymium-YAG and the argon-helium lasers require pigment, rather than water, for energy absorption and, therefore, tend to produce their effects deeper in the tissue. Recent experience with the argon laser suggests that if the power density is high enough, these differences are minimized and, therefore, it tends to behave similarly to the CO_2 laser, but with the added advantage that its beam may be focused by glass lenses and it may be passed through glass fibers. However, there is extensive damage to adjacent tissue secondary to light scather so that accuracy is sacrificed. At the present time, almost all clinical experience has been with the CO_2 laser.

Three systems for delivery of the continuous wave CO_2 laser energy to the target are available: 1) a hand-held system, 2) a bronchoscopic attachment, and 3) a micromanipulator coupled to a Zeiss operating microscope. Use of the first two requires a laser instrument equipped with an articulated arm, such as the original American Optical model 200.

Comments in this chapter will be confined to the use of the handpiece and the micromanipulator in the area of the head and neck. It should further be recognized that, since squamous cell carcinoma comprises at least 90% of the tumors in this area, most clinical experience has been with this malignant disease.

The hand-held instrument was the original delivery system available for the CO_2 laser. It has been used for many years by head and neck surgeons as a cold knife substitute whenever the coincidental attribute of hemostasis was highly desired. As such, it may be of some advantage in lesions such as carcinoma of the tip of the tongue, although it must be recognized that laser excision of large amounts of tissue is somewhat tedious and time-consuming. The electrocautery is equally hemostatic and much faster. The laser has been used as a knife for minor surgery such as excision of basal cell and squamous cell carcinoma of the skin, and for major surgery including radical neck dissections. However, we have found it to be of no particular advantage over the usual cold-knife or scissor techniques except for the unusual and unexplained fact that laser burns are relatively pain-free. Thus, if a tumor is excised with the Bovie electrocautery, postoperative pain may be severe; however, if the area of the electrocautery burn is promptly removed with the laser, postoperative pain is minimal. Further, healing is improved since it is not delayed by the usual slough of cauterized tissue. The electrocautery and the laser may thus be combined to some advantage.

This hand-held delivery system is not suitable when extreme accuracy is required or when the laser must be delivered to inaccessible regions such as the back of the oropharynx, to the larynx, to the interior of the nose, etc.

By coupling the CO_2 laser to the surgical microscope, one is provided with a magnified binocular view of the operative field and with fine control of the laser beam by means of a micromanipulator. This achieves exquisite accuracy and is, therefore, the most useful and commonly used of the delivery systems.

However, it should be first remembered that the laser is only an adjunct in the management of malignant disease in this area and that its proper use requires a well-grounded skill in microsurgery, especially transoral microlaryngoscopy, and also a basic understanding of the nature of squamous cell carcinoma of the mucous membranes of the head and neck.

Squamous cell carcinoma in the head and neck area may be of two types: 1) a nonkeratinizing carcinoma (poorly differentiated, lymphoepithelioma, Schmincke cell tumor, etc), with its cells of origin in the deep crypts of Waldeyer's ring at the interface of the mesenchymal and ectodermal tissue, and 2) a keratinizing carcinoma (differentiated) with clearly defined intracellular bridges and cells of origin in the mucous membrane of the head and neck. Further, there may be various etiologies of these tumors. The Epstein-Barr virus has been suggested as the etiologic agent in the nonkeratinizing tumors of Waldeyer's ring, and an unknown etiology for squamous cell carcinoma arising in the sinus complex. However, it is the tobacco-alcohol-induced keratinizing squamous cell carcinoma which comprises over 90% of the head and neck carcinoma in the United States and Europe. The carcinogens in tobacco tend to be applied over a long period of time and over a wide area of mucous membrane, although they do tend to concentrate in certain areas such as the larynx, piriform sinus, floor of the mouth, and palatine arch.

If a carcinogen is widely applied, one should expect and, in fact, one does find multiple tumors at the time of the first examination. If the carcinogen continues to be applied, subsequent tumors will develop. Because of this widespread application of a carcinogen, all exposed mucous membrane is diseased and, since all of the diseased mucous membrane cannot be removed, there is no such thing as a "cure." The most obvious and dangerous expression of this disease, namely, invasive squamous cell carcinoma, may be successfully removed surgically or destroyed with radiation therapy, chemotherapy, etc, but the remaining mucous membrane is subject to further development of cancer. This will certainly occur if the patient lives long enough.

This widespread "field cancerization" is easily recognized by the experienced clinician. It may be accurately defined by supravital staining with toluidine blue O. Proper treatment demands that all areas of atypia, whether it be carcinoma in situ, early invasion, or frank carcinoma, be completely removed while at the same time preserving maximal amounts of "normal" tissue. This is well achieved with the accuracy realized with the operating microscope combined with the fine control of the micromanipulator which guides the CO_2 laser beam.

In treating such malignancies, the CO_2 laser may be guided to any area that can be visualized either directly or with the use of a hand-held surface reflecting mirror. It has been used to excise and/or ablate lesions throughout the oral cavity, nasopharynx, hypopharynx, nose, etc.[3]

In such cases the hot or cold knife may be used to almost equal advantage, except that the cold knife is not hemostatic and, in such relatively confined spaces, any amount of bleeding is a significant problem. The electrocautery produces hemostasis and creates a variable, but always generous, amount of adjacent tissue death resulting in slow healing and considerable postoperative pain. The laser minimizes these problems. It has the further attribute of being more accurate.

Endoscopic application utilizes the advantages of the CO_2 laser to the maximum. It is here that the laser is most useful. The surgeon is working at a distance in a confined area and usually is attempting to preserve maximum function while removing all of the disease. This demands the great accuracy provided by the laser-microscope-micromanipulator system. These procedures also demand a surgical team skillful in the art of suspension laryngoscopy.

BASIC REQUISITES

Adequate Working Time

The procedures may take from minutes to hours to perform. General anesthesia with complete muscle relaxation is essential. An endotracheal tube is preferred since it immediately establishes a protected airway and tends to hold the vocal cords apart for easier observation in surgery. Since it lies between the arytenoids, it does not obstruct the vocal cords. Should an unusual tumor occur in the interarytenoid region, the tube can be displaced anteriorly or can be removed, and a venturi ventilating system substituted. Throughout the procedure, the patient must be continuously monitored electrocardiographically because suspension laryngoscopy frequently induces reflex changes in the cardiac rhythm.

Excellent Exposure

The anterior portion of the oral cavity may be exposed by assistants opening the mouth, retracting the tongue, etc; more posterior areas are best exposed by using the Dingman gag to which may be applied light carriers, suction tubes, etc. Exposure of the hypopharynx and larynx requires wide-aperture laryngoscopes such as the Jako-Pilling, the Dedo-Pilling, or the Kleinsassauer. These provide binocular vision and, therefore, depth perception and increased working room for bimanual surgery. The original Lynch suspension may also be used, but it has the disadvantage of requiring anesthesia by some method other than tracheal intubation, and most anesthesiologists are unhappy under such circumstances.

Laryngoscope Support

The Lewey and Kleinsassauer holder systems are generally available but are not recommended since their use requires hyperextension of the head or the neck. The best position for viewing the interior of the larynx, especially the anterior commissure, is the Boyce "sniffing" position advocated by Jackson, with the neck anteflexed and the chin extended. This requires true suspension laryngoscopy, as can be achieved by the Boston University—Pilling suspension system. This provides a lifting force away from the teeth and gums and is essential for difficult exposures.

Adequate Illumination

Distal illumination from the standard fiberoptic cables currently available is preferred. The microscope light should be turned off whenever possible as it tends to add reflection and, therefore, interferes with vision. This is especially true for laryngeal photography. For photographic documentation a xenon light source may be necessary, such as that supplied by Wolf (catalog No. D5008U) or Karl Storz (catalog No. 487).

ENDOSCOPIC APPLICATION[4]

Dysplasia

All dysplastic lesions and carcinoma in situ which can be visualized can be excised and/or ablated. The exact margins of the atypia are reliably defined with the use of supravital staining. The areas of excision and/or ablation should be confined precisely to the areas of excess dye uptake.

Excisional Biopsy for Cure

The laser can be used in localized, well-defined T1 carcinoma, especially verrucous carcinoma. Higher-staged tumors occasionally can be treated if the protective function of the larynx is not thereby compromised. It is always desirable to have the excised specimen show that the margins are free of tumor. However, if the margins are not free of tumor, this is of no great significance since at least 2 mm of margin are lost by laser vaporization of tissue in excising the specimen. The only important margins are those of the wound, following the surgical excision. Frozen section biopsies should be obtained from the wound bed. If such facilities are not available, we recommend that this type of transoral laser surgery for cure not be attempted.

Aid to Diagnosis for Accurate Staging

Bulky lesions can be reduced in order to determine their true extent. This is one of the most important applications of the CO_2 laser. We have found that clinical staging with indirect endoscopy and even direct endoscopy is frequently inexact and inaccurate. For instance, T_1 carcinoma by definition requires that the tumor be confined to the vocal cord and that these cords be mobile as determined by indirect examination, the implication being that the tumor is confined to the surface epithelium and has not invaded muscle. Our experience with laser surgery, however, has shown that vocal cord mobility is an extraordinarily inaccurate indicator of tumor invasion of the muscle. Many patients with tumors clinically staged as T_1 have been found at the time of excision biopsy to have deep muscle invasion and, therefore, should realistically be classified and certainly treated as T_3 tumors.

Not infrequently, bulky supraglottic tumors may obscure their point of origin, and it is not until large amounts of the bulk of the tumor have been removed that one can discover whether the patient is suitable for a supraglottic resection or may require total laryngectomy, etc. An even more difficult area to ascertain tumor extent is the region of the anterior commissure where a tumor with a mobile vocal fold may represent a T_1 carcinoma. If the tumor has broken through the thyroid cartilage, it may represent a T_4 lesion. By utilizing the laser, the tumor may be gradually vaporized and followed until its true limits can be determined. We are convinced that excision biopsy, which is easily done with the laser, is essential for precise staging and meaningful statistical evaluation.

Recurrent Carcinoma Following Radiation Therapy

This frequently presents a difficult diagnostic problem. Routine biopsy, utilizing a cup forceps, is often unrewarding until the carcinoma ulcerates the surface. By utilizing the laser, an entire vocal cord may be resected and the specimen studied histologically, again emphasizing the need for large tissue specimens which can be obtained only by excisional biopsy.

UNIQUE APPLICATIONS

The Severely Compromised Airway

Reestablishment of a severely compromised airway can be achieved transorally by utilizing the CO_2 laser to ablate the obstructing tissue. This avoids the need for preoperative tracheotomy and its manifold complications, including wound sepsis, possible tracheal injury, and possible peristomal seeding.

"Debulking" or Cytoreduction

Reduction of a significant amount of tumor mass prior to chemotherapy or radiation therapy is theoretically desirable in that the smaller the tumor burden, the more successful these modalities are likely to be. The removal of large amounts of laryngeal tissue with the CO_2 laser is somewhat tedious but can be accomplished with little or no morbidity if the sphincter function of the larynx is not compromised. The long-term effects of debulking as adjuvant therapy are as yet unknown. However, immediate improvement and the general well-being of many patients is achieved rapidly by removing tumor bulk that has interfered with respiration, deglutition, or speech.

Airway Protection

Occasionally, patients require artificial glottic closure for protection from aspiration, etc. This has been achieved transorally with minimal morbidity by denuding the mucous membrane overlying the true vocal cords and then sewing the cords together. This position may be further maintained by Teflon injection laterally into the substance of the vocal cords.

CURRENT TREATMENT PLAN

Any malignant lesion of the lips or oral cavity, including the palatine arch and pharynx, which is suitable for local excision, may be a candidate for excision with the CO_2 laser. For tumors that can be viewed endoscopically the treatment is as follows. In carcinoma clinically staged as T_1 or "in situ", patients undergo diagnostic endoscopy, including esophagoscopy, and supravital staining, as well as bronchoscopy in those patients who have suggestive findings on chest x-ray. Excisional biopsy is then carried out, utilizing the CO_2 laser. The entire specimen is sent to the laboratory for evaluation. Any questionable margins are controlled by frozen-section biopsy at the appropriate site *in the patient*. If the clinical staging has proved to be correct (T_1 or less), the patient may be discharged on the first postoperative day, and carefully followed. If the tumor is found to be larger than T_1, the laser can be used during diagnostic endoscopy and staining for excisional biopsy, if possible. This allows accurate staging and tumor cytoreduction prior to definitive radiation therapy or surgery; it may be curative if the margins are free. In cases of questionable postradiation recurrence of carcinoma, the laser can provide a large specimen with good exposure of the depths of the lesion. The procedure may be curative if the margins are free, but it allows further surgery if necessary.

This technique has the following advantages:

1. *Accuracy*. The limits of the tumor can be precisely defined, thus allowing maximal excision of the tumor and preservation of normal tissue.
2. *Minimal morbidity*. Gentle interreaction between biologic tissue and the CO_2 laser results in minimal inflammatory response with little postoperative pain and undelayed healing. The operative time is usually measured in minutes rather than hours. Major resections can be accomplished without skin incision or tracheotomy. The patient may be discharged with normal alimentation and a useful voice. This is highly cost-effective.

CURE RATES

Cure rates are difficult to describe in an aging population with a normal death rate from other causes over a five-year period of about 25% to 30%. Further, if one believes, as we do, that one is dealing with a diseased mucous membrane which cannot be replaced in its entirety, then *cures* are impossible. One should speak more accurately of "local control" of the most severe expression of this disease, namely, carcinoma in situ or invasive carcinoma.

Transoral treatment of malignant tumors has for many years been highly effective in terms of cost, lack of morbidity, and cure rate (local control). Lynch has reported the successful treatment of 39 patients utilizing suspension laryngoscopy.[5] New and Dorton reported a 90% cure rate with transoral excision and diathermy.[6] Lillie and De Santo reported on 98 patients; all were cured, although five required further treatment, generally additional transoral resection.[7]

We are not aware that the course of any patient's disease has suffered directly from the use of the CO_2 laser, although in three instances definitive treatment was unduly delayed because the patient would not consent to further therapy such as laryngectomy, preferring to "wait and see what happens."

In a study of our earliest patients, there were 31 who were at risk for more than three years. Of these, five had undergone CO_2 laser excision of the tumor prior to definitive laryngectomy; of these four were alive and well at three years. One patient had undergone a diagnostic excisional biopsy which subsequently led to a total laryngectomy, and was alive and well at three years.

Five had excision biopsies following radiation therapy because of possible recurrence following treatment. Of these, two were alive and well at three years with no further treatment. Two had undergone total laryngectomy and were alive and well; one continued to have multiple laser excisions on 12 occasions over the subsequent ten years. He remains alive with a functional voice, although he continues to produce "mini tumors" in his larynx and now has carcinoma of the lung.

Four patients were "debulked" prior to radiation therapy; of these three are alive and well. One died of leukemia, apparently free of recurrence at 18 months. Two were treated to reestablish airways prior to laryngectomy, and both were alive and well at three years.

Fourteen underwent laser excision as the primary mode of treatment. Of these, 13 were alive and well without disease; one eventually was further treated with radiation therapy. We now have treated over 200 patients over the past ten years and believe that the above experience remains typical.

COMPLICATIONS

Fire

Fire continues to present the possibility of serious complication. *If the energy of the CO_2 laser is absorbed by inflammable substances, the latter will ignite.* Any gauze in the operative field must be kept moistened with water or normal saline solution. The patient's eyes must be covered at all times, and the operating personnel should wear protective eyeglasses. Endotracheal tubes must be protected and be made of the least possible flammable material. Currently, the most acceptable tube is the flexible, metal, Norton endotracheal tube (V. Müeller, catalog No. VE5-25-1 through -6).

Bleeding and Obstruction

Neither postoperative bleeding nor airway obstruction requiring tracheotomy, has been observed. Intraoperative bleeding from vessels larger than 0.5 mm in diameter has been encountered on occasion. Experience has shown where to expect such vessels and how to control them with judicious use of diathermy cautery or vascular clips.

Aspiration

Aspiration leading to fatal pneumonia has been encountered experimentally in dogs deprived of their protective sphincter function by vertical hemilaryngectomy, ie, endoscopic removal of both the true and false vocal cords on one side with or without epiglottectomy. However, aspiration has not been encountered in several patients who have undergone horizontal partial laryngectomy, ie, excision of the epiglottis, aryepiglottic fold, or one or both false vocal cords, or, alternatively, excision of both true vocal cords if the arytenoids and false cords are preserved.

Lack of Experience

Inexperience on the part of the surgeon in the transoral approach and in working through the narrow confines of the laryngoscope while attempting to remove large amounts of laryngeal tissue are major operative problems. Crosby Green in 1920, while commenting on Lynch's transoral cordectomy using suspension laryngoscopy,[5] stated, "I think few of us are able to do this satisfactorily by means of the suspension method. I do not believe that the method is generally applicable." This probably remains true today, even with the added advantage of the CO_2 laser. Most laryngeal surgeons should not attempt these procedures until competence with this approach has been achieved by studious practice on experimental animals. The scope of surgical expertise may then be gradually applied to highly selected patients.

REFERENCES

1. Polanyi TG, Bredemeier H, Davis T: A CO_2 laser for surgical research. *Med Biol Eng* 8:541–548, 1970.

2. Vaughan CW, Homburger F, Shapshay S, et al: Carcinogenesis in the upper aerodigestive tract, *Otolaryngol Clin North Am* 13:405–412, 1980.

3. Strong MS, Vaughan CW, Jako G, et al: Transoral resection of cancer of the oral cavity: The role of the CO_2 laser. *Otolaryngol Clin North Am* 12:207–218, 1979.

4. Vaughan CW, Strong MS, Jako G: Laryngeal carcinoma: Transoral treatment utilizing the CO_2 laser. *Am J Surg* 136:490–493, 1978.

5. Lynch RC: Intrinsic carcinoma of the larynx with a second report of the cases operated on by suspension and dissection. *Trans Am Laryngol Assoc* 43:119–126, 1920.

6. New GU, Dorton HE: Suspension laryngoscopy and the treatment of malignant disease of the hypopharynx and larynx. *Mayo Clin Proc* 16:411–416, 1941.

7. Lillie J, De Santo L: Transoral surgery of early cordal carcinoma. *Trans Am Acad Ophthalmol Otolaryngol* 77:92–96, 1973.

16 Trachea and Bronchi

Albert H. Andrews, Jr., MS, MD
Steven F. Soltes, MD

Accuracy, reduced bleeding, immediate effect, minimal (adverse) reaction, and rapid healing are the advantages of surgery on the trachea and bronchi with the CO_2 laser. The first endoscopic delivery system for this purpose, attached to the articulated arm of the laser, was reported by Polanyi and his associates[1] and used by Jako[2] in animals. This endoscopic system was later modified to be used in conjunction with a standard ventilating bronchoscope.[3] This first adapter was bulky and heavy, and was followed in 1974 by a much smaller and lighter model of radically different design, well adapted for clinical work[4] (Figure 16-1). With the use of this coupler, suitable lesions within the lumen of the trachea or bronchus may be destroyed or removed by the CO_2 laser.

The principal problem with this apparatus is that precise aspiration of the trachea and bronchi requires disconnection of the coupler from the scope. A second problem is the time and effort required to shift from laryngeal application (micromanipulator) to tracheal or bronchial application (endoscopic coupler) and vice versa.

APPROACH TO THE TRACHEA

The upper trachea may sometimes be approached through the laryngoscope suspended in the conventional fashion. It is also possible at times to pass the bronchoscope through the suspended laryngoscope and thereby have access to the trachea. The tracheoscope may provide adequate exposure of the upper trachea; however, its small diameter and length make its use with the operating microscope practically impossible. The axial adapter, described by Andrews in 1976,[3] makes it possible to view the lumen of the tracheoscope with the axial adapter attached to the front of the micromanipulator (Figures 16-2, 16-3). The aiming light is still functional, but only one eye can be used. The lower trachea may be approached through a tracheotomy tract or a tracheostomy under local or general anesthesia through the bronchoscope or metal endotracheal tube. A nasal speculum of appropriate size and length may control a tracheostomy, so that good visualization and lasing are obtained. The micromanipulator and operating microscope are used in this application.

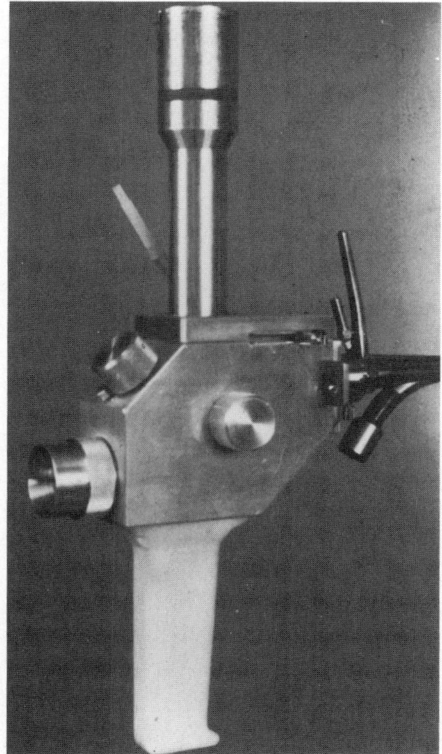

Figure 16-1 Bronchoscopic coupler attached to the articulated arm of the A0 model 200 laser.

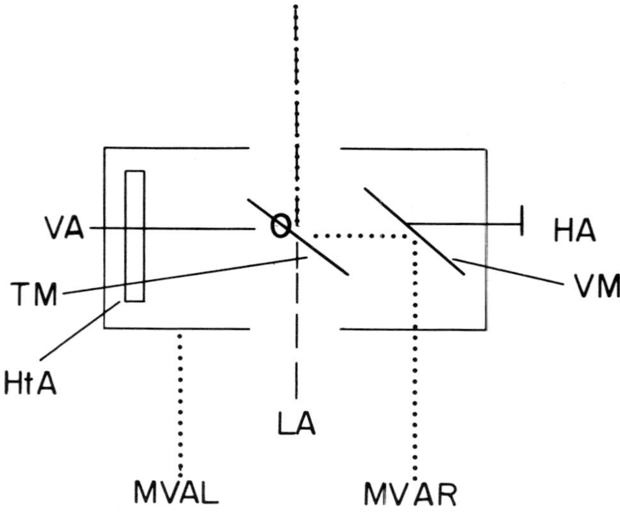

Figure 16-2 Diagram of axial adapter. MVAL: microscopic visual axis for left eye is blocked. MVAR: microscopic visual axis for right eye. Aiming light and area of burn are adjusted to coincide. LA: laser axis. TM: mirror for transmitting the laser beam and reflecting the visual beam. VA: adjustment of the aiming light in the vertical plane. HA: horizontal adjustment. HtA: heat absorber for the portion of the laser beam reflected by the TM.

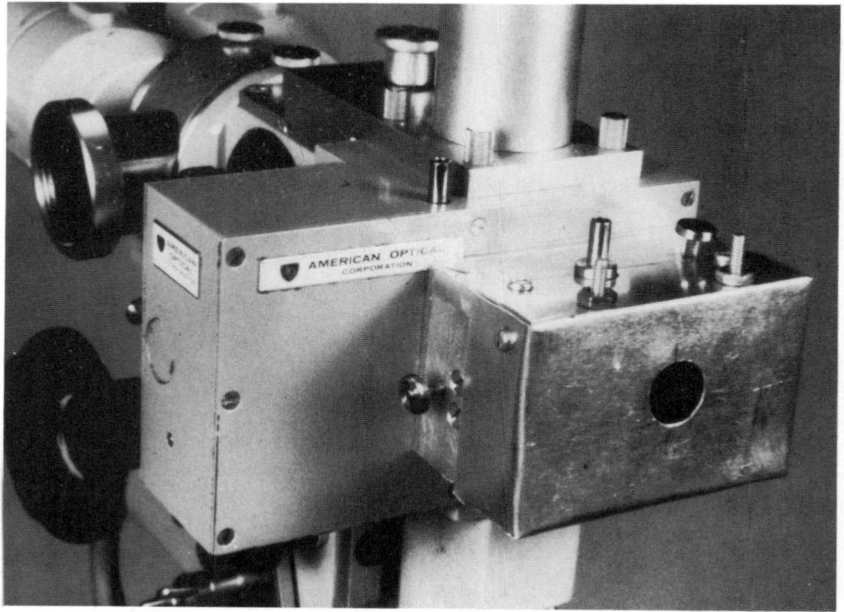

Figure 16-3 Axial adapter attached to the micromanipulator.

BRONCHOSCOPIC COUPLER

The bronchoscopic coupler (Figure 16-4) fulfills the following functions:

1. It enables the laser beam to have access to the bronchoscope.
2. It focuses the laser beam at the appropriate distance for the bronchoscope being used, usually 30 cm or 40 cm.
3. It attaches rigidly to the bronchoscope so that alignment can be maintained.
4. It seals the end of the bronchoscope so that controlled respiration can be given through the side arm of the bronchoscope, and also protects the interior of the coupler from being soiled by sputum.
5. It supplies vision on the axis of the bronchoscope.
6. It protects the surgeon's eye from the laser beam.
7. It can hold a 2X magnifier if needed.[4]

ANESTHESIA

General anesthesia is considered ideal for this purpose because it provides absolute stillness and tranquility of the patient. If the patient's dyspnea makes general anesthesia impossible, local anesthesia may be

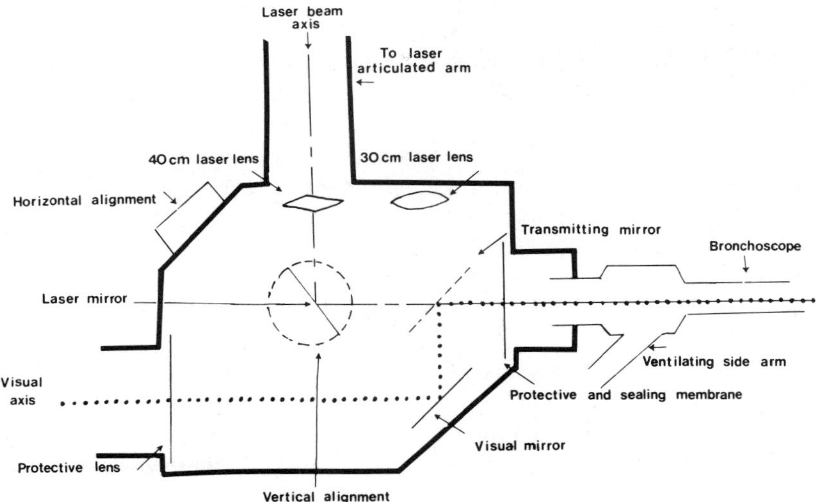

Figure 16-4 Diagram of bronchoscopic "coupler."

used. We prefer 2% tetracaine hydrochloride limited to 0.5 ml and 10% cocaine limited to 2 ml. If additional anesthesia is needed during a procedure, it may be applied by the bronchoscopic atomizer. If obstruction can be relieved by the procedure, anesthesia may be initiated locally and shifted to general anesthesia administered intravenously and through the side arm of the bronchoscope. Provided general anesthesia can be administered from the beginning, the bronchoscope can be introduced as soon as the pharyngeal and laryngeal reflexes are abolished. Anesthesia may then be given by the side arm of the bronchoscope with the window plug in place. When the bronchoscopic coupler is attached, it is still possible to continue controlled ventilation.

TECHNIQUE

Preparation

The appropriate diameter and length of bronchoscope are selected. The instrument is attached to the coupler in a fashion similar to that used when the bronchoscope is employed. Using the asbestos block, the alignment of the laser beam is checked vertically and horizontally, and the stops on the controls are adjusted so that the beam travel is limited to the lumen of the bronchoscope (Figures 16-5, 16-6). The bronchoscope is then sterilized.

Bronchoscopy

The bronchoscope is allowed to approach but not touch the lesion in the trachea or bronchus, thus lessening the likelihood of bleeding. Inspection is performed and a correlation is made between the bronchoscopic findings and those on the chest and tomographic x-rays. A biopsy may be taken, but this has usually been done previously; so it is not repeated and bleeding is thereby avoided. Aspiration of secretions is done very cautiously. The flexible bronchoscopic aspirators and velvet eye and open-end tubes may be used; the former is preferable.

Lasing Through the Bronchoscope

The window plug is removed from the bronchoscope and the coupler attached in a true and solid fashion. A test is made at relatively low power to be certain that the burn is as desired. It is frequently helpful to make appropriate marking burns at the junction of the normal mucosa and the

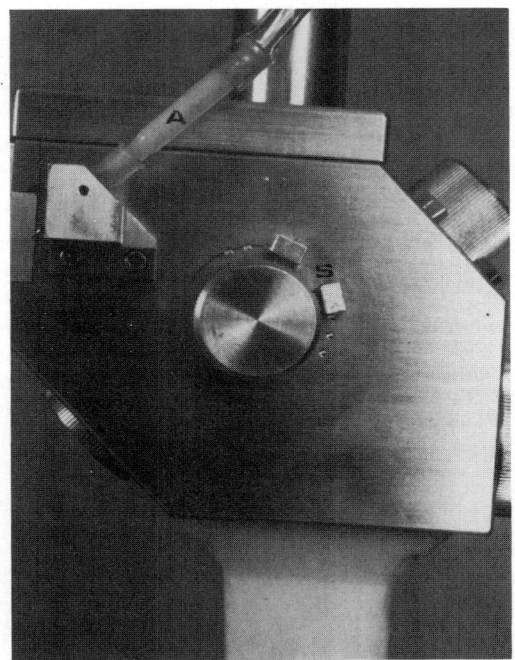

Figure 16-5 Bronchoscopic coupler, left side. A: air supply for cooling the membrane; S: stops for confining the beam to the lumen of the bronchoscope.

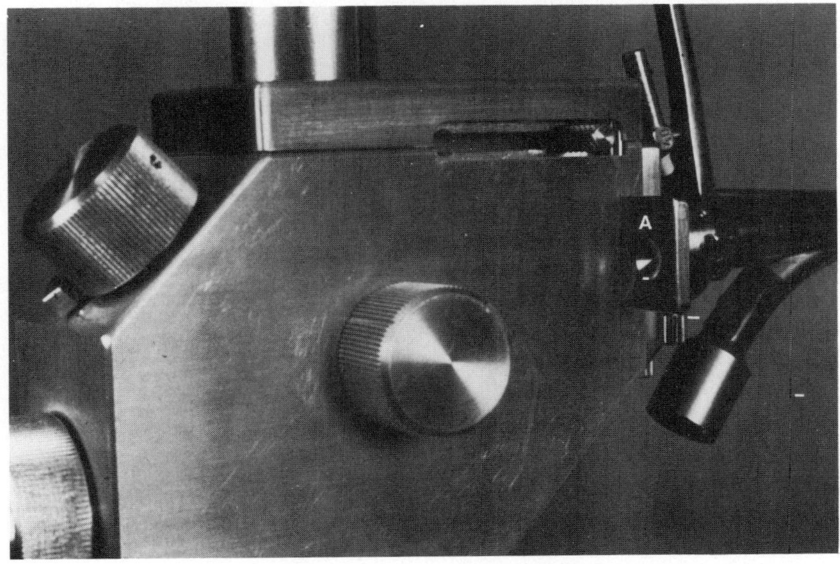

Figure 16-6 Bronchoscopic coupler, right side: A: holder for membrane which can be quickly changed during a procedure.

lesion. These can then serve as a landmark as the lasing proceeds. The lesion is vaporized rather than cut off, because the latter may result in the aspiration of fragments of removed tissue (Figures 16-7, 16-8).

The power and duration of exposure or manual mode are selected to fulfill the requirements of the individual patient. While it is probably advantageous to lase only during expiration so that the steam is blown away, this is somewhat impractical. Aspiration is done as required and can be used to remove the char. Lasing of the char is to be avoided because the char is oxidized tissue which can exceed the temperature of liquid water and may transmit more heat to the surrounding tissue. This is thought to increase the reaction to the lasing. Aspiration is kept to a minimum

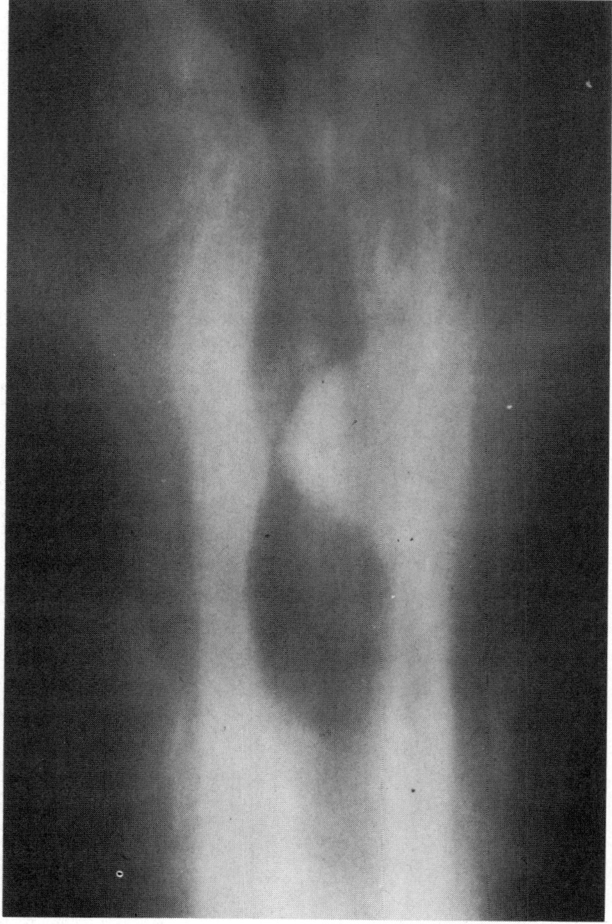

Figure 16-7 Intratracheal extension of carcinoma of left upper lobe following cobalt therapy; before lasing.

because it requires disconnection of the coupler and the insertion of the window plug except while aspiration is being done. A fine catheter can be passed through a side arm of the bronchoscope, but precise and rapid aspiration is not possible.

Protection of the mucosa beyond the area of burn is important. This requires that the surgeon know the status of the anatomy beyond the lesion. Tomography frequently supplies important information on this point. The bronchoscope may be angled to one side so that the beam does not go down the lumen. The beam may also be displaced to one side of the lumen of the bronchoscope in order to hit the lesion more adequately and avoid passage down the lumen. It is essential to recognize the importance of stopping the lasing before harm is done beyond the lesion.

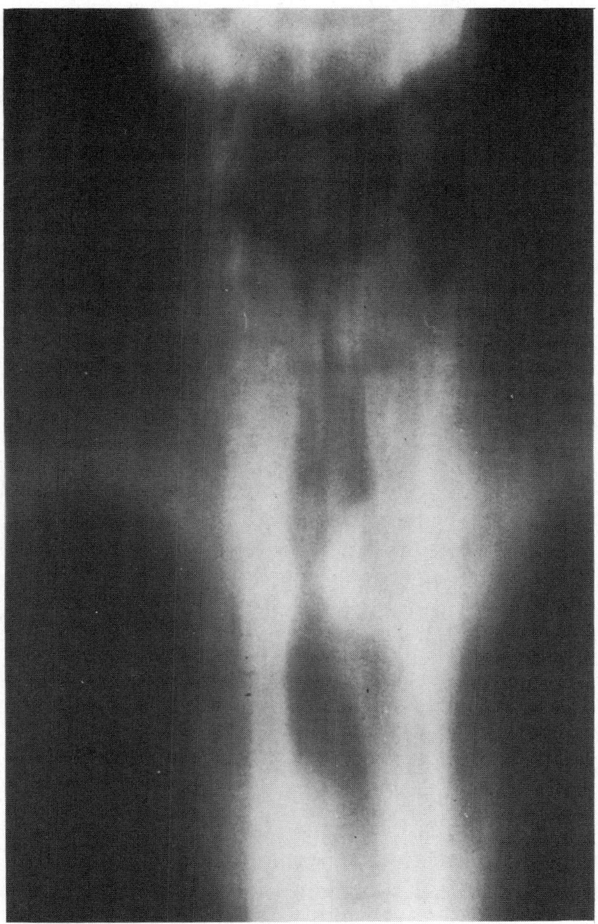

Figure 16-8 Same patient as Figure 16-7 after lasing.

PAPILLOMA OF TRACHEA AND BRONCHI

See Chapter 9.

GRANULOMA AND/OR FIBROSIS OF TRACHEA AND BRONCHI

Most of these conditions have been associated with oral-tracheal or nasal-tracheal intubation for respiratory control. The majority of granulomas resulting from this procedure can be cured by conventional bronchoscopy. Those that do not respond may be treated with the CO_2 laser, which is the ideal therapeutic approach to these sometimes severe problems. Care must be exercised not to lase through the tracheal or bronchial wall because of the likelihood of an air leak or mediastinitis. Repeated lasings may be required, but success can usually be achieved. Some patients may have loss of cartilaginous support. Two such patients have been successfully managed after relief of the granuloma by insertion of a T-tube as described by Montgomery.[5]

HEMANGIOMA

See Chapter 11.

CARCINOMA

Palliation of intraluminal extension[6] of these tumors is an important use of the CO_2 laser. The absence or reduction of bleeding is of great importance. Many patients are miserable because of dyspnea and coughing, and obtain relief following the lasing. There is usually recurrence of the dyspnea because the procedure is palliative rather than curative. Two fatalities have been associated with this procedure. One patient with carcinoma of the trachea had a tracheal resection followed by recurrence and intractable obstructive dyspnea. The tumor was lased away at the upper portion, but it was impossible to approach the lower obstruction. Adequate relief was not obtained and the patient died on the third postoperative day. The second patient had a carcinoma of the right main bronchus treated by radiation therapy with relief for three years. The CO_2 lasing was done because of dyspnea, and a good response was obtained. Three months later the dyspnea and cough recurred and another lasing was done. She died of cardiac arrest on the first postoperative day. Autopsy revealed the tracheal bronchial tree to be partially filled with mucopurulent secretions, the probable etiology of the cardiac arrest. This stresses the importance of vigorous aspiration of the tracheal bronchial tree.

Compression of the trachea or bronchus may result from growth of the extraluminal portion of the tumor. This, of course, cannot be lased away because mediastinitis would probably follow.

One patient with metastatic malignant melanoma of the trachea was successfully lased on two occasions. Previous bronchoscopies had been complicated by severe hemorrhage. He eventually died of pulmonary incompetence due to metastases to the lung, but without recurrence of the obstructive dyspnea.

GRANULAR CELL TUMOR

Two patients with this benign tumor (myoblastoma) have been treated with the CO_2 laser.[7] These bronchial tumors can cause atelectasis, pneumonitis, and excessive coughing. The symptoms were relieved after the lasing. One patient returned after two years because of symptoms of pneumonitis. Bronchoscopy revealed scarring at the sites of the first lasing, but no evidence of recurrence. A new tumor was present in the left lower lobe bronchus below the orifice of the superior segmental bronchus. This tumor was lased only partially because of the danger of involving the spur just below the nodule. Symptomatic relief followed the lasing.

SUMMARY

The CO_2 laser supplies technically easy access to the trachea and bronchi for the destruction of appropriate lesions. Absence of bleeding, accuracy, minimal reaction, and good visualization are the principal advantages of the CO_2 laser. These make the laser the instrument of choice for certain lesions of the trachea and major bronchi.

REFERENCES

1. Polanyi TG, Bredemeier HC, Davis TW Jr: A CO_2 laser for surgical research. *Med Biol Eng* 8:541–548, 1970.

2. Jako GJ: Laser surgery of the vocal cords. *Laryngoscope* 82:2204–2216, 1972.

3. Strong MS, Jako GJ, Polanyi TG, et al: Laser surgery in the aerodigestive tract. *Am J Surg* 126:529–533, 1973.

4. Strong MS, Vaughan CW, Polanyi TG, et al: Bronchoscopic CO_2 laser surgery. *Ann Otol Rhinol Laryngol* 83:769–776, 1974.

5. Andrews AH Jr, Bailey LL: Laser adapter for tracheoscopy. *Ann Otol Rhinol Laryngol* 87:625, 1976.

6. Andrews AH, Horowitz SL: Bronchoscopic CO_2 laser surgery. *Lasers Surg Med* 1:34–45, 1980.

7. Montgomery WW: Silicone tracheal T-tube. *Ann Otol Rhinol Laryngol* 83:71–75, 1974.

8. Laforet EG, Berger RL, Vaughan CW: Carcinoma obstructing the trachea: Treatment by resection. *N Engl J Med* 294:941, 1976.

9. Schwartzberg DG, Al-Bazzaz FJ, Cassel J, et al: Multiple granular cell tumors of the bronchi: Treatment with laser. *Am Rev Respir Dis* 120:193–196, 1979.

PART III
The CO_2 Laser in Gynecology

17 Cervix

Joseph H. Bellina, MD, PhD, FACOG

The laser is gaining in acceptance as a surgical tool by surgeons in all disciplines. As this energy transfer system is explored and tested, its potential applications in medicine become increasingly apparent. In gynecology the laser is being used with much success by colposcopists in the management of neoplastic disease of the cervix, vagina, and vulva.

Tissue ablation is accomplished both through excision and vaporization procedures. The several advantages of this modality over conventional surgery and cryotherapy include: 1) complete destruction and removal of the neoplastic process by vaporization of diseased cells; 2) precision of application; 3) an unobstructed operating field; 4) cauterization and coagulation of smaller vascular channels, thereby preventing bleeding; 5) minimal damage to adjacent normal tissue with reduced postoperative sequelae; 6) minimal operative side effects and postoperative complications; and 7) preservation of the reproductive, anatomic, and sexual integrity of the patient. Most importantly, laser therapy has been shown by several investigators to result in the highest success rates of all conservative management alternatives in certain lesions.[1-3]

INSTRUMENTATION

For application in lesions of the cervix, vagina, vulva, perineum, anus, and other selected sites, the CO_2 laser is coupled to an operating microscope or colposcope. In this way the operating field can be viewed with suitable magnification and the laser beam appropriately directed. Through "joystick" control via a micromanipulator, the helium-neon finder beam and the optically combined invisible laser beam are positioned to impinge upon the target site (Figure 17-1).

A standard electronic cabinet contains the gas supply, power packs, recirculating water-cooling source, operating controls, and safety interlocks. The laser head attached to the colposcope contains all the

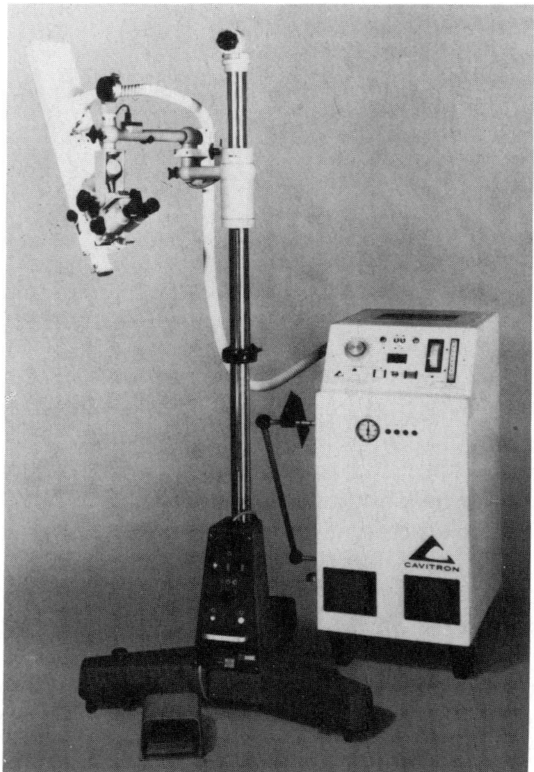

Figure 17-1 Surgical CO_2 laser used in gynecology.

elements necessary for laser action. A flexible "umbilical cord" carries gas, water, and electric current to the laser. A separate foot pedal controls the shutter mechanism, either in continuous or intermittent mode. When not in use, the beam is deflected into a heat sink by a reflective shutter. During application the beam is directed through any of several laser lenses ranging in focal length from 50 mm to 400 mm. These lenses and their resultant beam spot sizes, coupled with power settings from 0 to 100 watts, determine the power density delivered at impact, expressed in watts per square centimeter (W/cm^2).

BIOLOGICAL EFFECTS

Basically, CO_2 laser irradiation has a wavelength of 10.6 μ and is strongly absorbed by water so that the energy vaporizes and/or incises by heating the impacted tissue. Intra- and extracellular water boils and expands, causing cell disruption, and some particles which are blown free of the site are further carbonized by the beam. Thermal energy produces a crater-like lesion. Ninety percent of the incident laser energy is absorbed within an area 0.1 mm beyond the lased tissue; thus, very little tissue necrosis results from laser impact. Minimal continuous tissue damage facilitates healing and accounts for reduced scarring. Additionally, the impact tissue is concurrently sterilized and small blood vessels are sealed, resulting in hemostasis.

CLINICAL APPLICATIONS

General Principles

The CO_2 laser in the hands of an experienced colposcopist trained in the biophysics and gynecologic applications of the instrument, can vaporize or excise diseased tissue with a precision heretofore unavailable. Its effectiveness continues to be documented; however, careful patient selection, diagnostic accuracy, and appropriate instrument utilization is mandatory. Courses in gynecology laser surgery offer such training and supervised applications. Reading a text such as this cannot substitute for the type of training recommended for gynecologists who intend to use the CO_2 laser. However, some basic principles can be described here.

Laser therapy should be considered for patients with neoplastic lesions of the cervix, vagina, and vulva, after diagnosis by cytologic, colposcopic, and histopathologic procedures. All of these diagnostic methods must rule out microinvasive or invasive carcinoma. As with other conservative procedures, only those patients who will cooperate in the postoperative follow-up regimen should be treated with laser therapy.

Patients with lesions whose borders cannot be colposcopically identified should never be lased.

When conservative management is desirable for preservation of anatomic, sexual, and/or reproductive integrity, when surgery is contraindicated, and when correlation between diagnoses is established, laser therapy can be performed.

Cervix

The cervix is covered by squamous and columnar epithelium. The zone of transition or transformation between the two cell types is the site of potential neoplastic development. After abnormal cytology has been detected, colposcopically directed biopsies should be taken to confirm the condition. When conservative management is elected, laser therapy is the method of choice.

Intraepithelial cervical neoplasia, grades I to III, can be effectively treated with the CO_2 laser. Although other forms of treatment for cervical neoplasia have been and continue to be employed, each has its significant disadvantages. The cold-knife conization procedure requires hospitalization for one to three days, as well as the administration of a general anesthetic. Postoperative sequelae of hemorrhage, cervical incompetency, and cervical stenosis can occur. Although the residual tumor rate for this procedure is reported to range from 1% to 13%, the potential for severe complications cannot be ignored.[4] The risk factor of general anesthesia must also be considered.

Hot cauterization, to be effective, requires deep cauterization, also

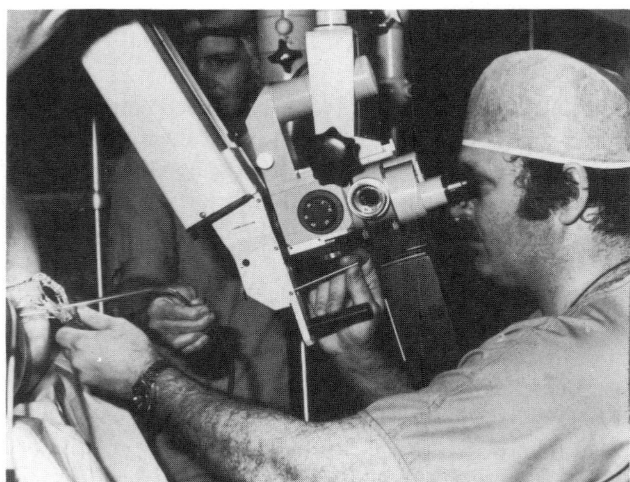

Figure 17-2 Instrumentation and configuration for laser removal of cervical lesion.

under general anesthesia. Postoperative sequelae are similar to those of cold-knife conization treatment. The residual tumor rate is reported to range from 2% to 60%.[5-8]

Cryosurgery has the advantage of not usually requiring a general anesthesic, but residual tumor rates are high, 12% to 48%.[9-11] Furthermore, the depth of the freezing is limited and difficult to monitor. Postoperative sequelae include cervical stenosis, heavy vaginal discharge, occasional hemorrhage, and the possibility of undetected residual disease manifesting itself as invasive carcinoma.

Tissue healing and repair with CO_2 laser surgery are superior to that observed with other destructive modalities. The epithelium is replaced with minimal scar formation and without cervical stenosis. Clinical observations also include low persistence rates, low treatment complication rates, superior tissue repair, and reduced healing time.[12]

METHOD OF APPLICATION

Patients are placed in the dorsal lithotomy position and encouraged to relax. Usually no anesthetic or analgesic is required. A nonflammable plastic or blackened speculum is introduced and the cervix exposed. A 3% solution of acetic acid can be applied to the cervix to clear any mucus and also to aid in reassessment of the lesion. The colposcope and laser head are positioned by the surgeon and the target site is identified (Figure 17-2). The colposcope is focused and the helium-neon finder beam is positioned (Figure 17-3). Vacuum tubes for elimination of smoke and steam can be

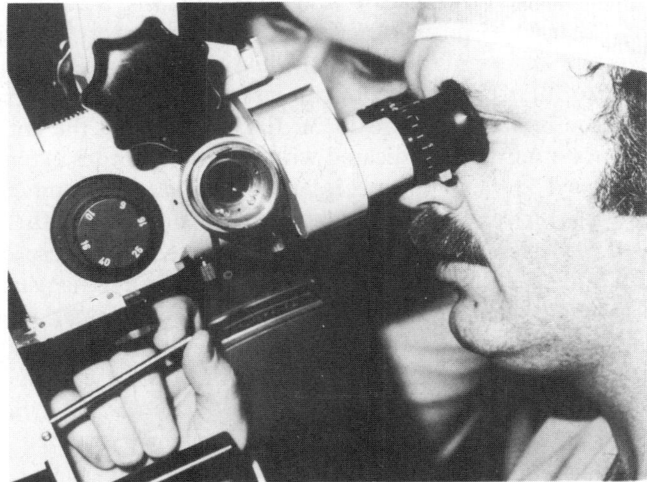

Figure 17-3 Close-up of instrumentation showing micromanipulator joystick beam control.

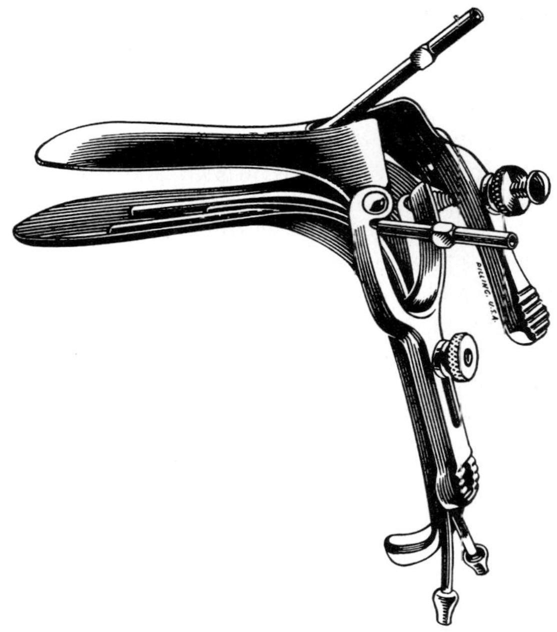

Figure 17-4 Speculum for CO_2 laser surgery with fiberoptic cables for illumination and tube for plume aspiration.

attached to the speculum (Figure 17-4) or hand-held by the surgeon or an assistant.

Then, in a continuous mode, with moderate power densities (500 to 700 W/cm^2 [BP15-35W]) contributing to hemostasis, a 2-mm spot-sized laser beam is used to outline the lesion(s) is directed in the x-, y-, and z-axes over the surface of the lesion(s). This method insures adequate and equal depth of destruction. Depth can be measured with a microruler to confirm tissue removal (Figure 17-5). Each lesion and the entire transformation zone must be eradicated with adequate border extension to a depth of at least 5 mm. This is necessary to eliminate aberrant cells which may reside in cervical crypts and glands existing at this depth.

When the lesion(s) has (have) been eliminated, the microscope with laser head and speculum are withdrawn. Since bleeding is usually not a problem, vaginal packing or dressings are applied. The patient can then be discharged with appropriate postoperative and follow-up instructions. These usually include prohibition of coitus for three days to three weeks, and caution against the use of tampons or douches. Some gynecologists recommend the use of a condom when intercourse is resumed.

Excisional conization can also be performed with the CO_2 laser for CIN lesions with endocervical extension. This method was developed and perfected by Dorsey and is accomplished via laser microsurgery in a fashion similar to vaporization procedures. Extremely high power density (over 1000 W/cm^2 [BP30W]) incisions result in tissue suitable for histopathologic examination. Since these power densities do not result in hemostasis, excisional conizations require administration of vasopressin and lateral cervical sutures. After removal of the cone, the power density can be dropped and the cone bed coagulated to reduce bleeding and the possibility of late postoperative hemorrhage.

The advantages of the laser procedure include less bleeding, both immediate and delayed, than with the scalpel; less necrosis than with the electrocautery; self-sterilization of the wound; reduced postoperative possibility of cervical stenosis; little postoperative pain;[13] elimination of the transformation zone; and the maintenance of the squamocolumnar junction which remains colposcopically visible postoperatively. The cure rate with this technique is approximately 98% when the pathologist confirms that cone margins are free of disease.

THE LASER LESION IN CERVICAL TISSUE

Tissue damage from CO_2 laser results from the transfer of energy, specifically heat, into the impacted tissue. Damage ranges from injury due to thermal conduction, to cell necrosis, to vaporization and expulsion of cellular debris from the impact site.[14] In cervical tissue the zone of injury is exceptionally small, estimated to be less than 100 μ from the crater rim.[15] The area of vaporization is actually a shallow crater, deeper at the

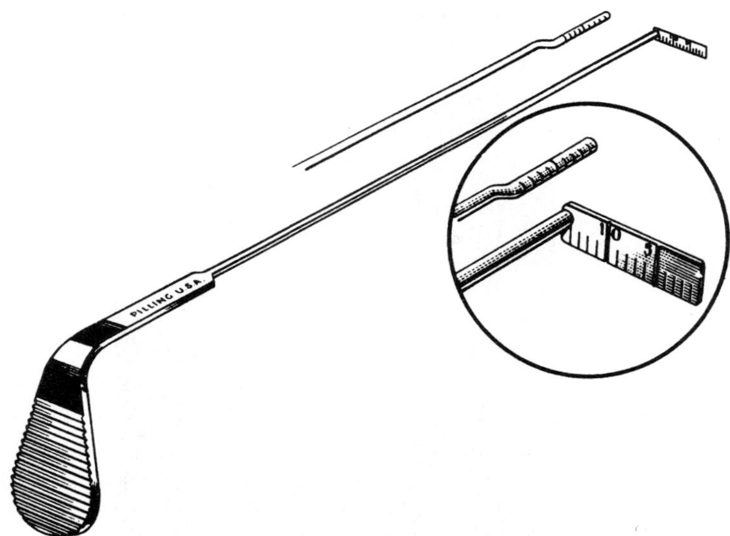

Figure 17-5 Microrulers for measuring depth and width of laser destruction.

center with tapering side walls. This can be demonstrated by scanning electronic microscope (SEM) analysis; the pattern is shown in Figure 17-6a, b, c. Internal portions of the crater contain no epithelial elements. The sides exhibit charring and the rims are slightly elevated. Adjacent tissue shows loss of architecture and coagulation necrosis. It is in this area that hemostasis can be demonstrated. Finally, thermal injury may be observed beyond the area of necrosis.

Absorption of laser energy and resultant tissue damage depend upon the water content of the impacted cells. Superficial squamous cells have relatively low water content. The deeper, intermediate parabasal, basal, and stroma cells have progressively higher water content. Therefore, tissue removal is greatest for any given power density in the superficial layer and rapidly diminishes as stromal layers are approached. Because energy is rapidly dissipated in these higher water content cells, adjacent tissue necrosis is minimal or absent.

HEALING

Few macrocytes and fibroblasts are present during the healing phase. The fibroblast, by depositing collagen, contributes to scar formation.

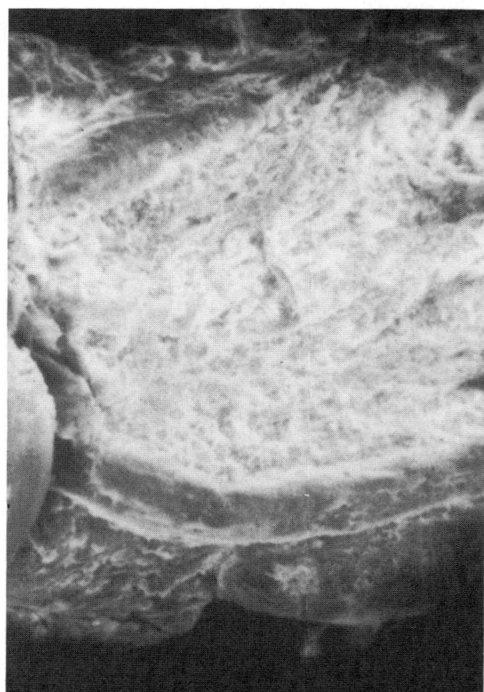

A

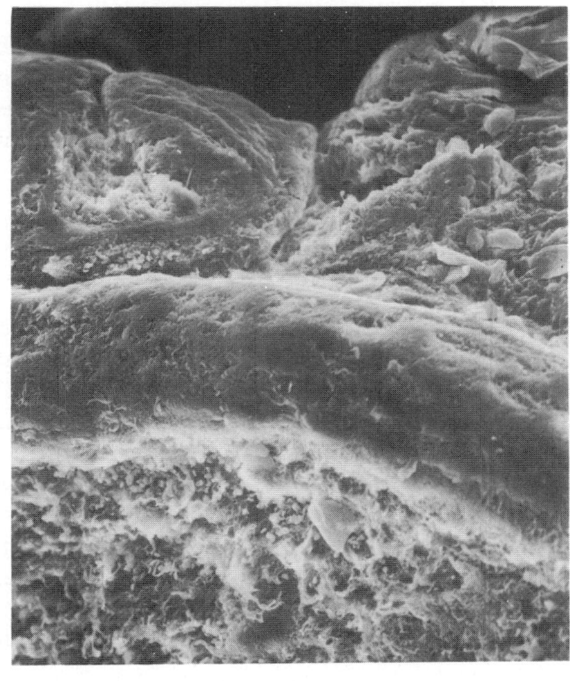

B

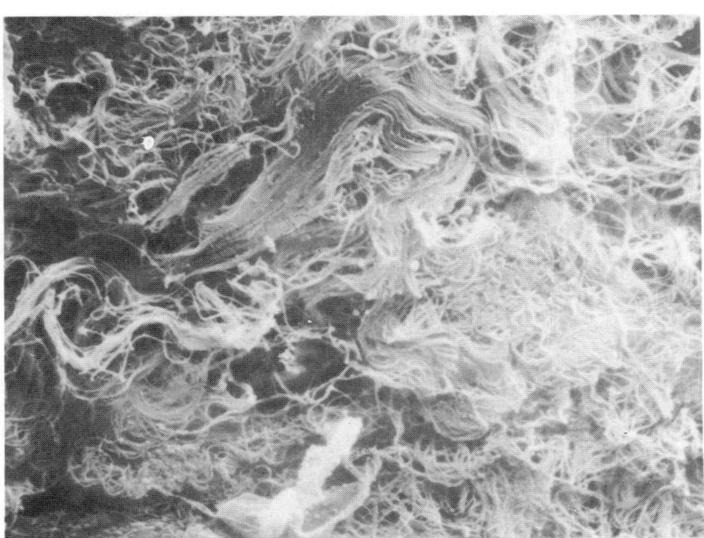

C

Figure 17-6 Laser lesion showing **A)** crater shape, **B)** crater rim, and **C)** absence of epithelial elements in the internal cavity. (Reproduced with permission from Bellina JH, Seto YJ: Pathological and physical investigations into CO_2 laser-tissue interactions with specific emphasis on cervical intraepithelial neoplasm. *Lasers in Surg and Med* 1:47–69, 1980.)

Also, certain proteins, notably alpha-2-macroglobulins, can prevent the enzyme collagenase from removing excess collagen. This leads to intense scar and synechiae formation. However, as the application of CO_2 laser energy to tumor cells creates minimal adjacent tissue necrosis, a lessened repair phase ensues. This may account for the minimal scar formation and rapid healing time observed clinically.

CYTOLOGIC DOCUMENTATION

Cytologic specimens obtained daily on patients demonstrate healing from the day of treatment to the 21st day. The cytologic pattern immediately after treatment reveals elongated columnar epithelial cells of the endocervix, closely resembling fibrocytes (Figure 17-7). Changes appear to be due to thermal coagulation with lengthwise destruction of the stromal cells. Epithelial cells are absent and only carbon residue remains.

A large number of acute inflammatory cells are seen on the day after treatment (Figure 17-8). However, by the 7th to the 9th day, this reaction subsides, and many multinucleated epithelioid cells can be noted (Figure 17-9). The appearance of giant cells heralds the rapid squamous cell replacement phase. By the 21st day, the cytologic smear returns to normal (Figure 17-10).

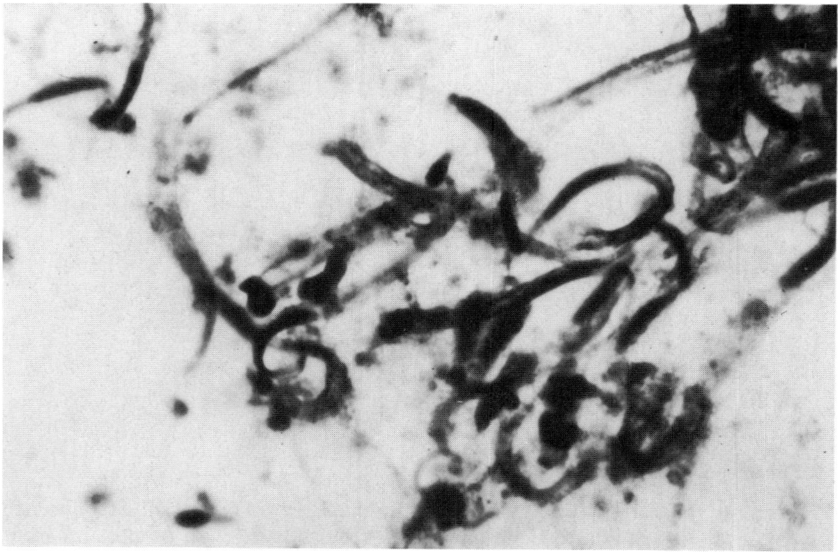

Figure 17-7 Cytology: post-laser day 0. The cells are stromal in origin, elongated for desiccation. Epithelial squamous cells are absent.

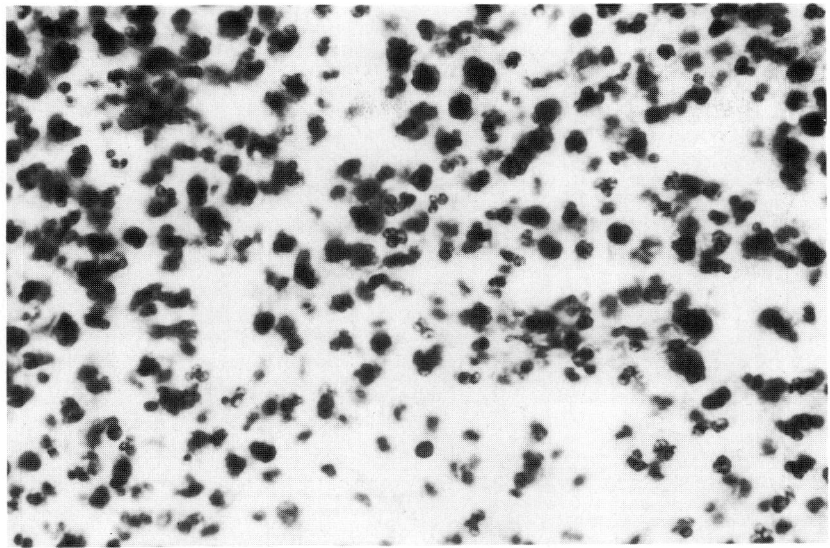

Figure 17-8 Cytology: post-laser day 1. Inflammatory cells predominate the smear.

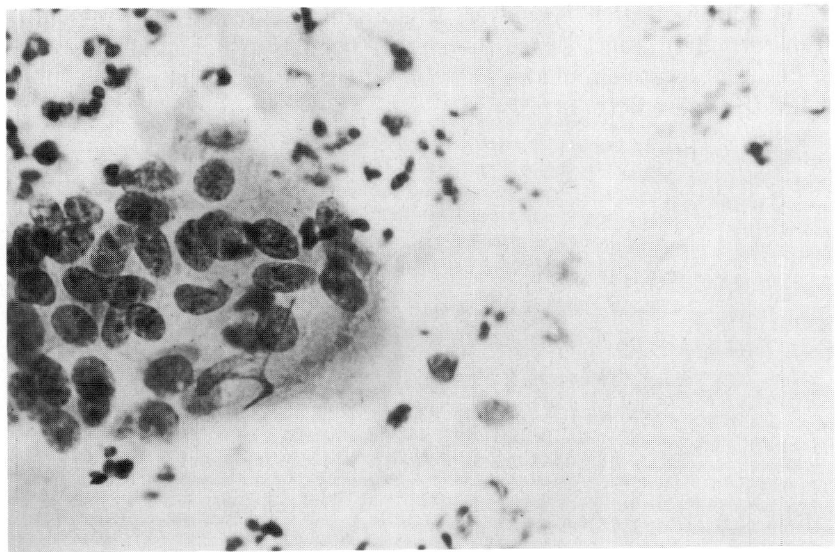

Figure 17-9 Cytology: post-laser days 7–9. Multinucleated giant epithelioid cells are noted. Inflammatory cell response is minimal.

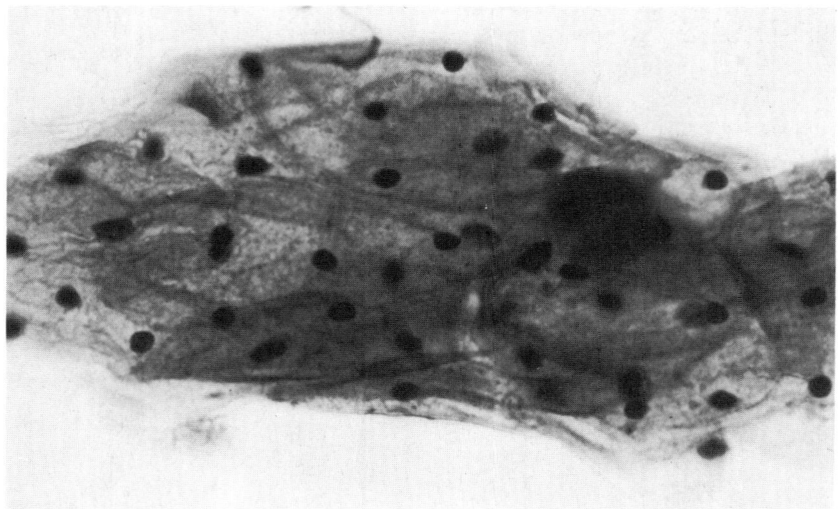

Figure 17-10 Cytology: post-laser 21. Normal superficial squamous cells are noted.

COLPOSCOPIC FINDINGS

The colposcopic appearance of the laser wound is shown in Figure 17-11. Carbonization is evident. It is important to note that the entire transformation zone, hence the site of neoplastic potential, has been eradicated. Depth should be uniform, at least 5 mm. Figure 17-12 illustrates the lesion before treatment.

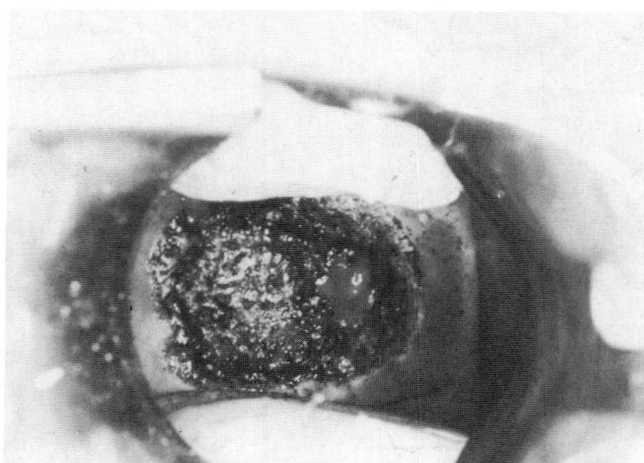

Figure 17-11 Cervical lesion during laser vaporization. (Reproduced with permission from Bellina JH, Voros JI and Riopelle MA: Cervical intraepithelial neoplasma in the reproductive female. *J La State Med Soc* 133:1–5, 1981.)

Following surgery, rapid healing commences (Figure 17-13). By day three, regenerating squamous epithelium begins to fill the vaporized cavity. Specks of carbonized cellular debris from the crater surface can still be seen. By day 17, new epithelium completely fills the cavity. Within three weeks most lesions are completely healed. Figure 17-14 shows the cervix 16 months after laser surgery.

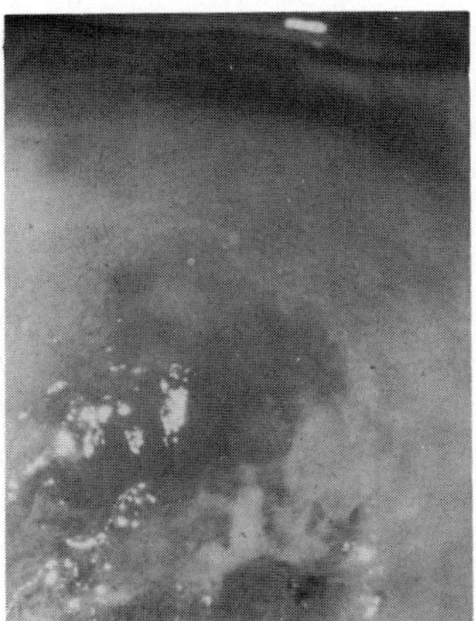

Figure 17-12 Cervical lesion—pre-laser, moderate cervical dysplasia with condyloma acuminata. (Reproduced with permission from Bellina JH, Voros JI and Riopelle MA: Cervical intraepithelial neoplasma in the reproductive female. *J La State Med Soc* 133:1–5, 1981.)

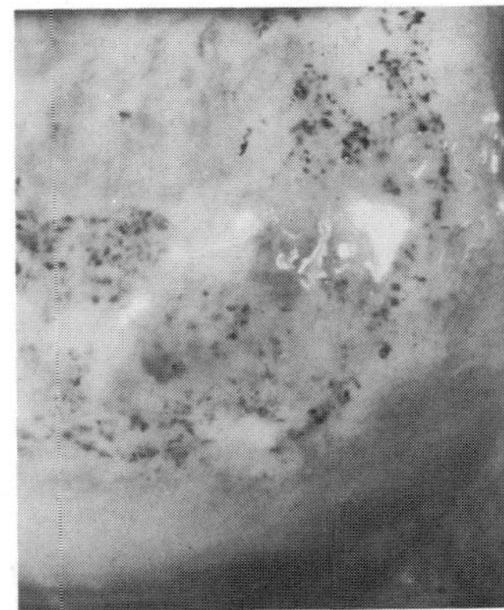

Figure 17-13

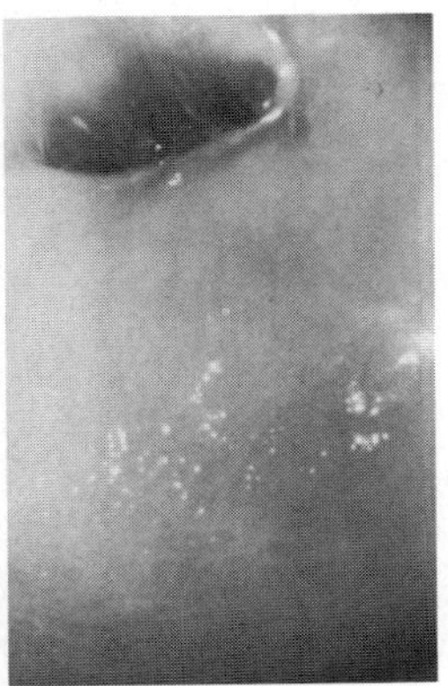

Figure 17-14

Figure 17-13 Laser lesion, postoperative day 3, showing regenerating epithelium and some remaining carbonization.

Figure 17-14 Cervix at 10 months. (Reproduced with permission from Bellina JH, Voros JI and Riopelle MA: Cervical intraepithelial neoplasma in the reproductive female. *J La State Med Soc* 133:1–5, 1981.)

Histologic Documentation

Histologic samples obtained on the day of treatment, the tenth day after treatment, and the 21st day after treatment with a Jako microlaryngeal biopsy forceps also document healing patterns. The histological pattern immediately after treatment reveals a total absence of epithelium (Figure 17-15). The lateral demarcation of tissue removal is sharp and perpendicular to the basal cell layer; adjacent normal epithelium remains undisturbed (Figure 17-15a). Occasionally, a small carbon residue is noted at the bottom of the shallow crater formed by the laser impact. Thermal injury can be observed for an additional 50 to 100 μ, which terminates abruptly in a plane contiguous to the stroma (Figure 17-15b).

The histologic pattern on the tenth day is one of normal reepithelialization (Figure 17-16). Along the surface of the new epithelium multinucleated giant cells are seen. Cellular maturation, polarity, and cytoplasmic-nuclear ratios are remarkably normal. However, this epithelium can be easily detached from the stroma.

Mature squamous epithelium is noted on the 21st day (Figure 17-17). The cellular polarity, maturation, and cytoplasmic-nuclear ratios are normal. There is usually an absence of inflammatory cells in the adjacent stroma. Tensile strength of this new tissue appears to be normal.

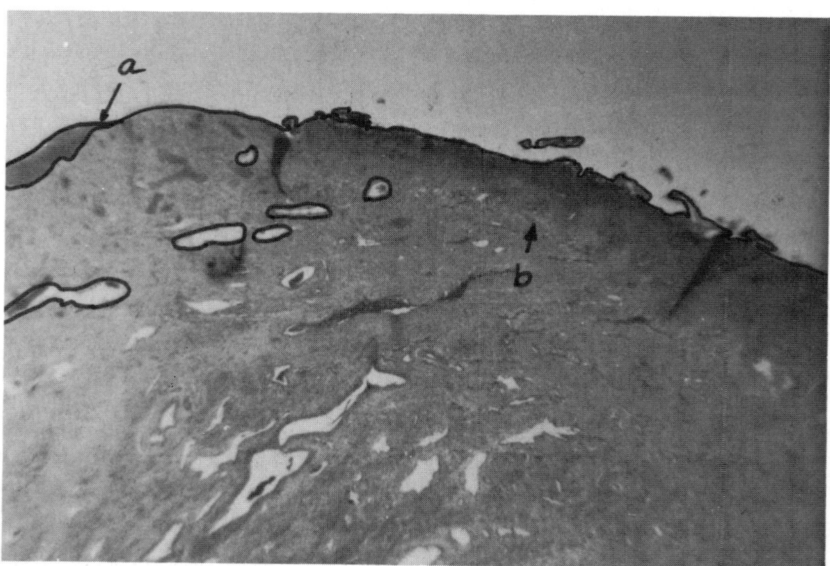

Figure 17-15 Histology: post-laser day 0; (a) normal epithelium junction; (b) thermal damage is limited to 50 to 100 μ. (Reproduced with permission from Bellina JH, Seto YJ: Pathological and physical investigations into CO_2 laser-tissue interactions with specific emphasis on cervical intraepithelial neoplasm. *Lasers in Surg and Med* 1:47–69, 1980.)

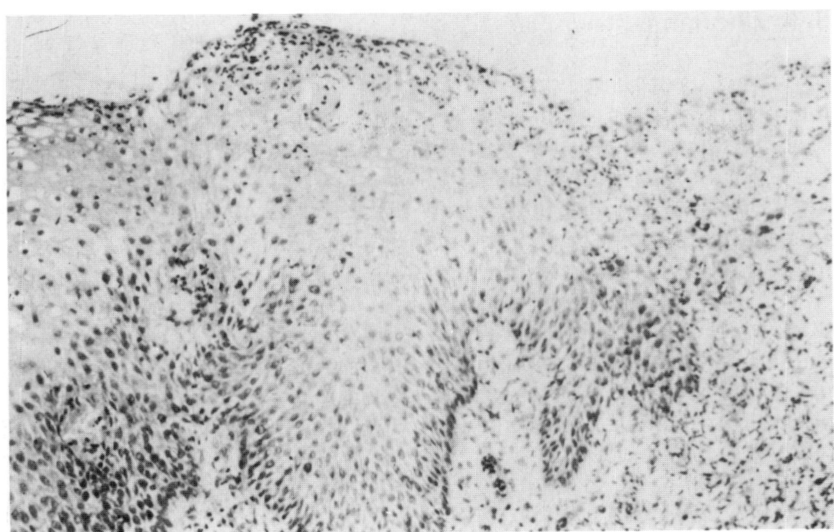

Figure 17-16 Histology: post-laser day 10. Normal maturation of epithelium. Minimal inflammatory response. (Reproduced with permission from Bellina JH, Seto YJ: Pathological and physical investigations into CO_2 laser-tissue interactions with specific emphasis on cervical intraepithelial neoplasm. *Lasers in Surg and Med* 1:47–69, 1980.)

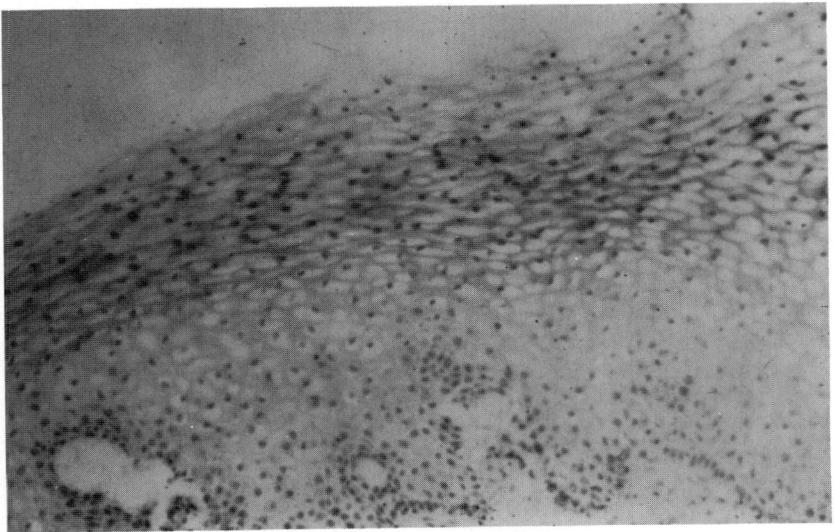

Figure 17-17 Normal mature epithelium, day 21. (Reproduced with permission from Bellina JH, Seto YJ: Pathological and physical investigations into CO_2 laser-tissue interactions with specific emphasis on cervical intraepithelial neoplasm. *Lasers in Surg and Med* 1:47–69, 1980.)

SEM Documentation

Analysis of samples obtained on the 10th day by scanning electronic microscope reveals a remarkably intact surface epithelium. Large, flat squamous epithelium with microridge formation and early intercellular bar formations are noted (Figure 17-18). Microvilli are seen in 30% of the scanned cells. The epithelium again reveals poor cohesiveness, and large tissue plaques can be seen. The plaques were avulsed during preparation, indicating low tensile strength.

On the 21st day after treatment the surface topography appears normal. Mature epithelial cells with well-defined microridges, prominent cellular bar formation, scant microvilli and small nuclear convexities are noted throughout the surfaces studied (Figure 17-19). The tensile strength appears normal, as free plaque formation is not seen.

OTHER CERVICAL LESIONS

The CO_2 laser has been used with similar success in eliminating various other cervical lesions. These have included condyloma acuminata, chronic cervicitis, cervicovaginal adenosis, ectopy, and cervical polyps. The hemostasis afforded with the laser permits successful removal of a large (5 cm × 7 cm) cervical capillary hemangioma encompassing the upper portion of the cervix in a 16-year-old girl, with a lesser

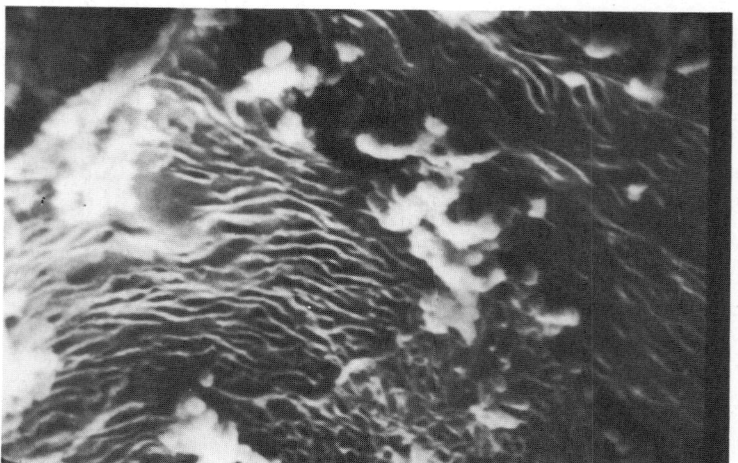

Figure 17-18 SEM: epithelial regeneration post-laser day 10. Metaplastic epithelium is present. (Reproduced with permission from Bellina JH, Seto YJ: Pathological and physical investigations into CO_2 laser-tissue interactions with specific emphasis on cervical intraepithelial neoplasm. *Lasers in Surg and Med* 1:47–69, 1980.)

(2 cm × 2 cm) lesion on the lower portion (Figure 17-20). Using low power densities (100–150 W/cm² [BP3–6.5W]), the large lesion was vaporized from the peripheral border inward. When the remaining central portion of the tumor mass was reduced to 1 cm × 3 cm, the mass was excised with a cold knife and sutures were placed, occluding the arterial sources. The posterior cervical lesion was not removed at this time. Blood loss was estimated to be 150 ml, which compares favorably to the four units of blood which were required at biopsy despite prednisone administration, sutures, and vaginal packs.

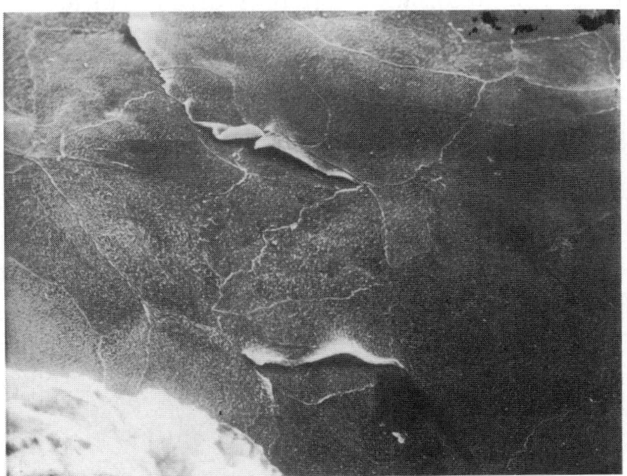

Figure 17-19 SEM: epithelial regeneration post-laser day 21. Normal, mature epithelium is present. (Reproduced with permission from Bellina JH, Seto YJ: Pathological and physical investigations into CO_2 laser-tissue interactions with specific emphasis on cervical intraepithelial neoplasm. *Lasers in Surg and Med* 1:47–69, 1980.)

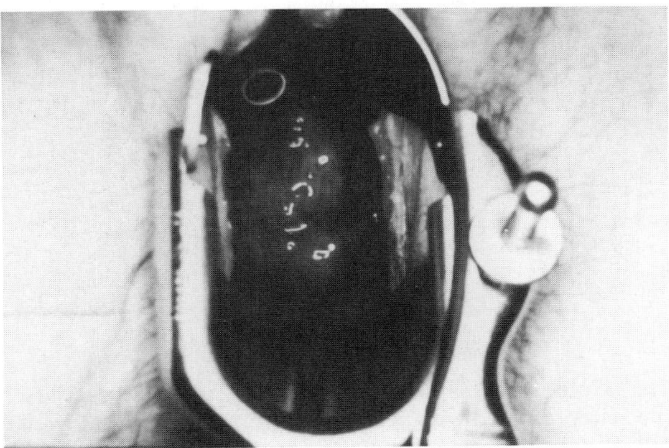

Figure 17-20 Gross appearance of capillary hemangioma lesion.

On day 21, the posterior lip bled, requiring sutures. The anterior lip healed without complications. At six months postoperatively, the patient was reevaluated. A small area of residual tumor in the anterior portion was removed. No bleeding occurred. Recovery was uneventful; healing was complete by the fourth week. The patient has had no apparent genital dysfunction 1.5 years after treatment (Figure 17-21).

This case can be used to demonstrate the remarkable hemostatic properties of the CO_2 laser. Prior to the availability of this instrument, such a lesion would have required surgical excision, cauterization or perhaps hysterectomy, compromising the fertility of the patient. The laser can remove such large cervical lesions with minimal blood loss, while preserving structural and physiological integrity of this reproductive organ.

COMPLICATIONS

Complications pre- and postoperatively can occur, although they are rare. These include pain, delayed bleeding requiring vaginal packs, and suture, with or without hospitalization, as well as vaginal discharge. No impairment of reproductive capability or other ill effects have been reported.

FOLLOW-UP OF PATIENTS WITH CERVICAL LESIONS

Consistent follow-up of patients with cervical lesions is mandatory in order to detect persistent or new lesions. This is particularly important in

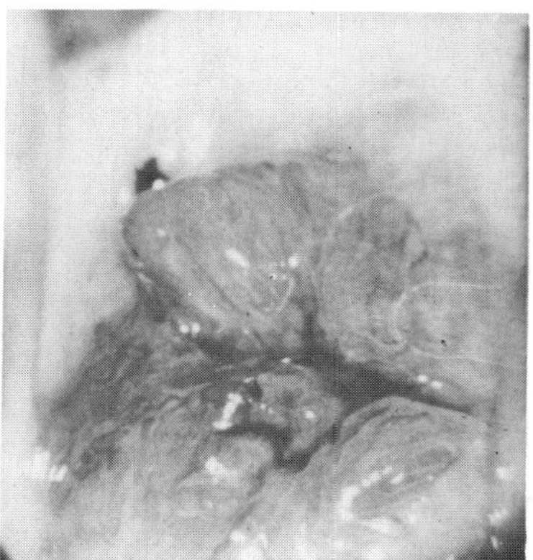

Figure 17-21 Colposcopic appearance of the cervix 1.5 years after removal of hemangiomas. (Reproduced with permission from Bellina JH, Gyer DR, Voros JI, et al: Capillary hemangioma managed by the CO_2 laser. *Obstet Gynecol* 55:128–131, 1980.)

intraepithelial cervical neoplasia because of the potential for this lesion to progress, if undisturbed, to invasive cervical carcinoma. Although rare, lesions do reappear. This may be expected to occur in approximately 4% to 6% of cases following adequate lesion destruction. Recurrence (persistent disease or new disease) is a function of the adequacy of tissue removal both in depth and lateral extent, and reinfection, eg, condyloma acuminata. Patients who are informed of the venereal nature of their disease can take steps to prevent reinfection by arranging for treatment of the consort, by using barrier methods of contraception, and/or by using spermatocides which destroy DNA.

The follow-up requirements vary with the gynecologist, but usually entail a postoperative visit at two to six weeks for evaluation of healing. During the first year the patient should be evaluated cytologically and colposcopically every three months. Persistent disease can be identified and retreated. After the first year, patients must be followed cytologically every six months, perhaps for life, until further study proves this to be unnecessary.

OTHER GYNECOLOGIC APPLICATIONS OF THE CO_2 LASER

The laser is currently being used to vaporize recurrent tumors as well as to treat the lesions described above. Several investigators contemplate utilization of high-power CO_2 lasers in removal of abdominal gynecologic malignancies. Recently, the laser has been employed in microsurgical reconstruction of Fallopian tubes for restoration of fertility.[15] When the laser is finally coupled to fiberoptic cables, many other lesions and sites will be able to be treated.

As is being experienced in many other surgical specialties, laser applications in gynecology appear to be increasing. This new surgical modality, with its hemostatic capability and precision of application, will increase the surgical capabilities of gynecologic surgeons.

ACKNOWLEDGMENTS

The author wishes to express his appreciation to the following individuals for their contribution to this chapter: Mary Ann Riopelle for her photographs and significant editorial assistance; Dr Jerome Kurpel for his assistance in the SEM analysis; V. Bewig, Jr., for photographic printing and Hazel Domingue and Donna Yost for their preparation of the copy.

REFERENCES

1. Bellina JH: Laser microsurgery in gynecology, *Intern Advances Surg Oncol* 1:227–236, 1978.

2. Wright VC: Observations regarding patients diagnosed with cervical intraepithelial neoplasia: The use of cryosurgery and the CO_2 laser, in Bellina JH et al (eds): *Gynecologic Laser Surgery.* New York, Plenum Press, in Press.

3. Popkin DR: The carbon dioxide laser in the treatment of cervical Intraepithelial neoplasia—Preliminary report, in Bellina JH et al (eds): *Gynecologic Laser Surgery.* New York, Plenum Press, in Press.

4. Holzer E: Behandlungsergebnisse bei Carcinoma in situ und frühinvasiven Stadien des Lervix Karzinoms an der, Universitats—Frauenklinik Graz von 1958 bis 1973. *Wien Med Wochenschr* 127:534–536, 1977.

5. Beard RW: Diathermy coning and cautery in the treatment of the eroded cervix. *J Obstet Gynecol Br Commun* 71:287–292, 1964.

6. Behney CA: Treatment of endocervicitis by cauterization. *Surg Clin North Am* 6:109–111, 1926.

7. Masson JC, Parson E: Cystic cervicitis, with special reference to treatment by cauterization: Clinical study of 1031 cases. *Am J Obstet Gynecol* 16:348–358, 1928.

8. Peyton FW, Rosen NA: Cervical cauterization and carcinoma of the cervix: Long-term study from a private gynecologic practice. *Am J Obstet Gynecol* 86:111–119, 1963.

9. Collins RJ, Pappas HJ: Cryosurgery for benign cervicitis with follow-up of six-and one-half years. *Am J Obstet Gynecol* 113:744–750, 1972.

10. Creaseman WT, Weed JC, Curry SL, et al: Efficiency of cryosurgery of severe introepitheliar neoplasia. *Obstet Gynecol* 41:501–506, 1973.

11. Jordan JA: The diagnosis and management of premalignant diseases of the cervix. *Clin Obstet Gynecol* 3(2):295–315, 1976.

12. Bellina JH, Seto YJ: Pathological and physical investigations into CO_2 laser-tissue interactions with specific emphasis on cervical intraepithelial neoplasm. *Lasers in Surg and Med* 1:47–69, 1980.

13. Dorsey JH: Cervical conization by the carbon dioxide laser. *The Pelvic Surgeon* 1(3):1–4, June 1980.

14. Hall RR, Hill DW, Beach HD: A carbon dioxide surgical laser. *Ann Coll Surg Engl* 48:181–187, 1971.

15. Bellina JH: Reconstructive microsurgery of the fallopian tube with carbon dioxide laser: Procedure and preliminary results. *Reproduccion* 5:1–17, 1981.

18 Excisional Conization of the Cervix

James H. Dorsey, MD, FACOG

Cervical conization was first described by Lisfrac in 1815 as an operation designed to cure invasive cervical cancer.[1] Unfortunately, because of the aggressive nature of the disease and its penchant for early lymphatic involvement, this procedure soon proved to be inadequate for treating even early invasive cervical cancer. Subsequently, the use of cervical conization was rarely reported in the literature until the concept of intraepithelial carcinoma was introduced into gynecology.[2,3] At that time, this preinvasive form of cervical neoplasia could only be accurately assessed by pathologic examination of an entire conization specimen. Thus, conization became a common diagnostic procedure for determining the presence of benign or malignant disease.

For many years, in the United States, hysterectomy was considered the procedure of choice for cervical carcinoma in situ.[4] However, a better understanding of the pathophysiology of cervical intraepithelial neoplasia, along with the development of the colposcope as a tool for identifying the limits of the disease and the proven success of more conservative therapy, have now led to the use of simpler forms of treatment.

Patients with significant intraepithelial neoplasia may be divided by colposcopy into two distinct groups. In Group I are patients who have a completely visible transformation zone, the intraepithelial neoplasia does not disappear into the endocervical canal, and endocervical curettage is negative for dysplastic cells. Thus, the lesion can be seen in its entirety, and evaluation by directed biopsy is possible.

Group II includes patients who have a transformation zone, which is not completely visible, and a lesion, which does disappear into the endocervical canal. This group also encompasses those who do not have colposcopically visible lesions, but who do show a positive endocervical curettage or suspicious cytology. For Group II patients, there is no possibility of accurate colposcopic biopsy.

CONIZATION OF THE CERVIX BY LASER

Conization of the cervix can be defined as a surgical procedure in which a cone-shaped volume of tissue is removed from the central longitudinal axis of the cervix. Not all conization operations yield specimens for pathologic evaluation. For example, electrosurgical conization usually produces so much tissue destruction in the specimen that the microscopic sections show only thermal artefact. When used to vaporize intraepithelial neoplasia, the CO_2 laser may destroy a cone-shaped volume that extends well down into the endocervical canal. If adequate biopsy has proven the completely intraepithelial nature of the disease, Group I patients may be treated by laser vaporization of the lesion and ablation of the transformation zone. This operation is referred to as a *vaporization conization.*[5]

Group II patients require a different approach to therapy. Intraepithelial neoplasia, which disappears into the endocervical canal, may be associated with an occult invasive squamous cancer that is not apparent until the cone specimen is examined microscopically. Thus, an excisional cervical conization must be performed in Group II patients so that the entire transformation zone and an adequate length of endocervical canal can be evaluated pathologically. Only when the pathologist is able to verify complete excision of an intraepithelial lesion does a diagnostic conization have therapeutic significance.

Cold knife conization has been associated with a relatively high morbidity, which includes hemorrhage, both immediate and delayed, as well as cervical stenosis and infertility.[6,7] This procedure usually requires inpatient hospitalization. Moreover, after healing, the new squamocolumnar junction often cannot be colposcopically identified because it is located too far up in the canal. Excisional laser conization was developed in an effort to reduce the incidence of such problems.

EXCISIONAL CERVICAL CONIZATION BY CO_2 LASER

Excisional laser conization of the cervix is a microsurgical procedure. The laser is mounted on a colposcope or an operative microscope, and the laser incision is directed by a micromanipulator located well outside of the surgical field. In over 90% of the cases, excisional laser conization can be performed on an outpatient basis because of the diminished risk of hemorrhage. General anesthesia is usually employed, since it is more convenient for the surgeon; however, sedation and local anesthesia may also give satisfactory results. Preoperative preparation includes gentle cleansing with povidone-iodine solution and, when indicated, painting the cervix with acetic acid solution in order to identify the ectocervical margins of the lesion.

POWER DENSITY AND SPOT SIZE

The power density selected for excisional laser conization is higher than that used for vaporization. Since the purpose of the operation is to produce a specimen for pathologic interpretation, only minimal thermal artefact should be present in the tissue sent to the laboratory. High power density and small focal spot size result in rapid cutting with minimal heat damage in the tissue lateral to the incision.[8,9] Thermal damage in the deep stromal side of the cone specimen is of no importance, for it is the interior of the specimen, the mucosa and the immediate stroma beneath the endocervical crypts that must be evaluated by the pathologist (Figures 18-1, 18-2).

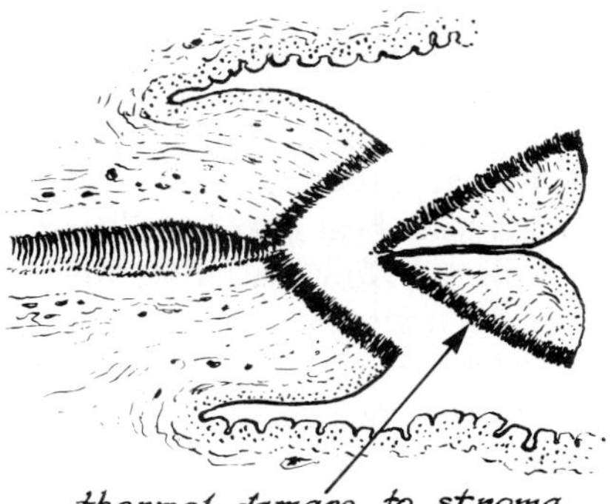

Figure 18-1 During cervical conization, thermal damage by laser energy is minimal. Damage occurs in the stroma, not in the mucosa. (Reproduced with permission from Dorsey JH: Cervical conization by the carbon dioxide laser, in Wheeless CR (ed): *The Pelvic Surgeon*. Baltimore, Northern Chesapeake Publishers, 1980.)

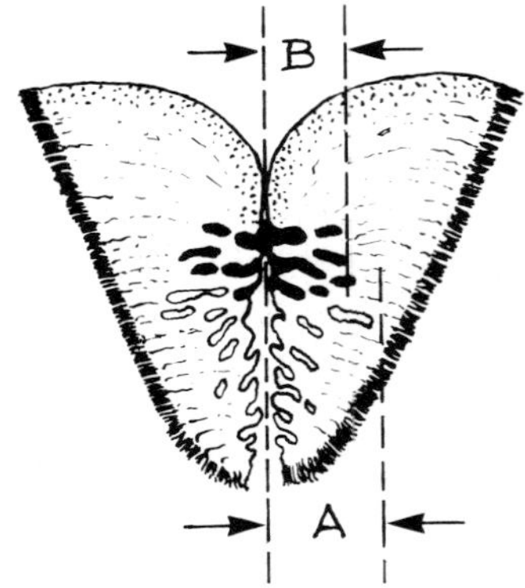

Figure 18-2 Endocervical crypt involvement by neoplasia (B) must be properly evaluated. Thermal artifact will not interfere with pathologic interpretation when cone is properly planned. (Reproduced with permission from Dorsey JH: Cervical conization by the carbon dioxide laser, in Wheeless CR (ed): *The Pelvic Surgeon*. Baltimore, Northern Chesapeake Publishers, 1980.)

It must be emphasized that the laser incision is three dimensional. In addition to length and depth, there is a width that is approximately equal to the focal spot size in diameter; the larger the focal spot diameter, the larger the cervical defect when the cone specimen is removed (Figure 18-3). For excisional conization, a spot diameter of 1.3 mm to 1.5 mm is recommended when a power density between 1,000 and 1,500 W/cm^2 (beam power 13 to 26W) is used. These values are obtainable with most of the commercially available CO_2 lasers.

HEMOSTASIS

When heat is retained in the tissue lateral to the laser incision, hemostasis is facilitated. The hemostatic effect of the CO_2 laser is mediated by heat energy and is inversely proportional to the power density. If high power densities are used, cutting becomes so rapid that vessels are transected with little laser heat energy transmitted laterally, and the hemostatic effect is reduced. However, when lower power densities are used, cutting is slower and more laser heat energy is dispersed laterally, resulting in better coagulation.

The cervix, particularly when chronically inflamed, contains vessels that may bleed profusely when transected by laser energy of high power density. Although there is always less blood loss with the laser incision than with the scalpel, injection of a dilute vasopressin solution (1.5%) into the cervical stroma (Figure 18-4) and placement of lateral cervical sutures to ligate the cervical artery reduce bleeding to an average loss of less than 5 ml during the entire operation (Figure 18-5). Attempting to

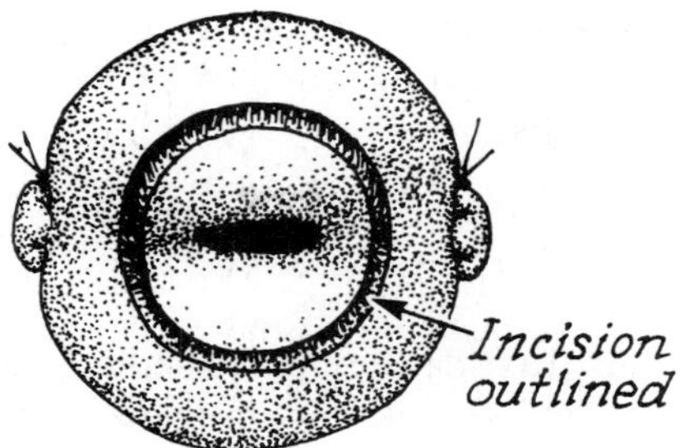

Figure 18-3 Laser incision has a width that is approximately equal to the spot size diameter. Larger incisions produce larger cervical defects when the specimen is removed. (Reproduced with permission from Dorsey JH: Cervical conization by the carbon dioxide laser, in Wheeless CR (ed): *The Pelvic Surgeon*. Baltimore, Northern Chesapeake Publishers, 1980.)

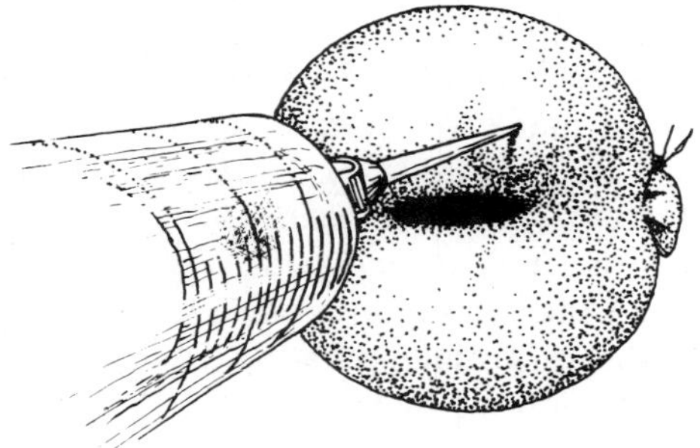

Figure 18-4 Ten ml of a dilute vasopressin solution are injected circumferentially around the cervical os. (Reproduced with permission from Dorsey JH: Cervical conization by the carbon dioxide laser, in Wheeless CR (ed): *The Pelvic Surgeon*. Baltimore, Northern Chesapeake Publishers, 1980.)

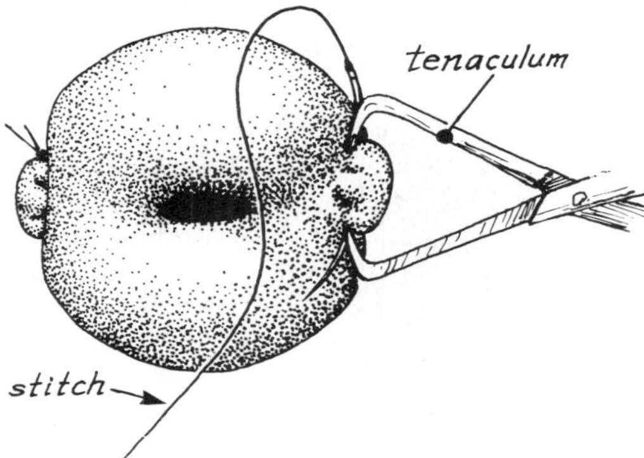

Figure 18-5 A lateral cervical suture may also be used to insure hemostasis. (Reproduced with permission from Dorsey JH: Cervical conization by the carbon dioxide laser, in Wheeless CR (ed): *The Pelvic Surgeon*. Baltimore, Northern Chesapeake Publishers, 1980.)

coagulate an actively bleeding vessel while removing a conization specimen can be very frustrating since much time will be expended in vaporizing a pool of blood.

THE INCISION

The surgeon must first decide upon the diameters and the depth of the cone. Often, it is helpful to visualize the endocervical canal with a contact endoscope.[10,11] This instrument accurately locates the internal cervical os from which the exact location of the cone apex can be estimated.[12] If a contact endoscope is not available, an attempt should be made to locate the internal os with a uterine sound. The upper limits of the conization incision should, of course, stop short of the internal os.

When making the incision, the anterior portion of the cervix is first grasped with a single tooth tenaculum, and the circumference of the cone is outlined on the cervix with a burst of laser energy (Figure 18-6). A circular incision is then made by connecting the *dots* and the incision is deepened to about 2 mm (Figure 18-7). The cone edge can then be grasped with fine tooth forceps. The laser beam is angled toward the predetermined cone apex in the endocervical canal (Figure 18-8). Gentle traction on the lateral part of the cone greatly aids rapid cutting and directional control of the laser beam. By manipulating tissue into the line of fire, the angle of the laser incision may be changed. The incision is most easily developed by a *four quadrant* technique (Figure 18-9), whereby the incision is deepened and carried almost to the apex in each respective quadrant. This minimizes repositioning of the laser tube and colposcope (Figure 18-10). In some instances, it may be desirable to remove the apex of the cone with a scalpel to eliminate the possibility of thermal artefact at the upper margin of the cone (Figure 18-11). If the cone is well planned, however, this maneuver is usually not necessary.

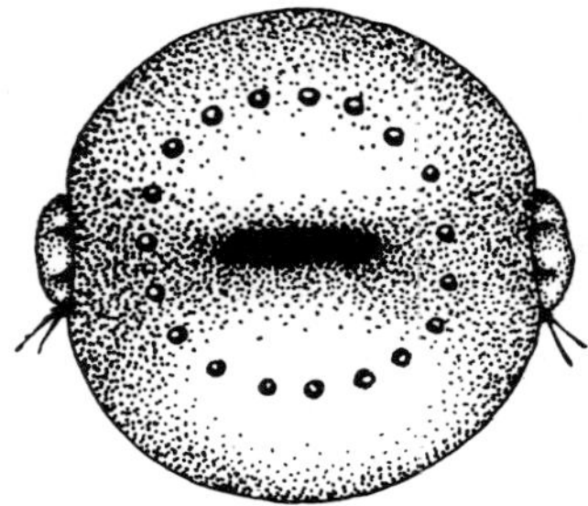

Figure 18-6 The incision is first outlined accurately with short bursts of laser energy. (Reproduced with permission from Dorsey JH: Cervical conization by the carbon dioxide laser, in Wheeless CR (ed): *The Pelvic Surgeon.* Baltimore, Northern Chesapeake Publishers, 1980.)

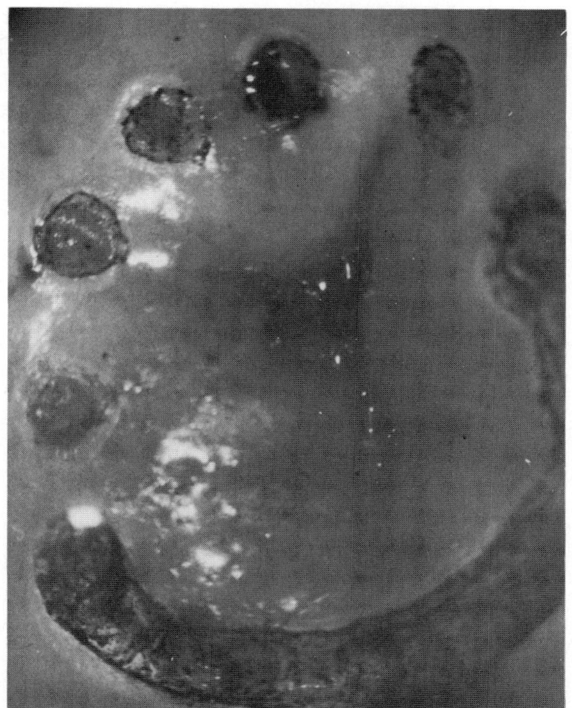

Figure 18-7 This colpophotograph shows how the incision is made by connecting the dots. Note the lack of bleeding.

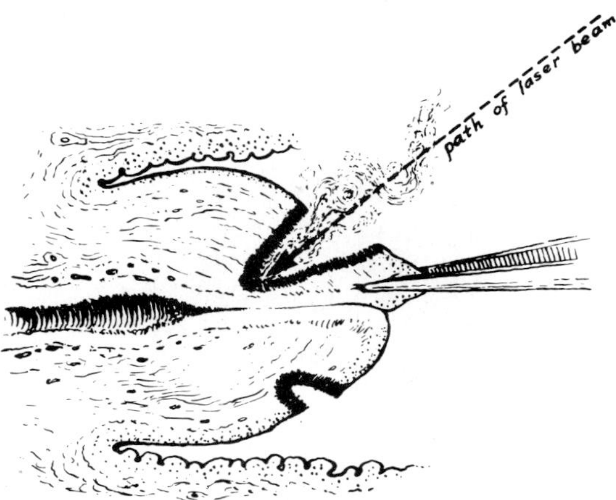

Figure 18-8 The laser beam is directed toward the apex of the cone. Traction on the specimen aids in developing the cone by moving the tissue in or out of the path of the laser beam. (Reproduced with permission from Dorsey JH: Cervical conization by the carbon dioxide laser, in Wheeless CR (ed): *The Pelvic Surgeon*. Baltimore, Northern Chesapeake Publishers, 1980.)

Following removal of the cone specimen, the problem of hemostasis is reassessed. Power density is dropped to approximately 100 W/cm² (beam power 1.5W) and, if possible, spot size is increased by defocusing the beam or changing the laser focusing lenses. The entire area of the cervical cone bed is then superficially coagulated (Figure 18-12). The end result is thus equivalent to a deep vaporization procedure. This maneuver seems to have significantly reduced the incidence of delayed postoperative hemorrhage by sealing cervical stromal vesicles.

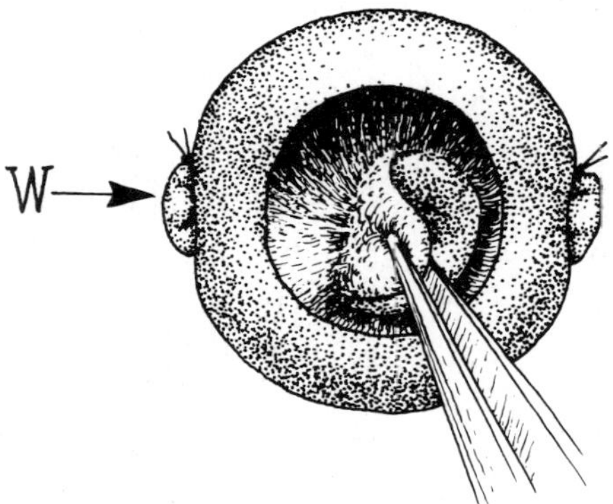

Figure 18-9 The incision is deepened and carried almost to the cone apex in each of the four cervical quadrants. (Reproduced with permission from Dorsey JH: Cervical conization by the carbon dioxide laser, in Wheeless CR (ed): *The Pelvic Surgeon*. Baltimore, Northern Chesapeake Publishers, 1980.)

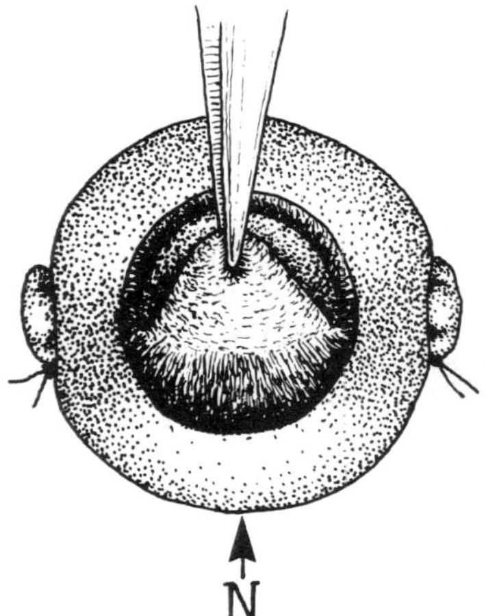

Figure 18-10 Using continuous power, the superior portion of the incision has been carried almost to the cone apex. (Reproduced with permission from Dorsey JH: Cervical conization by the carbon dioxide laser, in Wheeless CR (ed): *The Pelvic Surgeon*. Baltimore, Northern Chesapeake Publishers, 1980.)

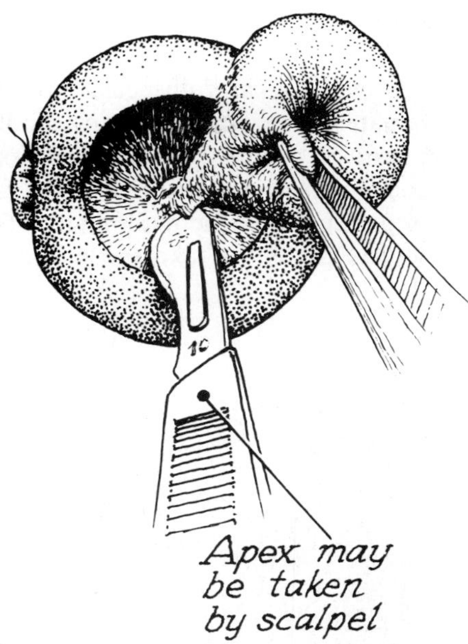

Figure 18-11 In order to avoid thermal damage at the apex of the cone, it is sometimes necessary to excise the endocervical canal with a scalpel. (Reproduced with permission from Dorsey JH: Cervical conization by the carbon dioxide laser, in Wheeless CR (ed): *The Pelvic Surgeon.* Baltimore, Northern Chesapeake Publishers, 1980.)

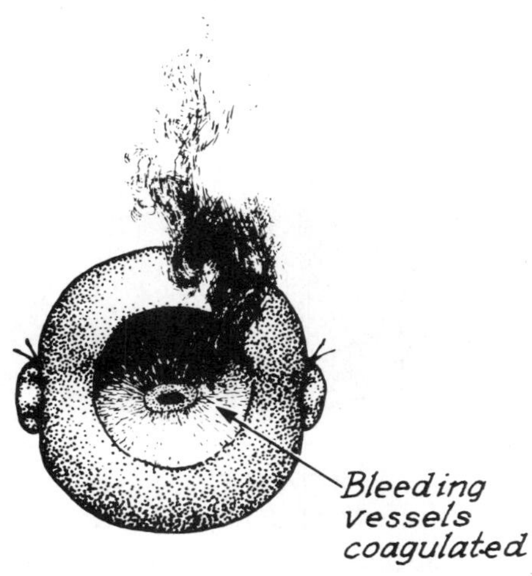

Figure 18-12 The entire cone bed is now thoroughly coagulated with low power density laser beam. The end result is thus equivalent to a vaporization. (Reproduced with permission from Dorsey JH: Cervical conization by the carbon dioxide laser, in Wheeless CR (ed): *The Pelvic Surgeon.* Baltimore, Northern Chesapeake Publishers, 1980.)

THE CONE SPECIMEN

The cone specimen must be carefully sectioned so that the pathologist can properly evaluate its margins. The cone should be opened and pinned flat on cardboard or a cork before immersion into a fixative (Figure 18-13). The cone is then sectioned in a radial fashion so that its true margins will be represented on the pathologic slide (Figures 18-14, 18-15). Some pathologists prefer to take the entire upper and lower margins separately.

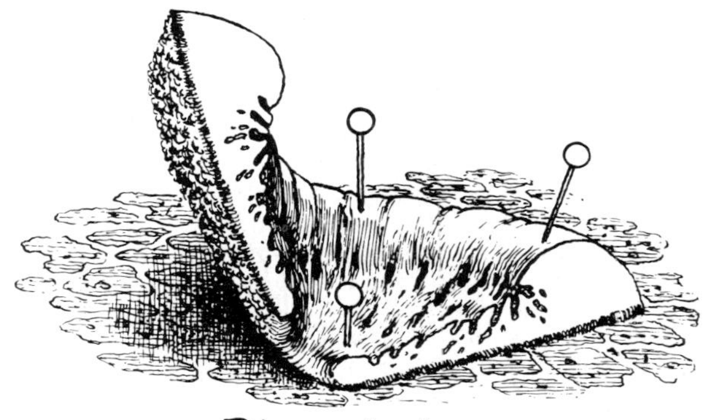

Figure 18-13 Prior to fixation, the cone specimen should be opened and pinned on a flat piece of cardboard or cork. This enables the pathologist to establish important landmarks and correct borders. (Reproduced with permission from Dorsey JH: Cervical conization by the carbon dioxide laser, in Wheeless CR (ed): *The Pelvic Surgeon*. Baltimore, Northern Chesapeake Publishers, 1980.)

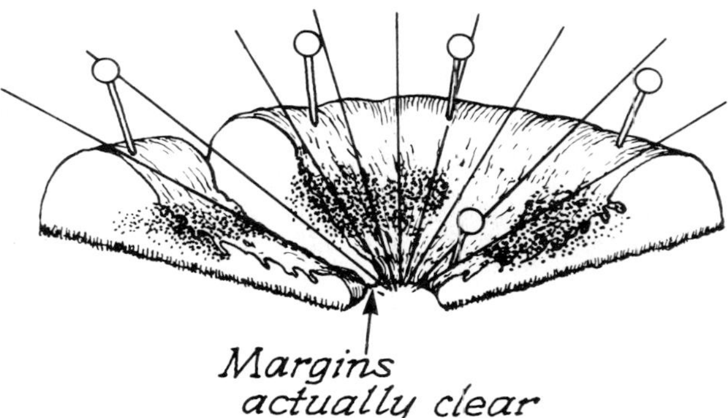

Figure 18-14 The cone specimen must be sectioned in a manner that will allow proper evaluation of the margins. This technique, in which the sections are angled to the apex of the cone, is one method of accomplishing the objective. (Reproduced with permission from Dorsey JH: Cervical conization by the carbon dioxide laser, in Wheeless CR (ed): *The Pelvic Surgeon*. Baltimore, Northern Chesapeake Publishers, 1980.)

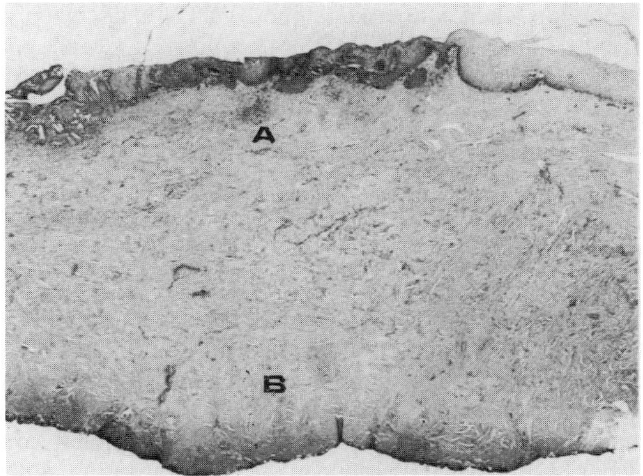

Figure 18-15 This photomicrograph shows clear cone margins with normal ectocervix separated from normal endocervix by an area of intraepithelial neoplasia (A). The stromal side of the cone (B) shows minimal thermal damage which does not interfere with pathologic interpretation of the specimen (35 ×). Reproduced with permission from *Obstet Gynecol* 54:565, 1979.

HEALING

By the end of the first postoperative week, a white necrotic pseudomembrane covers the entire cone bed. Careful daily observation and frequent biopsies of the cervical cone bed have shown that ectocervical squamous epithelium does not proliferate down into this site. The pH of this area is intensely alkaline and squamous metaplasia does not occur. Reserve cells from the cone bed apex gradually replace the debris and form a new endocervical lining along the surface of the healing stroma. These reserve cells eventually differentiate into columnar cells which migrate toward the incised edge of the ectocervix. This important process of reepithelialization results in a visible squamocolumnar junction and makes subsequent colposcopy meaningful. Often the columnar epithelium can be seen meeting the squamous epithelium very near the original incision.

RESULTS

In our series of over 100 excisional laser conizations, intraoperative blood loss averaged less than 5 cc. Delayed hemorrhage requiring suturing of bleeding points occurred in approximately 4% of the patients, a striking reduction when compared to the 10–20% incidence of this complication reported in the literature for cold conization. Healing, as judged by cervical biopsies, is usually complete within four to six weeks. Cervical stenosis is rare. When cone margins are clear of neoplasia, two-year *cure rates* in patients followed by cervical cytology, colposcopy and biopsy are 96% to 98%.

SUMMARY

Cervical intraepithelial neoplasia may be treated by either vaporization conization or excisional conization with the CO_2 laser, as indicated by the colposcopic and pathologic findings. Strict attention must be paid to spot size and power density, since vaporization and excisional procedures require different ranges of values. With excisional conizations, morbidity has been reduced by utilizing the laser both as a scalpel and as a technique for achieving hemostasis. When high power density and small spot size are used, the surgical specimen is very suitable for pathologic interpretation.

REFERENCES

1. Lisfrac J: Memoire sur une nouvelle methode de practique l'operation de la taille chez les femmes. *Gaz Med France* 2:835–846, 1815.
2. Galvin FA, TeLinde RW: The present-day status of noninvasive cervical carcinoma. *Am J Obstet Gynecol* 57:15–36, 1949.
3. Galvin GA, Jones HW, TeLinde RW: Significance of basal-cell hyperactivity in cervical biopsies. *Am J Obstet Gynecol* 70:808–821, 1955.
4. TeLinde RW: Hysterectomy for carcinoma in situ, in Meigs (ed): *Surgical Treatment of Cancer of the Cervix.* New York, Grune & Stratton, 1954, pp 130–136.
5. Dorsey JH, Diggs ES: Microsurgical conization of the cervix by carbon dioxide laser. *Obstet Gynecol* 54:565–570, 1979.
6. Leimen G, Harrison NA, Rubin GR: Pregnancy following conization of the cervix: Complications related to cone size. *Am J Obstet Gynecol* 136(1):14–8, 1980.
7. Onroos M, Liukko P, Kilkku P, et al: Pregnancy and delivery after conization of the cervix. *Acta Obstet Gynecol Scand* 58(5):477–80, 1979.
8. Verschueren R: *The CO_2 Laser in Tumor Surgery.* Assen/Amsterdam, Van Gorcum, 1976, pp 38–47.
9. Mihashi S, Jako GJ, Incze J, et al: Laser surgery in otolaryngology: Interaction of CO_2 laser and soft tissue. *Ann NY Acad Sci* 267:263–294, 1974.
10. Baggish M: Contact hysteroscopy: A new technique to explore the uterine cavity. *Obstet Gynecol* 54:350–354, 1979.
11. Dorsey JH, Diggs ES, Baggish MS: Cystourethroscopy with the direct view contact endoscope. *Obstet Gynecol* 57:115–118, 1981.
12. Baggish M, Dorsey JH: Evaluation of the endocervical canal with the contact endoscope as an adjunct to colposcopy (submitted for publication).

19 Vagina and Vulva

Rocco V. Lobraico, MD, FACS, FACOG
Joseph H. Bellina, MD, PhD, FACOG

VAGINA

Lesions in the vagina were generally overlooked by the gynecologist until the advent in recent years of colposcopy but are now receiving the attention they warrant. With concentrated efforts employing the colposcope and 3% to 4% acetic acid followed by Lugol's solution, precisely defined suspicious areas can be recognized for biopsy. The vagina with its many rugae makes close scrutiny a task, but careful manipulation and spreading of the rugae with the vaginal speculum are essential. A bright light source is also required for proper visualization.

Since the cervix and upper 80% of the vagina originate from the Müllerian ducts, lesions affecting the cervix also appear in the vagina. Benign as well as malignant lesions can be found extending from the cervix into the vagina or arising in the vaginal tissue. These may also appear in multicentric areas involving both squamous and glandular elements.

Conventional surgical treatment of lesions in the vagina is difficult because of the limited space and unapproachable angles. A rigid scalpel hinders the surgeon's ability to remove lateral lesions. Bleeding also obstructs vision.

The CO_2 laser solves many problems by allowing the reflection of the beam through the use of mirrors. This allows the lateral walls and fornices to be reached (Figure 19-1). Vaporization of polypoid lesions can also be affected. The laser's bloodless tissue destruction is particularly valuable, and scarring is not a problem following this method of tissue removal.

The CO_2 laser has been used effectively to eradicate condylomata acuminata on the vaginal walls and vulva as well as on the portio vaginalis. Recurrent or obstinate condylomatous lesions on the vulva can often be attributed to untreated lesions on the cervix and vagina.[1] Therefore, meticulous exploration of the vagina through the colposcope is necessary (Figure 19-2). All lesions must be destroyed. Viral papillomas also may occur in these sites and should be eliminated.

Vaginal adenosis is usually an asymptomatic lesion which occasionally causes a serosanguinous vaginal discharge. This can be corrected by laser ablation of the adenosis (Figure 19-3). Repeat biopsy of adenosis must be done prior to initial laser surgery and any subsequent laser surgery in order to detect malignant epithelial changes.

Dysplasia of the vagina progressing from mild to severe stages is a fragile lesion that can be removed. The lesion, identified with 3% to 4% acetic acid, can be seen through the colposcope as flat to slightly raised islands with an increased vascular pattern. Directed biopsy will confirm

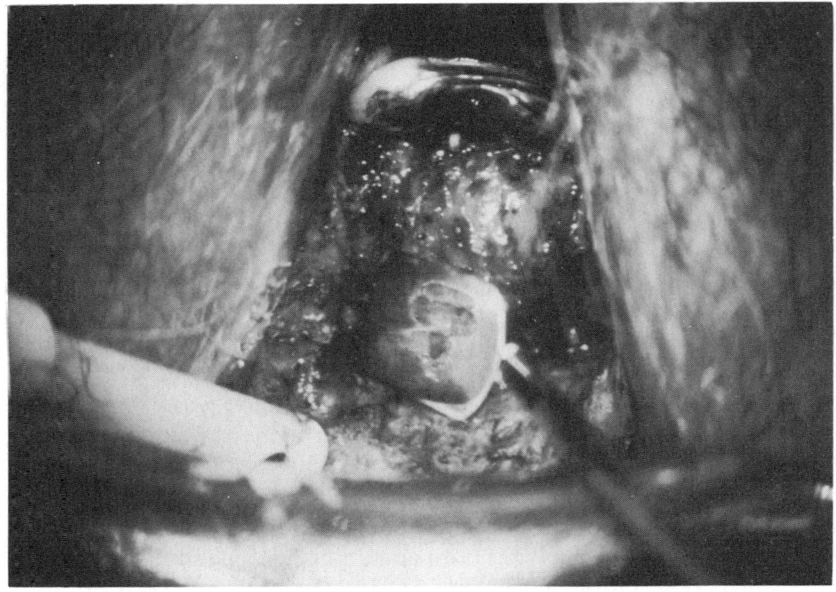

Figure 19-1 Mirror reflection of laser beam to lateral wall of vagina.

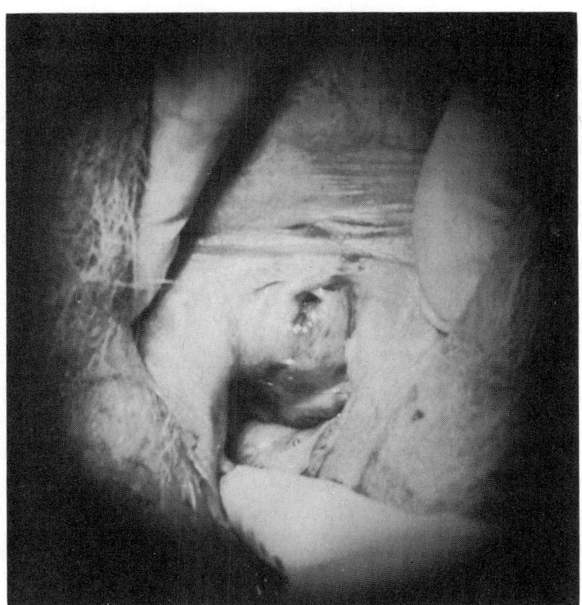

Figure 19-2 Suburethral metastasis from adenocarcinoma of the uterus.

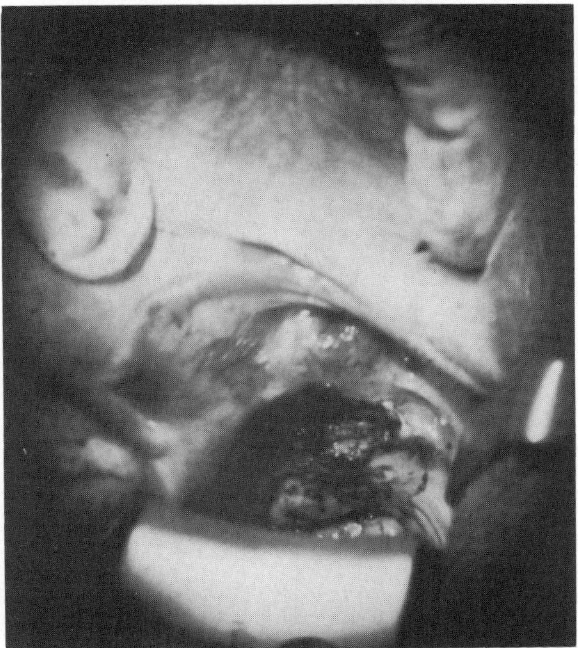

Figure 19-3 Laser ablation of suburethral metastasis.

the diagnosis. Papillomas of viral origin may be associated with dysplasia. These will be identified histologically through biopsy. The severe dysplasias that border on carcinoma in situ are difficult to cure since these lesions tend to recur. Although similar recurrence rates follow scalpel excision and laser vaporization, these recurrent lesions can be retreated, as many times as necessary without deformity or significant scarring. Carcinoma in situ of the vagina is often associated with cervical carcinoma in situ. Therefore, cervical examination and treatment is required to reduce the chance of recurrence.

The use of CO_2 laser therapy for herpes simplex hominis II lesions is considered investigational at this time but has offered some patients symptomatic relief. Vaginal cuff granulomas after hysterectomy have been successfully removed using laser vaporization, as have polyps and cysts of the vagina. Chronic inflammatory ulcers caused by foreign bodies imbedded in the walls of the vagina also can be vaporized, but these respond only when the offending factor has been removed.

Metastatic carcinoma to the vagina may be lased for palliation (Figures 19-3, 19-4). Repeated applications have controlled the serosanguinous discharge.

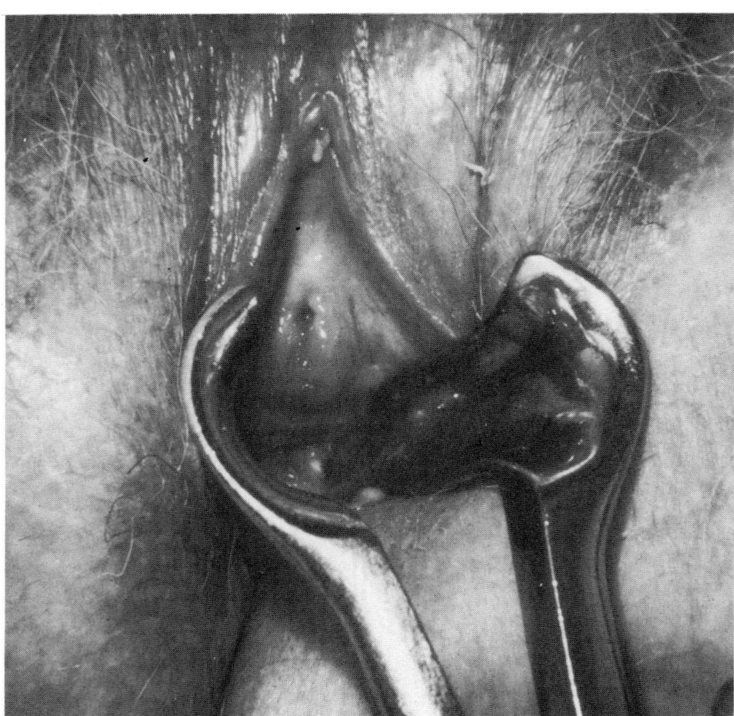

Figure 19-4 Healed suburethral metastasis – postlaser.

Methods of Applications

The patient is placed in the dorsal lithotomy position. A nonreflective metal or nonflammable plastic speculum is inserted into the vagina. Lesions are visualized through the colposcope with an adequate light source and further defined with Lugol's solution. Anesthesia may not be required in the upper 80% of the vagina. Local or general anesthesia is necessary for the lower 20% of the vagina, depending upon the patient's pain threshold.

Application of laser energy to the vaginal lesions is identical to that in cervical disease. The laser beam is directed to the target tissue by a micromanipulator and can be manipulated to reach all areas of the vagina. A highly polished, stainless steel mirror can be used to deliver the beam orthogonal to the lateral wall of the vagina. Careful observation through the colposcope with recognition of intervening tissue planes is important. Varicose veins in the vagina are not uncommon and must be approached with care. Hemorrhage may occur from a varix but can be managed by applying the usual methods of hemostasis.

Postoperative care usually requires minimal analgesia. There can be a serosanguinous discharge which may be odorous. The use of antiseptic vaginal creams is advisable to reduce secondary infections. Adhesive bands may form and should be disrupted digitally. If extensive lasing is performed, insertion of a vaginal dilator may be essential. Granulation tissue has been observed and can be removed with a chemical cautery or repeated lasing. Healing time varies from four to six weeks. Vaginal douching and intercourse should be avoided for at least one to two weeks after complete healing. Follow-up Papanicolaou smears and colposcopy should be done every three months for the first year and every six months to a year thereafter.

VULVA

The vulva is prone to many problems arising from infections, irritants, injury, and cellular changes. Unfortunately, care is often requested by the patient late in the disease process because of embarrassment or fear of surgical intervention with disfigurement. With laser surgery, however, even extensive vulvar disease can be cured or controlled without disfigurement. Injuries may be the underlying cause of some vulvar problems, but it is the viral growths and progressive cellular changes that present the challenge to the gynecologist.

Condylomata acuminata of the vulva are an increasingly common gynecologic problem. Therapy prior to the CO_2 laser was either ineffective or dangerous, and caused discomfort and formation of scar tissue.

Laser ablation eliminates these difficulties and has been demonstrated to be the most effective treatment method. Both persistent disease and recurrences are rare when adequate destruction of all lesions is done. Patients must be cautioned against reinfection by the consort and advised of venereal transmission of this viral tumor.

By introducing the vaginal speculum and observing the cervix and vaginal surface through the colposcope, many associated condylomata can often be identified. A search with the anoscope also may reveal anal condylomata which could account for lesions in the perianal region. All such growths must be ablated before the patient can be freed from condylomata.

Dysplasia of the vulva may be recognized through the colposcope. The continuum of cytologic changes, from mild through moderate to severe, is the same as in the cervix and vagina. The diagnosis with the Keyes biopsy punch can be performed safely in the office under local anesthesia. Instruments for these procedures are shown in Figure 19-5. Suspicious areas can be identified for biopsy with 1% toluidine blue washed with 3% acetic acid to bleach the benign areas and define the deeper stained parakeratotic nuclei.

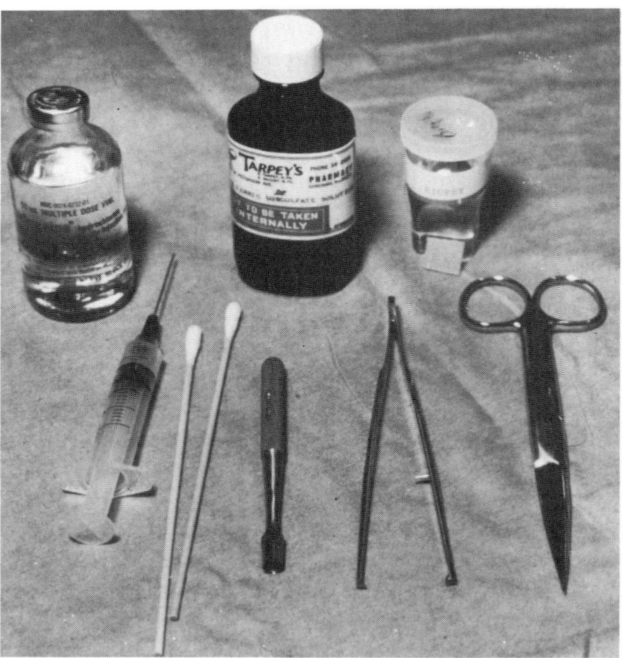

Figure 19-5 Vulvar biopsy tray containing: 1% mepivacaine, formalin, thin cardboard square for specimen, scissors, forceps to snip off tissue, cut for biopsy by the Keyes punch and ferric sulfate for hemostasis.

Carcinoma in situ of the vulva may be associated with severe dysplasia or with condylomata acuminata. Multiple biopsies should be taken after using 1% toluidine blue to define the suspicious area. The frequency of diagnosis of carcinoma in situ of the vulva is increasing because more attention is being paid to vulvar lesions and because of more sophisticated diagnostic techniques. Perhaps the incidence of this disease is also increasing.[2] Although the diagnosis of carcinoma in situ must be considered serious, conservative measures in removing the lesions are advised because of the effectiveness of newer therapeutic measures and because of the slow development of this tumor. Laser surgery is particularly valuable for this condition because extensive lesions can be destroyed without sequelae.

Vulvar dystrophy including hyperplastic dystrophy lichen sclerosis[3] and mixed dystrophy is characterized by disorders in epithelial growth resulting in alterations of the surface epithelium. This occurs with or without atypia. Questions concerning the malignant potential of these dystrophies have been raised and the matter remains controversial. The probability that a superimposed carcinoma will develop is in the range of 1% to 2% over a long period of time. This condition is also amenable to laser therapy and relief without mutilation can be attained even when repeated applications are required.[4,5]

Other lesions readily eradicated by ablation and coagulation are hemangiomas and urethral caruncles. Benign pigmented nevi are removed by undercut excision, sealing the lymphatics with the laser cut. This gives a total specimen for study of the nevus. Molluscum contagiosum has been successfully managed with the CO_2 laser, and symptomatic relief of recurrent herpes progenitalis is also possible.

Method of Application

The surface extent and depth of tissue destruction required for vulvar lesions vary according to the type and extent of the lesion. For large lesions, the surface is first encircled with the laser 5 mm beyond its margin. The lesion is then divided into smaller areas. Each is individually ablated to a predetermined and uniform depth until the entire lesion has been vaporized. Moving the laser beam in the XYZ axes allows complete and uniform removal of tissue. If hillocks of diseased epithelium remain, the incidence of recurrence is higher. Depth of penetration must attain 3–4 mm to be effective in dystrophy and dysplasia. More superficial ablation can be used in condylomata. Rapid movement of the beam and utilization of as high a power as can be handled by the surgeon (10-25W) reduces the carbonization. Keeping the operative field clean reduces the thermal effect on adjacent tissue. Carbonized tissue is removed from the operative site during vaporization with a wet sponge or irrigation. This is helpful since the carbon residue transmits heat when the laser passes over it, and will cause increased thermal damage to the underlying tissue. Neglecting this results in excess necrosis, poorer healing, and deeper scarring.

When the diagnosis is carcinoma in situ, it is recommended that the entire lesion(s) be available for histologic study. To accomplish this, each lesion and 5 mm beyond its periphery is undercut with the laser to a depth of 5–7 mm or more, depending upon the individual case (Figure 19-6). This tissue is excised with the laser beam using a beam power of 25–40 watts, lifted off with Allis forceps and submitted for microscopic evaluation (Figure 19-7). If necessary, definitive therapy for microinvasive or frank invasive carcinoma can be scheduled. The depth of tissue destruction or removal determines the success of the surgery, and adequate depth is important for cure.[6] It must be recognized also that, in the vulva, excess depth of destruction produces complications, lengthens healing time, and increases scarring (Figure 19-8).

The lateral extent of tissue destruction accomplished at one operation depends upon the condition of the patient and the judgment of the surgeon. The labia majora, minora, clitoral area, perineum, and perianal region can be done at one application. However, this may be too extensive for some patients' tolerance. Removing the lesion in stages may be preferable for most patients with either local or general anesthesia.

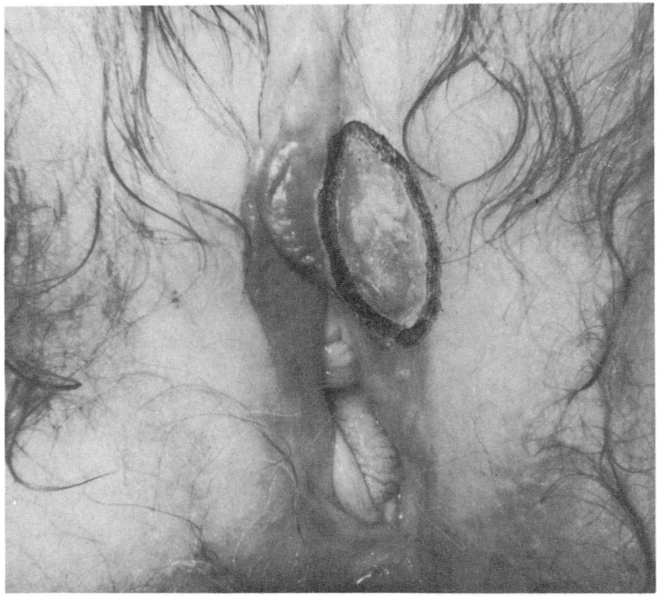

Figure 19-6 Margin of carcinoma in situ lesion encircled by laser.

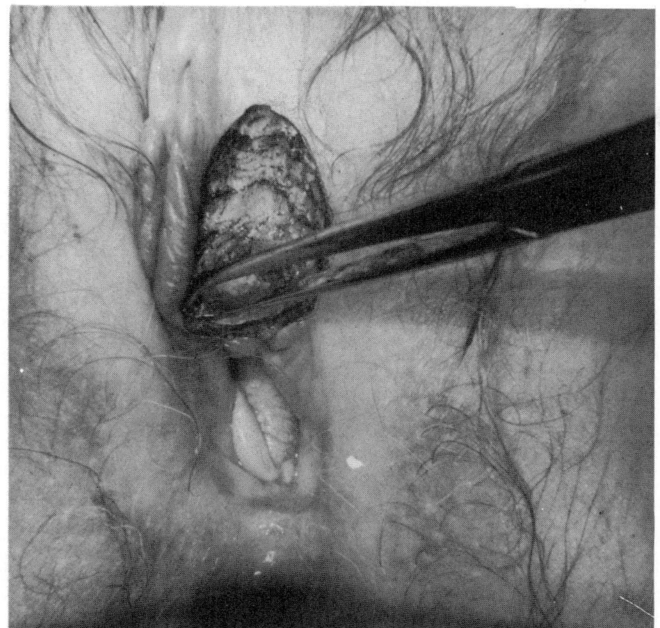

Figure 19-7 Lesion undercut by laser and lifted off by Allis forceps.

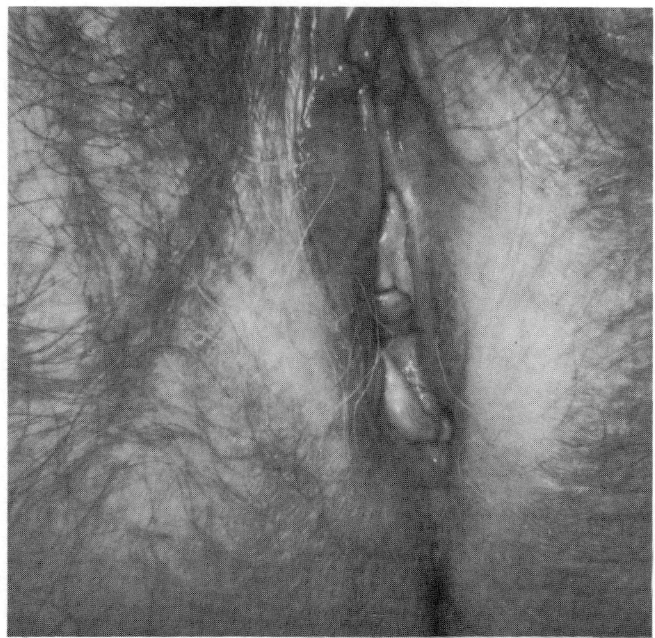

Figure 19-8 Healed area after lesion excised by laser.

Tissue Reaction

The immediate appearance of the vulva at the operative site is one of desiccated tissue with charring. Induration, exudation, and edema follow after 24 hours. On the third day a gray necrotic membrane forms over the operative area. Some investigators have reported that when both sides of the introitus have been lased at the same time, the tissue may agglutinate with fine adhesions. This complication is probably a reflection of excessive depth of destruction and, in addition to agglutination, scarring may occur. Digital separation facilitates proper healing and drainage of exudate retained in the vagina. Topical estrogen can be applied to the adhesions, and gentle traction will separate the tissue.

Postoperative Management

The lased site should be considered as a thermal burn even though the heat coagulum zone may only extend 600 μ below the impact site. Various medications have been employed to encourage primary healing but isotonic saline soaks in a whirlpool or pulsator apparatus are now recommended. Patients may experience moderate discomfort for the first 24 hours. In cases of extensive dissection for severe vulvar disease, micturation may become difficult. Occasionally, catheterization has been required to alleviate the dysuria.

With complete reepithelialization there is restoration of the normal anatomic architecture. Strictures, when they do occur, are minimal. When this technique is properly executed, scarring is not a problem. Edema and induration subside in 10 to 12 days. Sloughing of the eschar with complete healing takes four to six weeks. As with cervical and vaginal lesions, recurrence of disease depends on adequate eradication of all foci of the principal and associated lesions. Rates of persistent disease following laser therapy vary with the type and extent of the disease, but the effectiveness of treatment with this modality is in each instance comparable or superior to conventional treatment.[6] Additionally, the preservation of normal anatomic configuration and the absence of disfigurement and scarring are important benefits of laser therapy for vulvar disease.

FOLLOW-UP OF GYNECOLOGICAL LESIONS

Consistent follow-up of patients with gynecological lesions is mandatory in order to detect persistent or new lesions. This is particularly important in intraepithelial neoplasia because of the potential for this lesion to progress, if undisturbed, to invasive carcinoma. Although rare, lesions do reappear approximately 4% to 12% of the time following *adequate* lesion destruction. Recurrence (persistent disease or new disease) is a function of adequacy of tissue removal, both in depth and lateral extent, and reinfection, eg, condyloma acuminatum. Patients who are informed of the venereal nature of their disease can take steps to prevent reinfection by arranging treatment for the consort(s), by using barrier methods of contraception, and/or by using spermatocides which destroy DNA during intercourse.

The follow-up regimen required varies with the gynecologist, but usually entails a postoperative visit at two to six weeks for evaluation of healing. During the first year the patient should be evaluated cytologically and colposcopically every three months. Persistent disease can be identified and retreated. For the first year following treatment, patients must be followed cytologically every six months, perhaps for life, until further research proves this to be unnecessary.

OTHER GYNECOLOGIC APPLICATIONS OF THE CO_2 LASER

The laser is presently being used to vaporize recurrent tumors as well as to treat the lesions described above. Several investigators contemplate utilization of high power CO_2 lasers in debulking abdominal gynecologic malignancies, and recently the laser has been successfully employed in microsurgical reconstruction of Fallopian tubes for restoration of fertility. When the laser finally is coupled to fiberoptic cables, many other lesions and sites may benefit from this surgical modality.

Laser applications in gynecology appear to be increasing. This new form of surgical management, with its hemostatic capability and precision of application, will expand the capabilities of gynecologic surgeons.

REFERENCES

1. Baggish MS: Carbon dioxide laser treatment for condylomata acuminata infections. *Obstet Gynecol* 55:711–715, 1980.
2. Woodruff JD: Vulvar atypia and carcinoma in situ. *J Reprod Med* 17:155–163, 1976.
3. Friedrich EG: Lichen sclerosis. *J Reprod Med* 17:147–153, 1976.
4. Mering JH: A surgical approach to intractable pruritus vulvae. *Am J Obstet Gynecol* 64:619–627, 1952.
5. Langley LL, Hertig AJ, Smith GS: Relation of leukoplakia vulvitis to squamous carcinoma of the vulva. *Am J Obstet Gynecol* 62:167, 1951.
6. Bellina JH: Carbon dioxide laser in gynecology. *Obstet Gynecol Ann* 6:371–391, 1977.

20 Reconstruction of the Fallopian Tube

Joseph H. Bellina, MD, PhD, FACOG

Increased demand for sterilization reversal and surgical treatment for tubal occlusion, has resulted in a developing and explosive interest in microsurgery. Results of microsurgical repair of the fallopian tube are far greater than with gross surgical techniques. There remains, however, substantial room for improvement. The need for perfect hemostasis, reduced operating time, exceptional revascularization in anastomosis and cornual reimplantation, reduction of postoperative adhesions, and reduction in postoperative tubal occlusion from scarring prompted the experimental use of the CO_2 laser by this author in reconstructive microsurgery from 1974 to 1979.[1] The results of the first 14 cases were encouraging: live births in five women and conceptions in nine. Two ectopic pregnancies occurred. Unfortunately, results of the other pregnancies are unknown, and some of the original 14 cases preferred not to attempt pregnancy.

Subsequently, other investigators, notably in France and West Germany, began utilizing the laser fertility enhancement microsurgery.[2,3] Animal models, conducted abroad and in the United States, confirmed the increased postoperative patency, and demonstrated that laser-induced tissue necrosis prevented secondary adhesion formation. All investigators confirmed the intraoperative hemostasis and reported reduced operating time.[4-6]

In 1980, a large series of patients was begun by this author at the Reproductive Biology Center of F. Edward Hebert Hospital in New Orleans. All preoperative laparoscopy procedures, all microsurgical procedures, and all second-look laparoscopies are being video recorded for documentation and teaching reasons. Follow-up will determine the live birth rates in these cases, but patency and conception rates observed to date are encouraging.[7]

INSTRUMENTATION

A 40-watt (maximum output) continuous wave CO_2 laser, the Sharplan 791, was adapted to the OPMI 1 Zeiss operating microscope (Figure 20-1). An articulation arm contains a series of mirrors, and

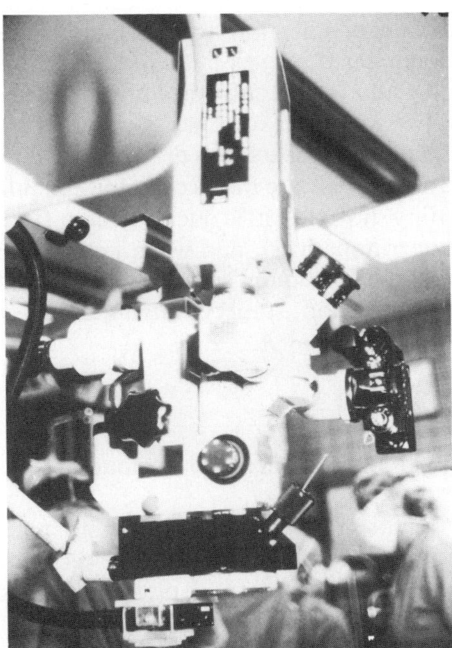

Figure 20-1 Instrumentation for gynecologic laser tubal microsurgery. Twin viewing system, lighting and recording devices, micromanipulator and CO_2 laser coupling mechanism are shown. (Reproduced with permission from Bellina JH: Reconstructive microsurgery of the fallopian tube with the carbon dioxide laser: Procedures and preliminary results. *Reproduccion* 5:1–17, 1981.)

delivers the laser beam to a coupling device attached to the operating microscope. Through the OPMI 1, the beam is optically coupled with both the surgeon's viewing system and a helium-neon finder beam of the CO_2 laser. A micromanipulator is attached below the microscope and delivers laser energy under the control of the laser surgeon. A visual lens with a focal length of 300 mm is used for intra-abdominal laser microsurgery. Power control settings of the laser allow the surgeon to employ power densities (PD) from 500 W/cm^2 to 10,000 W/cm^2 with a spot diameter (SD) of 550 μ and a beam power (BP) of 1 to 24 W. The hand-held laser scalpel is an alternative delivery system of the Sharplan 791 and can deliver up to 5×10^5 W/cm^2 with an SD of 125 μ and BP of 60 W.* The delivery systems can be changed as needed.

CANDIDATES FOR LASER MICROSURGERY

Candidates for tubal microsurgery with the CO_2 laser and their mates are subject to intense fertility evaluations. Tubal factors are identified by laparoscopy and hysterosalpingograms, and the site and extent of occlusion are identified. Contraindications to laser microsurgery are similar to those of conventional microsurgery and include active pelvic inflammatory disease, tuberculosis, and suspected malignancies. The absence of adequate reproductive structures for successful surgery are considered as relative contraindications. Patients who are at surgical risk, or for whom pregnancy is contraindicated, are not acceptable candidates.

When the fertility dysfunction is due to a tubal factor (with or without correctable endocrinopathies), and when both patient and mate are properly informed of the procedure, success, failures, and complications, and they still desire correction, surgery is undertaken.

SURGICAL PROCEDURES

Surgical Preparation and Intraoperative Evaluation

The patient is taken to the surgical suite and under general anesthesia, aerobic and anaerobic cultures of the cervical canal are made. The vagina is prepared with an antiseptic solution. The endometrial cavity

---

*Editors' comment: The relationship between PD, SD, and BP is as follows:

$$\text{BP in W/cm}^2 = \frac{\text{BP in W}}{\text{Area in cm}^2}$$

$$\text{Area in cm}^2 = \frac{\text{SD in mm}^2}{10 \times 2} \times \pi = \frac{\text{SD in }\mu^2}{10{,}000 \times 2} \times \pi$$

is distended via a Humi* cannula, and a catheter is inserted into the urinary bladder. The vaginal pack is inserted to help elevate the corpus uteri. An intraoperative hysterosalpingogram is performed with methylene blue dye added to the water soluble radio-opaque media to determine intra-abdominal spillage.

Standard laparoscopic examination findings are noted and filmed (Figure 20-2 and 20-3). At this point, the procedure can be aborted or advanced to the microsurgery phase. The surgeon may consult with a family member via an audio/video relay to a private consultation room. Permanent audio and visual recordings are made of this discussion, including the surgeon's recommendations and the additional consent of the appropriate family member. This phase concludes the intraoperative evaluation.

---

*Humi: United Marketing Resources—Harris Kronner Uterine Manipulator Injector—UNIMAR.

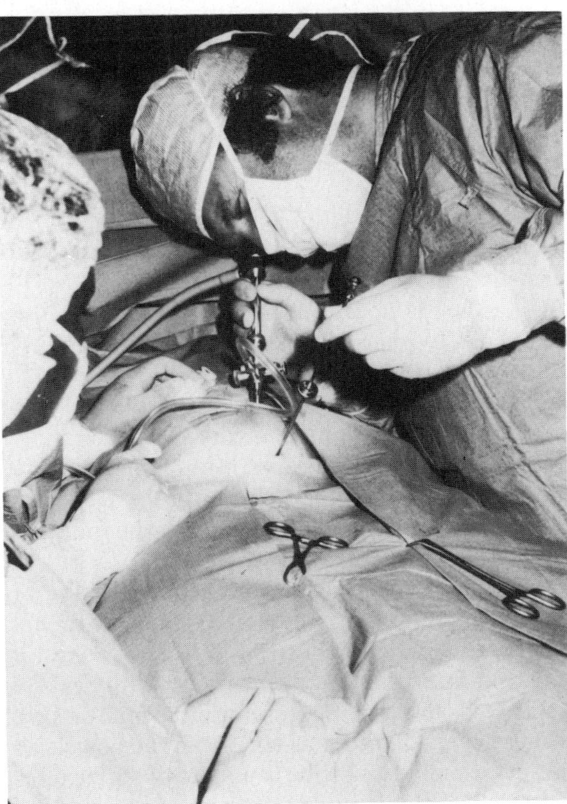

Figure 20-2 Preoperative laparoscopy to confirm the exact tubal disease before opening the abdomen.

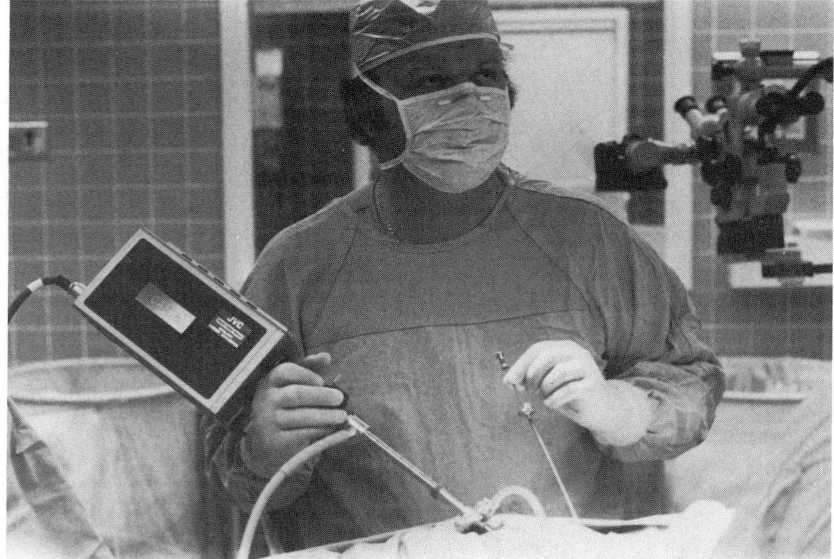

Figure 20-3 A videotape record is kept on each preoperative microsurgical case.

Microsurgical Preparation

A 50 mm focal length, handheld CO_2 laser is used to incise the skin, fat, and fascia, with power densities ranging from 1×10^5 W/cm² to 5×10^5 W/cm² (SD 125 μ, BP 12 to 60 W) (Figures 20-4, 20-5). The peritoneum is opened by sharp dissection and blood vessel coagulation is accomplished with the HF* bipolar current.

An O'Conner-Sullivan self-retracting retractor and intra-abdominal packing are placed in the abdominal cavity. The operating microscope, with laser micromanipulator, is draped with a sterile polyethylene bag, and positioned over the incision (Figure 20-6). Depending upon the pathology of the case, one, or a combination, of the following procedures may be done.

Adhesolysis Adhesive processes are removed using a micromanipulated laser beam with power densities (PD) ranging from 2×10^3 W/cm² to 1×10^4 W/cm (SD 550 μ, BP5 to 24 W). Each adhesion is removed from its origin and insertion. Adjacent tissue injury is minimal particularly at high power densities, because laser energy dissipation is finite and limited. Therefore, adhesions arising from the bowel can be removed on the serosal surface. A glass probe is used to absorb excess energy. The adhesions separate cleanly if gentle traction is applied (Figure 20-7).

*H.F.—2 MHz generation with microcoagulation forceps using unipolar electrical circuitry.

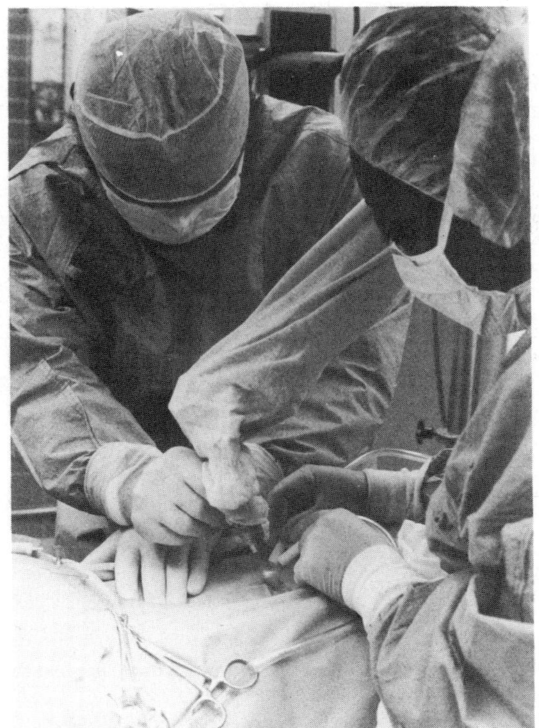

Figure 20-4 Handheld CO_2 laser used to open the abdomen.

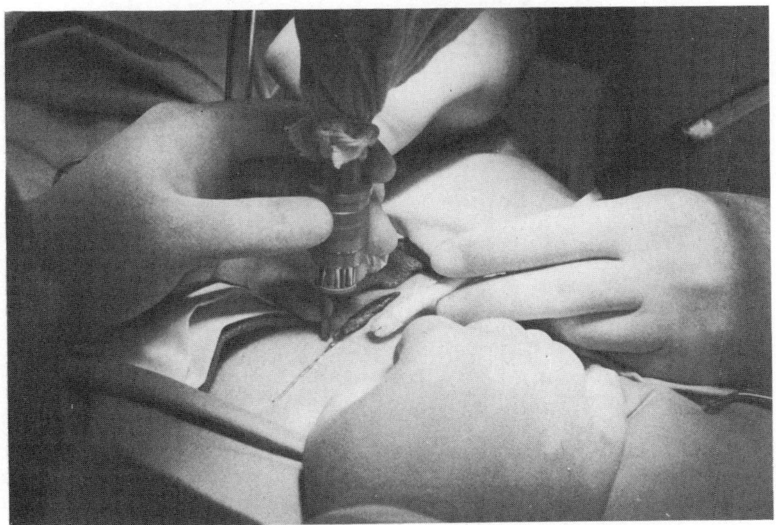

Figure 20-5 Close-up of skin incision using the CO_2 laser.

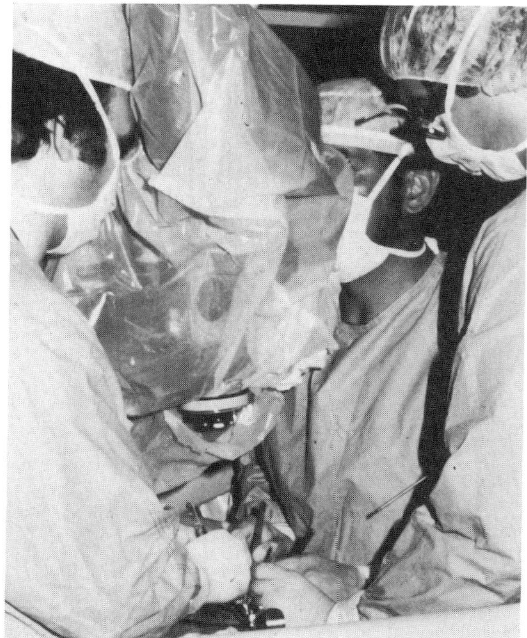

Figure 20-6 Microscopic and binocular surgical field.

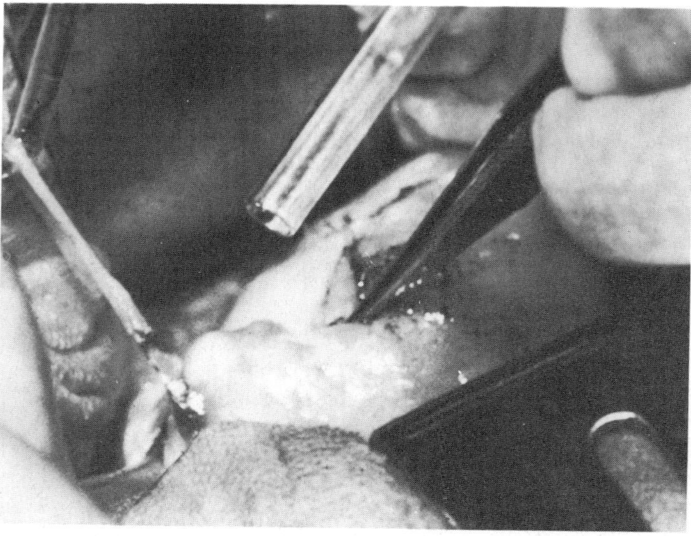

Figure 20-7 Separation of adhesions from origin. Glass rod is used to apply gentle traction. (Reproduced with permission from Bellina JH: Reconstructive microsurgery of the fallopian tube with the carbon dioxide laser: Procedures and preliminary results. *Reproduccion* 5:1–17, 1981.)

All serosal surfaces giving rise to an adhesive process are relasered with PD = 800 W/cm^2 to 1,000 W/cm^2 (BP 2 to 2.5 W), thereby reducing postoperative adhesion formation. This has been confirmed on second-look procedures and by other investigators.

Because the laser beam is electromagnetic energy, it behaves according to the laws of physics. The surgeon uses this behavior in the abdominal cavity by directing the beam with metallic mirrors. Thus, the surgeon can operate under structures, such as the ovary (Figure 20-8) and around corners. A front surface silvered mirror with an integrated light bundle* is used to remove adhesive processes inferior and lateral to the ovary by reflected energy. The utilization of energy in this fashion is a major advance made possible by this new technology. (Adhesolysis has been performed 42 times.)

Fimbrioplasty The diseased fimbria are examined and placed on saline-soaked Telfa.† Adhesive processes are removed with the use of the micromanipulated laser with PD $\cong 2 \times 10^3$ W/cm^2 to 1×10^4 W/cm^2 (BP 5 to 24 W). The tubal ostia are identified directly and/or by transillumination. If necessary, a neo-ostia can be created with the handpiece by exposing the dependent *dimple* to 1×10^5 W/cm^2 (BP 12 W) for 0.5

*Bellina front surface silvered mirror with integrated light bundle—Narco-Pilling Company.
†Telfa—The Kendall Company, Bauer and Black Division.

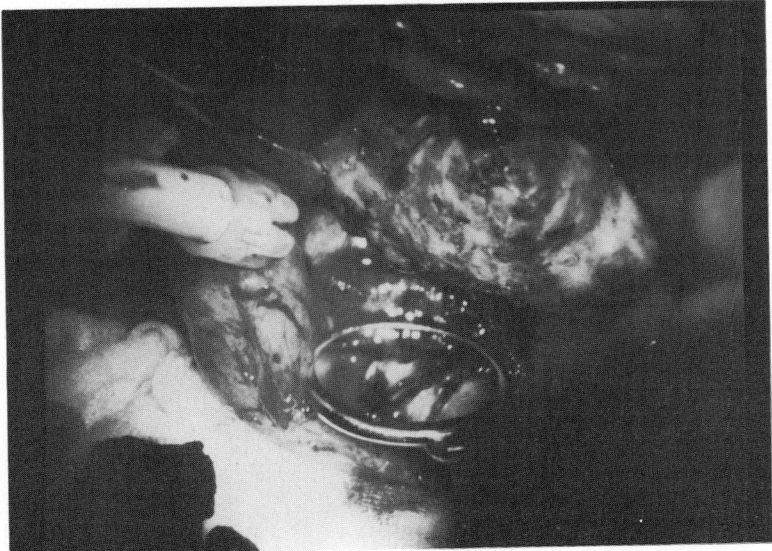

Figure 20-8 Utilization of a front surface silvered mirror to deflect beam to underside of ovary during adhesolysis. (Reproduced with permission from Bellina JH: Reconstructive microsurgery of the fallopian tube with the carbon dioxide laser: Procedures and preliminary results. *Reproduccion* 5:1–17, 1981.)

seconds. The neo-ostia is cannulated with a tapered glass probe and transilluminated. Radial incisions are made in the serosal surface as the vascular radiations are identified. Tubal distortion, tubal neovascularization, and ovarian location affect the geometric configuration of the radial incisions. The preferred geometry places the fimbrial ostia in juxtaposition to the ovarian surface.

The radial incisions are made with PD $\cong 5 \times 10^3$ W/cm^2 to 8×10^3 W/cm^2 (BP 12 to 20 W), which create precise lines of tissue separation with minimal thermal injury. The zone of thermal necrosis usually is sufficient to seal microcapillaries. Arterioles of greater than 1 mm in diameter may require HF microcoagulation. Liberal irrigation of incised surfaces with isotonic saline removes loose debris and carbonized tissue.

The serosal surface adjacent to the radial incisions are then irradiated at 100 to 300 W/cm^2 (BP 0.2 to 0.7 W). The surface heating causes linear protein contraction and tubal mucosal eversion. Usually three or four #8/0 Polyglactin 910 sutures are placed serosa to serosa to produce eversion (Figure 20-9).

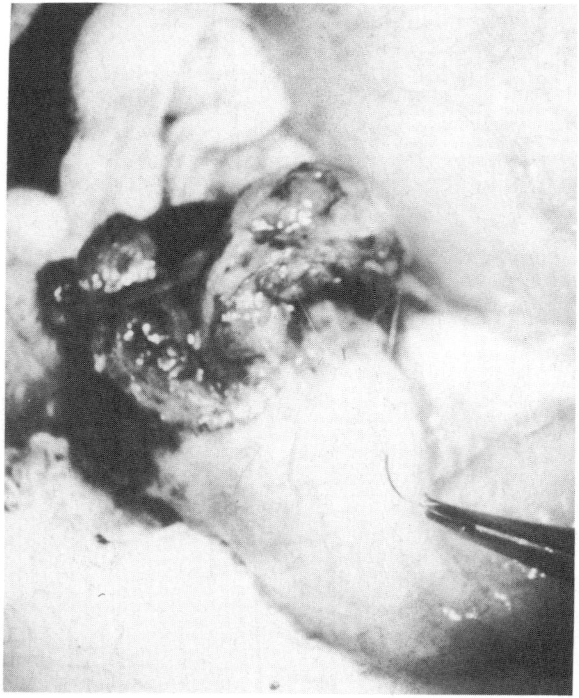

Figure 20-9 Sutures are placed in lasered fimbria to produce eversion. (Reproduced with permission from Bellina JH: Reconstructive microsurgery of the fallopian tube with the carbon dioxide laser: Procedures and preliminary results. *Reproduccion* 5:1–17, 1981.)

Mucosal surfaces are carefully evaluated for microadhesions and if found, can be removed using PD $\cong 1 \times 10^3$ W/cm^2 to 5×10^3 W/cm^2 (BP 2.5 to 12 W). Glass probes are used to absorb excess and deflected energies. Irrigation with normal saline removes loose debris and carbonized matter. Tubal patency is evaluated by hyperosmolar chromopertubation.[7] (Fimbrioplasty has been performed 24 times.)

Tubal reanastomosis The proximal and distal segments are prepared first, in similar fashion, as follows: the serosal layer is vaporized with PD $\cong$ 800 W/cm^2 to 1,000 W/cm^2 (BP 2 to 2.5 W), thereby exposing the muscular coat. The muscular coat is then incised to the mucosa with PD $\cong 5 \times 10^3$ W/cm^2 (BP 12 W) (Figure 20-10). Mucosal division is performed by cold instruments. Each segment is irrigated free of debris and carbonized matter with isotonic saline. Patency is assured by antigrade H:chromo-pertubation and retrograde chromo-pertubation. Retrograde chromo-pertubation is performed by cannulating the fimbria with a #18 gauge Jelco Silastic catheter. A standard isotonic chromo-pertubation solution is used to assure luminal patency in the distal segment.

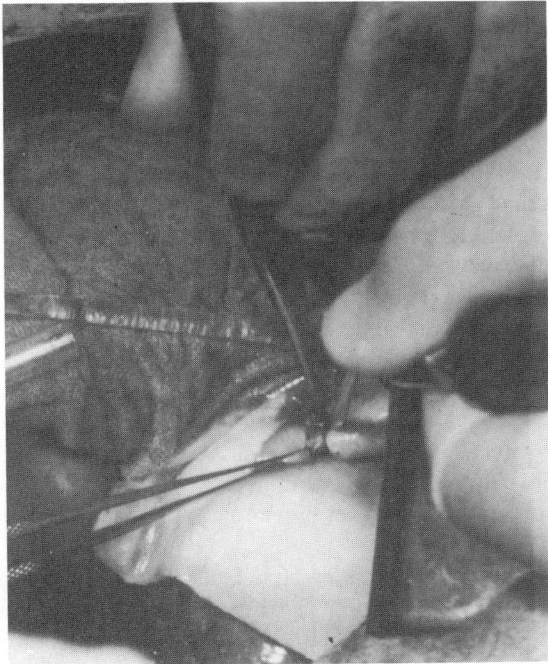

Figure 20-10 Muscular coat of fallopian tube is incised only to the mucosa. (Reproduced with permission from Bellina JH: Reconstructive microsurgery of the fallopian tube with the carbon dioxide laser: Procedures and preliminary results. *Reproduccion* 5:1–17, 1981.)

Anastomosis of the tubal segments is accomplished by microsuturing, not laser welding. The mesosalpinx is approximated with #6/0 Polyglactin 910 suture and four #8/0 Polyglactin 910 sutures are placed at 6, 9, 12, and 3 o'clock in the muscular coat. Care is exercised to avoid mucosal suturing. A final layer of #8/0 Polyglactin 910 is placed at 4, 8, 10, and 2 o'clock in the serosal layer. No guides or stints are used. Luminal apposition is demonstrated by gentle H:chromo-pertubation.

In certain sterilization cases, the ampullary segments have been severed leaving a terminal fimbrial cul-de-sac arrangement. In these special cases, a glass probe is placed in the fimbrial cul-de-sac, with transillumination and pressure applied. Under direct microscopic view, the avascular fibrotic site is vaporized in a drill fashion. This aperture is enlarged to accommodate the proximal ampullary segment. Suturing is then performed in the muscular and serosal layers. (Tubal reanastomosis has been performed 12 times.)

Cornual reimplantation This procedure is technically the most difficult of all fallopian tube microsurgical procedures and therefore, must be performed with extreme care. After appropriate abdominal preparation, the fundus is exposed. The site for reimplantation is chosen to avoid venous and arterial plexus, if possible. The myometrium is then infiltrated with vasopressin (1 ml of 1:2,000 vasopressin in 5 ml normal saline) through a #30 gauge needle. The uterine cavity is distended with hypertonic solution at a pressure of >150 mm Hg. This solution compresses the endometrium and absorbs the extra laser energy. A cornual neo-ostia is created using the 50 mm handheld laser applicator with PD $\cong 5 \times 10^5$ W/cm^2 (SD 125 μ, BP 60 W) (Figure 20-11). A cylindrical incision is completed, and the excised myometrium submitted for histopathologic examination. Aerobic and anaerobic cultures are now taken of the neo-ostia. Intrauterine fluid pressure is reduced to stop transabdominal flow. The diameter of the neo-ostia is enlarged sufficiently to accept the distal tubal segment. A microruler is used to assure proper calibration.

The distal tubal site is prepared by vaporizing the serosal surface with PD $\cong$ 800 W/cm^2 (BP 2 W). This process exposes the tubal muscle. The terminal tubal fimbriotic cap is incised with PD $\cong 1 \times 10^5$ W/cm^2 (BP 12 W) to the mucosa level by the handheld scalpel. The mucosa is incised with cold instruments.

After the lased sites are irrigated free of all debris and carbonized matter, the distal tubal segment is transfixed into the cornual neo-ostia with #6/0 and #8/0 Polyglactin 910 sutures (Figure 20-12). This technique assures mucosa-to-mucosa, muscle-to-muscle, and serosa-to-serosa closures. A water tight seal is not necessary and no splinting is used. Final aerobic and anaerobic cultures are taken at the fimbria segment, and patency is tested by pressurizing the intrauterine hypertonic solution. (Cornual reimplantation has been performed eight times.)

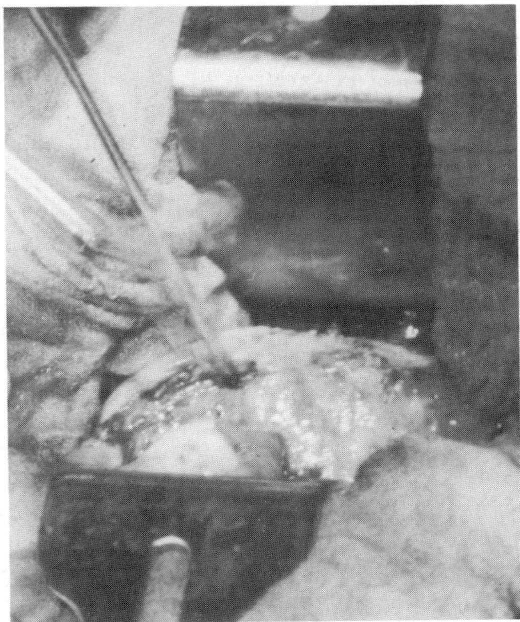

Figure 20-11 Drilling the cornual neo-ostia with the handheld CO_2 laser for cornual reimplantation. (Reproduced with permission from Bellina JH: Reconstructive microsurgery of the fallopian tube with the carbon dioxide laser: Procedures and preliminary results. *Reproduccion* 5:1–17, 1981.)

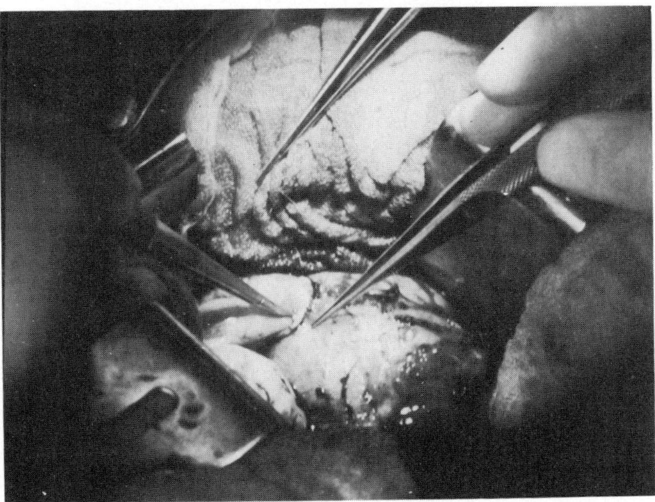

Figure 20-12 Sutures are placed for the cornual reimplantation. (Reproduced with permission from Bellina JH: Reconstructive microsurgery of the fallopian tube with the carbon dioxide laser: Procedures and preliminary results. *Reproduccion* 5:1–17, 1981.)

POSTOPERATIVE MANAGEMENT

During microsurgical procedures, all patients receive methylprednisolone sodium succinate at a rate of 100 mg/hr. The same medication and dose is continued for the first 24 hours, then replaced by methylprednisolone 15 gm/24 hrs for five days with declining doses over the next five days. Doxycycline 100 mg/12 hrs is administered intravenously, then orally for ten days. Adjustment in antimicrobial therapy is based upon cultures taken at surgery. At the termination of all surgical procedures, the abdomen is irrigated with 1,500 ml to 2,000 ml of normal saline, then 100 ml of 70,000 molecular weight (mol wt). Dextran is added and the peritoneum closed. The patients are usually ambulatory the first day postoperatively and are placed on a regular diet.

Postoperative danazol 800 mg/24 hrs for three months has been used to suppress endometriotic nodules in cases of cornual reimplantation. Suppression for 30 days prior to surgery and continued suppression for 60 days following surgery is currently being used in those cases in which endometrial spillage is expected.

Hysterosalpingographic studies with cinefluorography using atraumatic techniques are done prior to discharge on the fifth to seventh day. Hysterosalpingograms are performed using water soluble contrast media mixed with 100 mg of hydrocortisone succinate and 25 mg of 1% lidocaine. The total mixture is 30 ml. Cinefluorography is used in all hysterosalpingograms in an attempt to prevent needless pressure upon suture lines with excessively high instillation rates. X-rays are taken according to standard procedures, labeled, and kept for future follow-up. The video record is similarly processed.

At one, three, and six months patients complete a follow-up questionnaire about complications, menstruation, general health, and personal gynecologist's evaluations. If the patient has not conceived by the third month a repeat of the hysterosalpingogram and second-look laparoscopy is performed.

Should conception be suspected, patients are instructed to obtain confirmation via serum beta subunit pregnancy test. If positive, echograms are immediately ordered to document conception and to determine placement of the conceptus. This serves as an early detection for ectopic pregnancy.

RESULTS

The status among the 73 cases performed during 1980 is shown in Table 20-1. A large portion (68%) of the patient population is not at risk of conception for various reasons. These include postoperative danazol therapy or endocrine therapy. Some husbands are currently undergoing treatment, and some patients are voluntarily not at risk for reasons relating to their marital situations. A significant proportion of these cases are expected to be at risk in the near future. Continuing follow-up will monitor their conception status.

Table 20-1
Status Among 73 Cases Performed in 1980

Status	No.	%
Not at risk of conception	50	68.5
At risk of conception	23	31.5
Total	73	100.0

Ten of the 23 cases at risk of pregnancy (43.5%) have conceived as of March 1981 (Table 20-2). Four tubal pregnancies resulted and seven intrauterine pregnancies were documented. Considering the limited exposure to pregnancy of this sample population, the conception rates can be considered encouraging.

Table 20-2
Conception Status Among 23 Patients at Risk

Status	No.	%	No.	%
Not conceived	13	56.5		
1–3 months at risk			7	53.8
4–6 months at risk			3	23.1
7–12 months at risk			3	23.1
13+ months at risk			0	00.0
Conceived*	10	43.5		
Tubal pregnancy			4	36.4
Intrauterine pregnancy			7	63.6
Total conceptions			11	100.0
Total patients	23	100.0		

*One patient experienced two pregnancies.

Among the patients who have not conceived, more than half (53%) have been at risk only one to three months. Longer follow-up will be required in order to determine their conception potential.

The status of the seven intrauterine pregnancies is detailed in Table 20-3. One spontaneous abortion was experienced; another abortion resulted from an automobile accident (this patient is now pregnant for the second time); one live birth was documented and four intrauterine pregnancies are continuing.

Table 20-3
Status of Seven Intrauterine Pregnancies Following Laser Microsurgery as of March 1981

Outcome	No.	%
Spontaneous abortion	1	14.3
Traumatic abortion*	1	14.3
Continuing pregnancy	4	57.1
Live birth	1	14.3
Total	7	100.0

*Automobile accident.

It is important to note that the patients in this series required complicated combinations of procedures to reestablish patency and fully reconstruct the pelvic anatomy. Many of the 73 cases had extensive endometriosis and multiple dense adhesions, and some presented with the sequelae of previous failed conventional microsurgery. The conception rates must be interpreted with these facts in mind.

A profile of the ten patients who experienced conception following laser tubal microsurgery is exhibited in Table 20-4. The difficulty of reconstruction is evident. The fact that these patients conceived is

Table 20-4
Profile of Patients With Conceptions and Type of Conception

	Patient Number									
Procedures	*1*	*2*	*3*	*4*	*5*	*6*	*7*	*8*	*9*	*10*
Left										
Cornual implant						*		*		
Anastomosis			*							
Adhesiolysis	*	*	*	*	*	*	*	*	*	*
Neosalpingostomy										
Fimbrioplasty	*	*		*			*			*
Other						*				
Right		X	X							
Cornual implant						*		*		
Anastomosis										
Adhesiolysis	*			*	*	*	*	*	*	*
Neosalpingostomy										
Fimbrioplasty	*			*	*		*			*
Other				*		*				
Ablation of endometriosis	*								*	
Myomectomy									*	
Type of conception*	U	U	T	U	U	T	T	T	U	U

X = No tube preoperatively or salpingectomy and/or oophorectomy
*T = Tubal pregnancy
*U = Uterine pregnancy

evidence of the value of laser microsurgery for surgically correctable fertility dysfunction. Further evidence will accumulate as most patients in this series become at risk and experience conceptions. Replication of these results can be expected to occur as other experienced laser surgeons begin to use this instrument.

SUMMARY

Laser tubal microsurgery is still in its infancy. Methods will continue to undergo refinement as well instrumentation. The success with which this approach has been employed, however, even in extremely difficult cases, is encouraging. The diminished operating time which results from reduced bleeding is particularly beneficial to the patient. Obliteration of extensive dense adhesions and endometriotic implants is impressive. This surgical modality, in the hands of a trained laser surgeon and competent microsurgeon, may increase the probability for successful outcome of tubal reconstruction in various clinical situations. This author's experience with over 100 cases and the reported experience of other laser surgeons suggests this modality is of benefit in microsurgery.

ACKNOWLEDGMENTS

The author wishes to express his appreciation to Mary Ann Riopelle for editorial assistance and photographs, to V. Bewig, Jr., for his photographs and masterful darkroom work. Sincere thanks is extended to Donna Yost for excellent typing of this manuscript.

REFERENCES

1. Bellina JH: Reconstructive microsurgery of the fallopian tube using the CO_2 laser: Results of the first 46 cases. Presented at the Mainz Congress of Gynecological CO_2 Laser Surgery, Mainz, W. Germany, May 1980.

2. Bruhat MA, Mage G, Pouly JL: Use of the CO_2 laser in neosalpingostomy. Presented at the International Congress on Laser Surgery, Gratz, Austria, 1979.

3. Bruhat MA, Mage G, Jacquetin B, et al: Laser CO_2 in tubal surgery in Bellina JH, et al (eds): *Gynecologic Laser Surgery*. New York, Plenum Press, 1981 (in press).

4. Klink F, Grosspietzsch R, Klitzing LV, et al: Animal in-vivo studies and in-vitro experiments with human tubes for end-to-end anastomotic operation by a CO_2 laser technique. *Fertil Steril* 30:100–102, 1978.

5. Grosspietzsch R, Inthraphuvasak I, Klink F, et al: Experiments on CO_2 laser techniques for operative treatment of tubar sterility, in Bellina, et al (eds): *Gynecologic Laser Surgery*. New York, Plenum Press, 1981 (in press).

6. Grosspietzsch R, Schulz BO, Klink F, et al: Experiments on salpingolysis during refertilization operations by CO_2 laser technique, in Bellina JH, et al (eds): *Gynecologic Laser Surgery*. New York, Plenum Press, 1981 (in press).

7. Bellina JH: Reconstructive microsurgery of the fallopian tube with the carbon dioxide laser: Procedure and preliminary results. *Reproduccion* 5:1–17, 1981.

21 Intra-Abdominal Use in Gynecology

Michael S. Baggish, MD

Although the CO_2 laser has had extensive application in gynecology and several reports describing its therapeutic effects have appeared in contemporary literature,[1-3] very few publications have been written about the intra-abdominal use of this instrument.

Initial studies employing the CO_2 laser for experimental oviductal anastomosis and adhesiolysis were presented at the International Society for Laser Surgery Congress in Graz, Austria, 1979 and at the First World Congress of the Gynecologic Laser Society, New Orleans, 1980.[4,5] The results of animal and human microsurgical techniques on the uterine tube utilizing the CO_2 laser have only recently appeared in the current gynecological literature.[6] Investigations on intra-abdominal laser surgery were initiated at Mt. Sinai Hospital in 1979. Several operations are now considered routine, but patients are selected carefully for this type of laser surgery. All women receive suitable informed consent prior to the laser procedure; emphasis is placed on the newness of the technique and the lack of long-term follow-up.

The principal factors responsible for the growth of CO_2 laser technology in gynecology relate to: 1) precision for cutting tissue, 2) relative hemostasis, 3) ability to reach otherwise poorly accessible areas, and 4) beneficial unobstructed vision when directed through the microscope (ie, does not take up space in the operative field).

Although laser wounds do not heal as rapidly as fresh scalpel incisions,[7] the absence of ligatures in laser-treated tissue helps to promote rapid healing with minimal scar formation. The latter property makes laser surgery particularly advantageous for microtubular anastomosis and adhesion vaporization. As with any fine, skilled technique, the experience of the operator is of paramount importance. Certain precautions peculiar to the intra-abdominal operative site need to be implemented in conjunction with the use of the CO_2 laser. Special instruments and tissue handling techniques are required.

INSTRUMENTATION

Two types of laser machines were employed for these results. Early in the program, a Coherent model 400 CO_2 laser (two cases were performed with a model 450) was used for animal experiments and human microsurgical procedures. This laser delivered power up to 40 watts (W). At a focal distance of 300 mm, it produced a spot measuring 1.5 mm in diameter. A Sharplan, model 733 CO_2 laser has been used recently for seven months and has been coupled to a Zeiss OPMI 7 double-headed microscope with fiberoptic illumination. This laser provides power up to 38 W and delivers a spot of < 1 mm when focused at 300 mm. Both CO_2 lasers operate with a coincident helium-neon laser, which provides a visible red aiming beam. These two lasers produce a beam with an obvious fundamental difference; ie, the spot produced by the Coherent laser is donut-shaped (TEM 01 STAR MODE) whereas, that of the Sharplan laser has the characteristic point of TEM 00. Both instruments have proven to be highly dependable apparatuses with adequate safety features.

ADDITIONAL EQUIPMENT

In order to properly manipulate delicate structures during microsurgical procedures, specialized instruments are required. Rather than sponging tissues, irrigating solutions, eg, balanced Ringer's irrigation, warmed to 98° F and delivered via a 10 cc syringe with an 18-gauge blunt Luer-lock cannula, are used. Number 2 to 7 jeweler's forceps and Barraguer-type needle holders, together with 6-0 Vicryl and 8-0 nylon sutures, replace standard gynecologic operative instruments and suture material. Initially, we employed moistened tongue depressors behind tissue to be treated in order to protect neighboring structures from stray laser beams. Although the tongue blades absorbed the light energy advantageously, they were unwieldy. Tissue was next manipulated with glass rods, which were placed behind the adhesions and tubes prior to cutting with the laser. Unfortunately, the impact of the laser energy on the glass led to material fatigue and, on one occasion, a glass rod fractured and had to be retrieved from the abdomen. We now employ stainless steel, Teflon-coated manipulating rods of various sizes and shapes (Figure 21-1). Not only are these Teflon rods useful to manipulate tissue, but serve to absorb stray energy from the laser beam. Most recently, we have employed quartz rods to manipulate tissues.

ANIMAL STUDIES

Prior to using the CO_2 laser for humans, it was advisable to study the effects of the laser beam on animal tissues. We opened the abdomens of several animals, including dogs, rabbits, and rats, with the laser and studied healing after laser treatment. In all animals, the laser-induced skin incision healed more slowly than the knife wounds. Laser incisions were also cut into the uteri and tubes of rabbits and the healing effects noted. Initial investigations on rabbits who were sterilized, reopened, and then subjected to tubal reanastomosis, recently have been reported.[8]

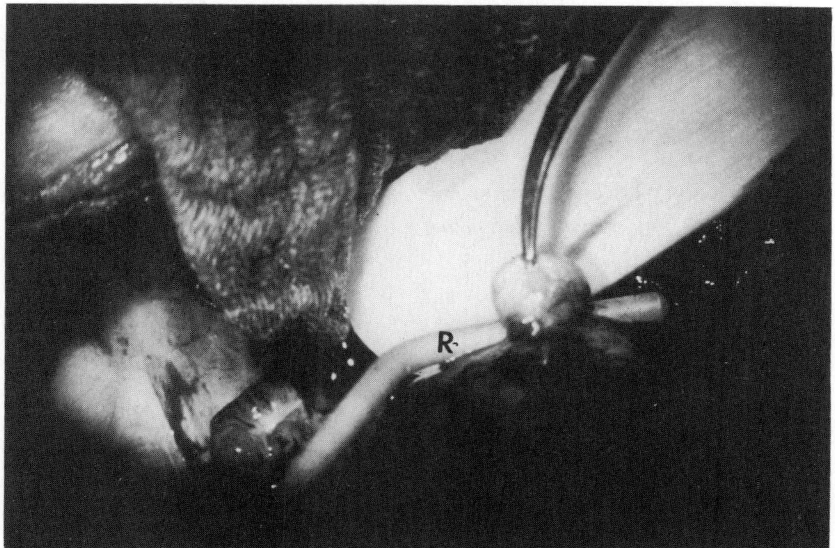

Figure 21-1 Teflon-coated stainless steel manipulating rod (R) placed behind a uterine myoma prior to laser excision.

Another timely experiment was conducted on an additional five rabbits who underwent sterilization, relaparotomy, and laser excision of the obstructed segments (Figure 21-2). Six weeks later, these animals were sacrificed and their tubes examined. The reunited tubes had healed and merged imperceptibly with the remainder of the tube. No adhesions were seen. The principal benefit of the laser over conventional scalpel microsurgery was the hemostasis produced by the laser, which in turn diminished manipulations of the tube prior to anastomosis. The precision of cutting by means of a micromanipulator was of substantial advantage.

HUMAN TUBAL AND ADHESIOLYSIS SURGERY

Initial studies on the application of CO_2 laser microsurgical techniques for women in the United States have recently been published[8] (Figures 21-3 to 5).

The preceding cases, as well as recent laser tuboplastic procedures, are always preceded by a complete infertility investigation. This workup includes a preoperative hysterosalpingogram, diagnostic laparoscopy,

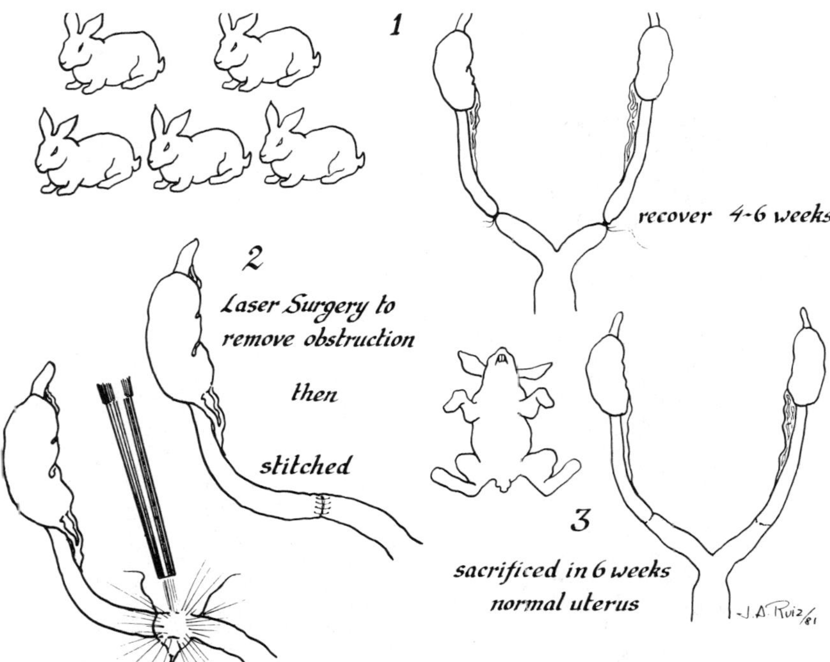

Figure 21-2 Schematic outline of second series of rabbit experiment utilizing the CO_2 laser.

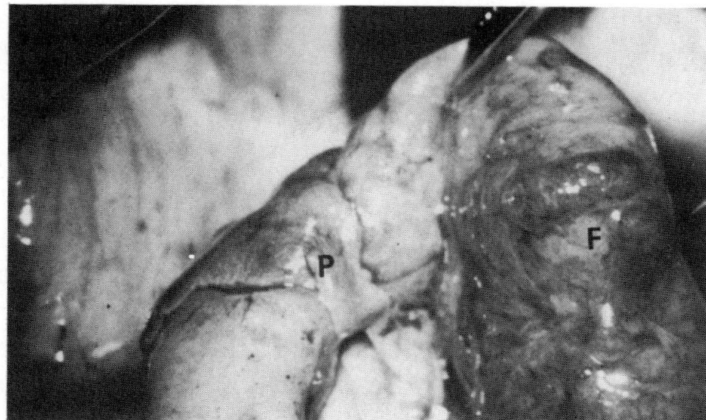

Figure 21-3 The tube has been anastomosed and a flap of peritoneum (P) is "welded" to the adjoining serosa of the oviduct. The fimbriated end of the tube is in the foreground (F).

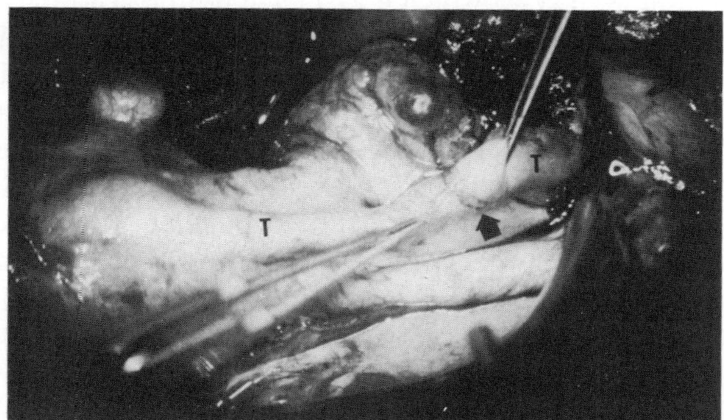

Figure 21-4 The tube (T) has complete obstruction of the isthmus secondary to pelvic inflammatory disease. A laser incision (arrow) is made at the level of the ampulla.

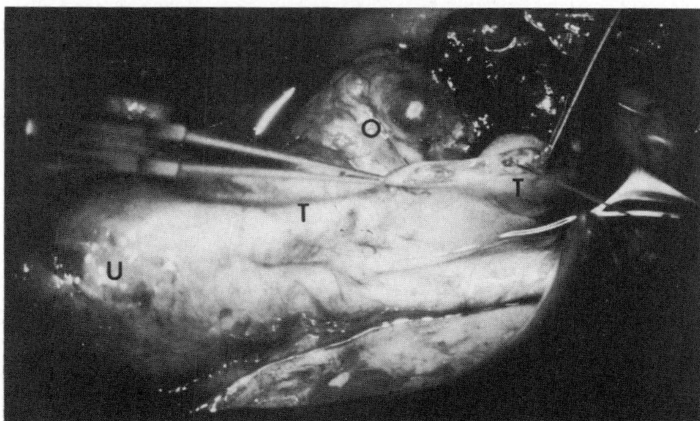

Figure 21-5 The incision is complete. The distal tube (T) in the forceps shows occlusion whereas the proximal tube has a probe in the lumen. (uterus, U and ovary, O)

and chromatubation. Women complaining of pelvic pain underwent complete investigations to exclude intestinal, urinary tract, or other system etiology. These women also underwent diagnostic laparoscopy prior to laparotomy.

Following CO_2 laser microsurgery, 200 ml of 32% dextran 70 is placed into the peritoneal cavity to reduce adhesion formation. Although the high molecular weight of dextran's action is unknown, several animal studies have shown it to diminish the development of postoperative adhesions. It has been postulated the slippery material coats the tissue and thereby prevents the structures from adhesing together. Others suggest the dextran floats the intraperitoneal structures (ie, hydroflotation) and thus prevents adhesions from occurring.

During operative procedures, all manipulations are accomplished by means of Teflon-coated stainless steel rods. Another adjunct to providing additional hemostasis is the injection of a 1:30 solution of vasopressin via a 1 cc tuberculin syringe to which a 27-gauge needle is attached (Figures 21-6 to 8). The laser plays a dual role as a cutting and hemostatic instrument. Cutting is accomplished most effectively at power densities of 1000 to 2000 W/cm^2.

To obtain hemostasis, irrigation is first carried out with Ringer's lactate, then a cotton-tipped applicator is rolled away while the laser (time interval at 0.2 sec) is activated and microcoagulation is accomplished (Figure 21-9). For larger vessels, subserosal pitressin produces additional vasoconstriction before laser coagulation. The laser has been useful to open "clubbed" tubes (ie, fimbrioplasty), to excise obstructed segments for end-to-end anastomosis, and for cornual shaving.

Fifteen patients with chronic pelvic pain had CO_2 laser lysis of peritubal, periovarian, utero-ovarian, uterotubal, and utero-enteric adhesiolysis. One major advantage was the ability to precisely separate

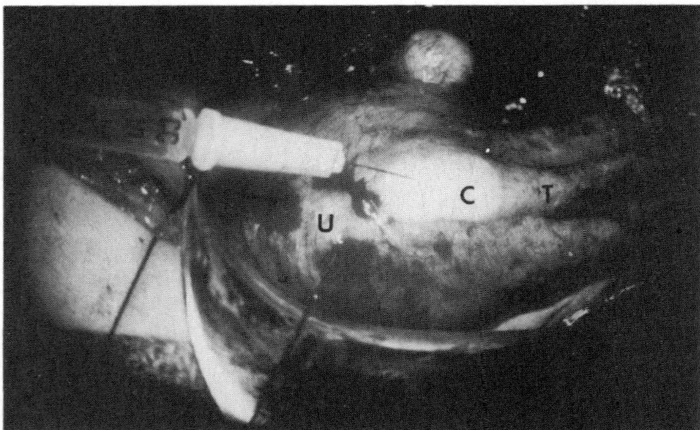

Figure 21-6 Cornual shaving is initiated by an injection of a 1:30 solution of vasopressin into the cornua (C) of the uterus (U). The tube (T) proximal to the cornua (C) is occluded.

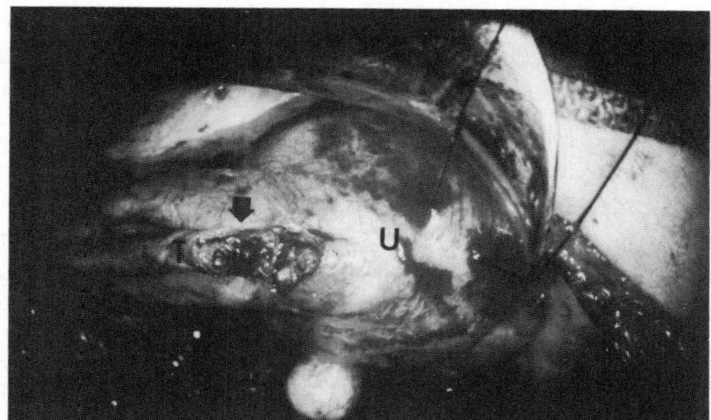

Figure 21-7 A laser incision has been made into the cornua and a small vessel is oozing blood (arrow).

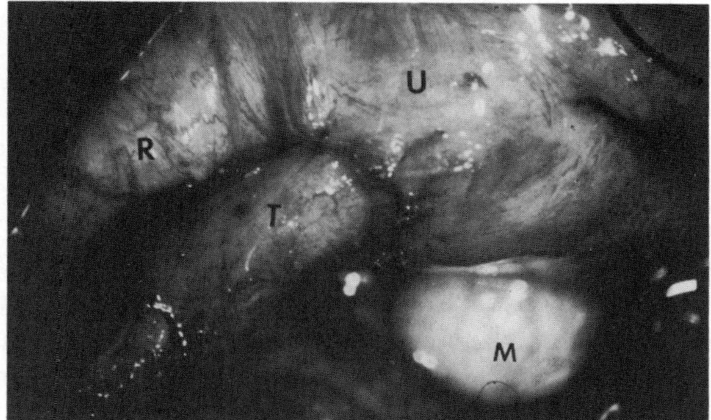

Figure 21-8 An ampullary-cornual end-to-end anastomosis has been completed (T). The round ligament (R), posterior uterus (U) and a small myoma (M) are clearly seen.

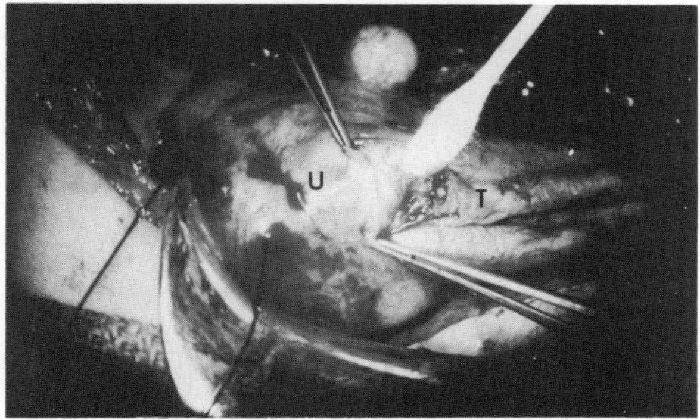

Figure 21-9 The vessel is tamponaded by a cotton-tipped applicator. As the applicator is rolled away, the laser beam (at low power density) coagulates the vessel.

the adhesions bloodlessly under microscopic control. The advantage of magnification to appreciate proximity of vessels, direction of adhesive bands, and appearance of tissue planes is substantial (Figures 21-10 to 13). The laser technique does not take up additional space in the limited field as is the case with conventional operative methodology. In four patients who had repeat diagnostic laparoscopy subsequent to laser adhesiolysis, none had reformation of adhesions and all were free of pain. As with the tuboplastic group of patients, 200 ml dextran 70 was instilled into the pelvis prior to closing the abdomen.

Emphasis must be directed toward securing neighboring structures from stray laser beams. Protective rods placed behind the target tissue and isolation of the field with wet abdominal pads have prevented inadvertent injury to date. Smoke evacuation has been carried out with the standard suction apparatus used for microsurgery. A small odor-evacuating cartridge was placed between the suction line and the pump.

TREATMENT OF ENDOMETRIOSIS

Ten women with pelvic endometriosis were treated by means of the CO_2 laser. Table 21-1 details the extent of endometriosis based upon stage of severity. It was thought the CO_2 laser might prove useful for therapy of this disorder because the laser is precise, affords accessibility to obscure areas, vaporizes in a bloodless field, and is superbly suited to preserve surrounding normal tissue. Half of the ten cases were performed with the free arm and handpiece; the other 50% were done with the microscope. Small spots of endometriosis (ie, up to 3 mm) were treated at 300 W/cm^2; whereas 700 W/cm^2 was employed for larger implants and endometriomas. Initially, as the laser beam hits the endometrial implant, brownish fluid exits the lesion, sizzles, then vaporizes completely (Figures

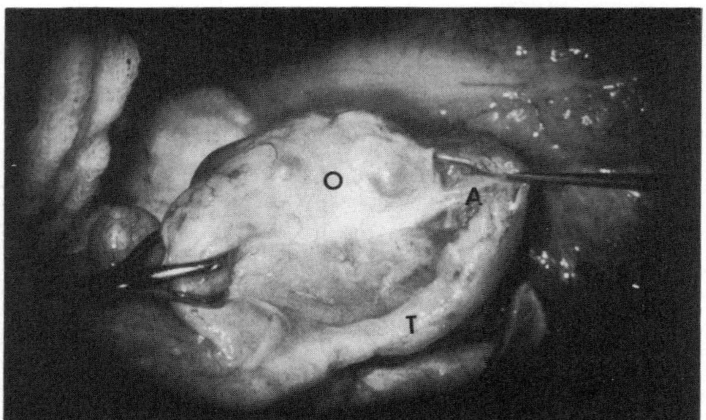

Figure 21-10 Series of four photographs (Figures 21-10 to 13) shows the tube (T) adhered to the ovary (O) by adhesions (A).

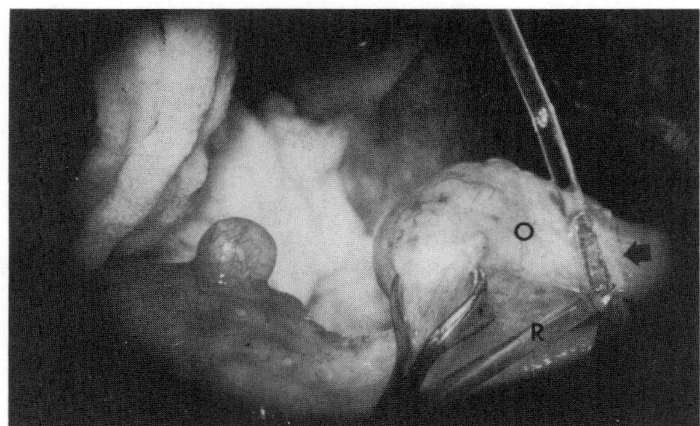

Figure 21-11 A glass manipulating rod (R) has been placed behind one layer of adhesions and the CO_2 laser beam begins to separate the scar tissue (arrow).

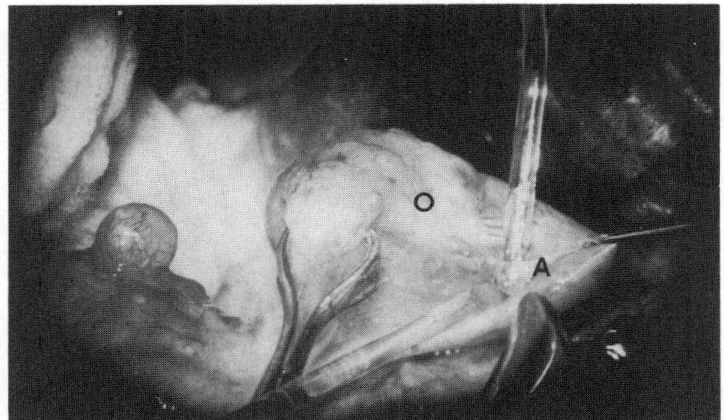

Figure 21-12 The adhesion (A) is almost completely separated. Note the cleavage plane is precise. There is both a lack of bleeding and charring.

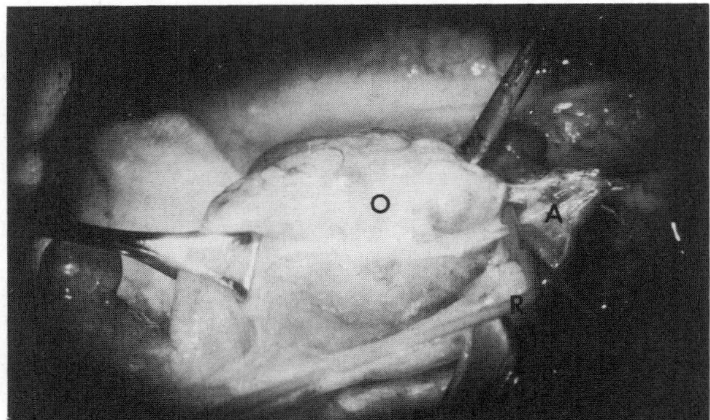

Figure 21-13 A Teflon-coated stainless steel rod (R) has been inserted between the final adhesive band (A) joining the ovary (O) to the tube.

21-14 to 17). The proper depth has been reached when no further fluid or sizzling is observed. Biopsies, which were carried out after treatment, have indicated the endometriosis was completely destroyed.

Table 21-1
Classification* of Patients Treated for Endometriosis with the CO_2 Laser

Classification	Number	Percent
Mild	3	30%
Moderate	5	50%
Severe	2	20%
Total	10	100%

*American Fertility Society.

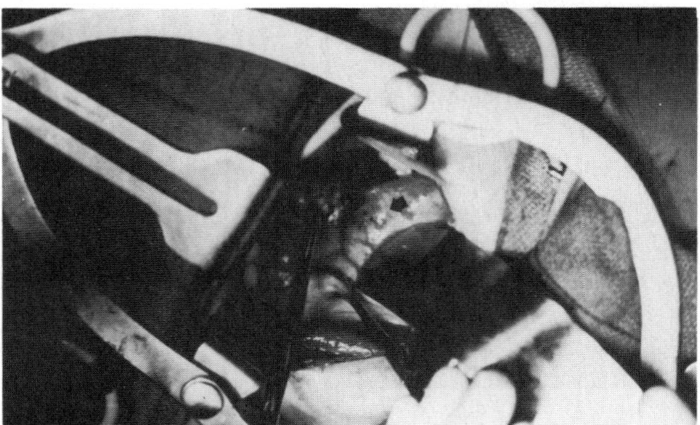

Figure 21-14 The ovary is exposed revealing several spots (arrow) of endometriosis.

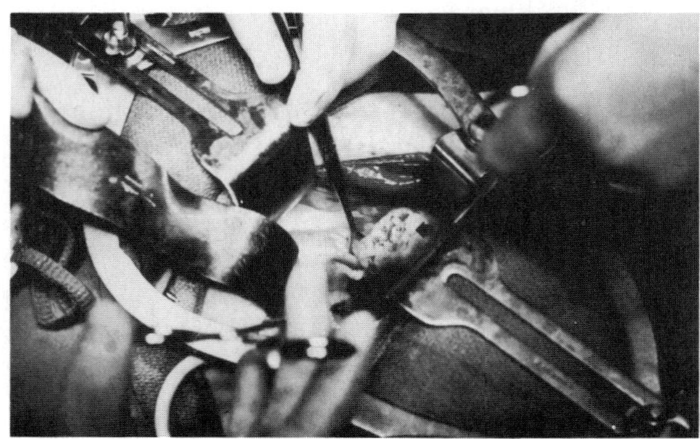

Figure 21-15 The ovarian endometrial implants have been vaporized (arrow) by a laser beam directed by the free arm and hand piece.

The fine laser beam is very well suited to reach spots in the cul-de-sac of Douglas, on and around the uterosacral ligaments, and in other recessed regions of the abdominal cavity (Figure 21-18). The surrounding intestine must be protected by a thorough dousing with water and protective moist packs. We have utilized the laser to drain and/or excise endometriotic cysts (Figure 21-19). This methodology was proven most helpful when such lesions were stuck in the cul-de-sac, making sharp dissection very difficult.

The goal of endometriosis surgery is to remove the ectopic endometrial tissue while maintaining assiduous hemostasis. Postoperatively, all patients were placed on danazol or oral contraceptive therapy in order to inhibit recurrence of the disorder.

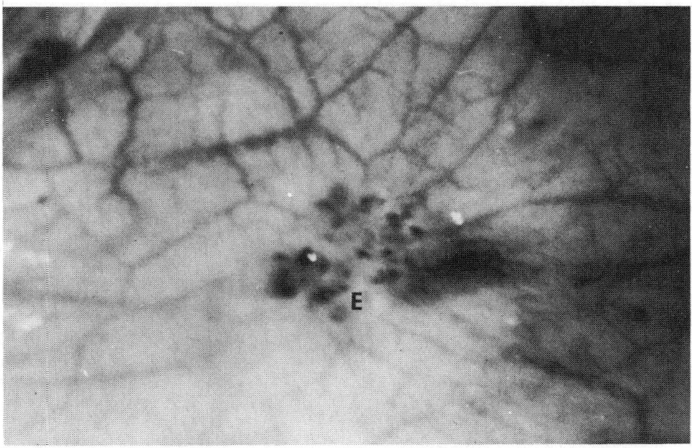

Figure 21-16 Deep in the cul-de-sac several foci of endometriosis (E) are visualized through the microscope.

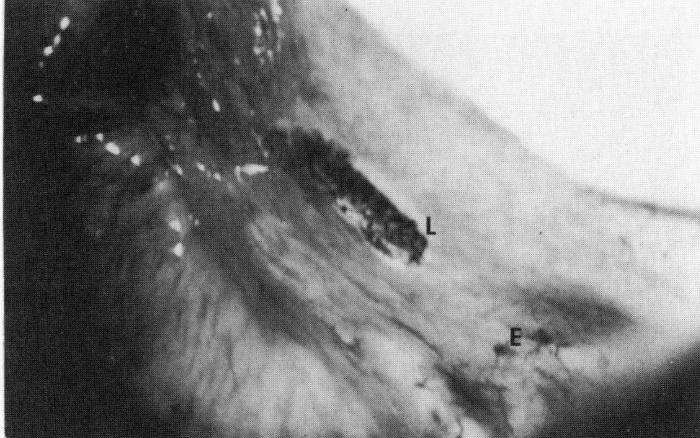

Figure 21-17 Several foci of endometriosis have been vaporized (L), but two tiny remnants remain to be destroyed (E).

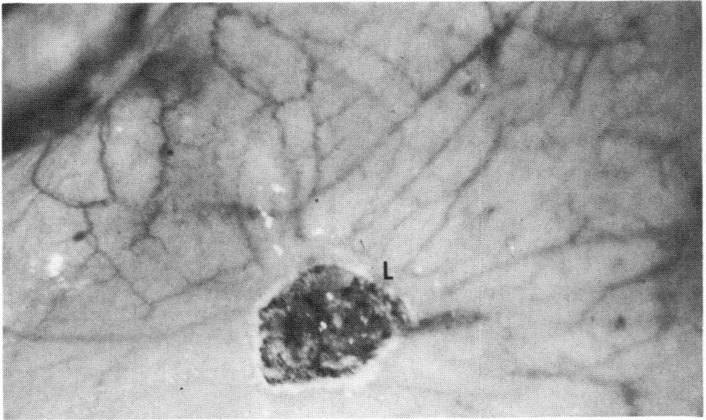

Figure 21-18 Highly magnified view of endometriosis partially vaporized. Some brownish fluid emits from the center of the lesion (L).

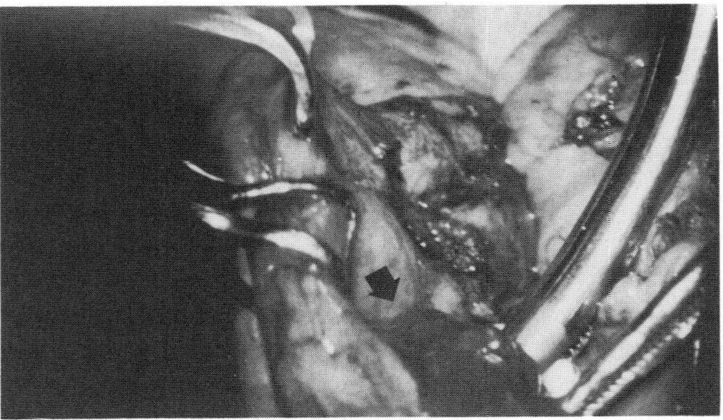

Figure 21-19 A fixed endometriotic cyst is drained (arrow) by drilling a hole into the mass with the CO_2 laser. Viscous chocolate fluid emits at the arrow.

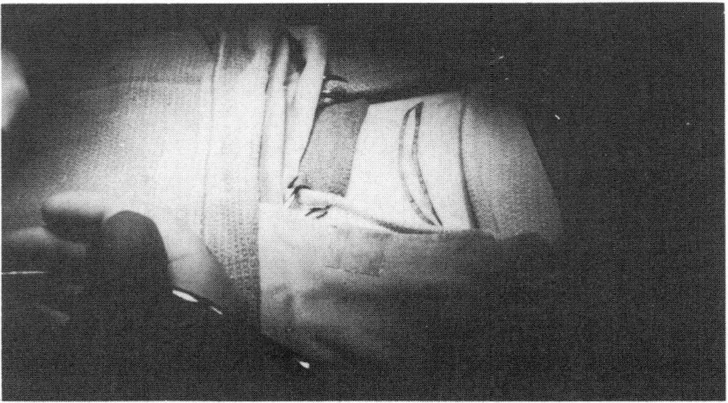

Figure 21-20 CO_2 laser incision into the anterior abdominal skin removes a previous scar. The principal advantage of the laser at this site relates to complete hemostasis.

LASER TO OPEN THE ABDOMINAL WALL

The free arm laser has been used to open the skin and deeper tissues of the abdominal wall (except the peritoneum) in 25 women. Although this technique requires more time than opening with the scalpel, the hemostasis obtained probably saves 10 to 15 minutes of operating time. We have also used the laser to our advantage for cutting and dividing the rectus muscles with low transverse incisions. The wounds are virtually bloodless and the incision line is sharp (Figures 21-20, 21). It is not advantageous to close these wounds with a subcuticular technique. Similarly, the skin seems to heal more slowly following laser incision, and we, therefore, allow sutures to remain in place an extra 72 hours.

MICROSCOPIC STUDIES

The question arises as to what effect laser energy has on oviductal tissue. Since the success of reanastomosis depends on minimizing scar formation, the answer is critical. Obviously, the thermal effect of the laser beam will produce tissue necrosis. Scar formation is dependent on the extent of necrosis, as well as the intensity of the foreign body reaction secondary to suture material. Poor control of bleeding points invariably leads to adhesion formation. Hematoxylin and eosin sections and scanning electron microscopic studies of the laser-treated uterine tube indicate substantial tissue destruction at the impact zone.[8]

Recent transmission electron microscopic (TEM) studies of the human oviduct after laser excision reveal discrete structural changes. At 500 μ from impact the mitochondria are swollen, the cells show sparse cytoplasmic elements, and there is electron transparency. At 1000 μ, the cells are normal (Figures 21-22 to 25).

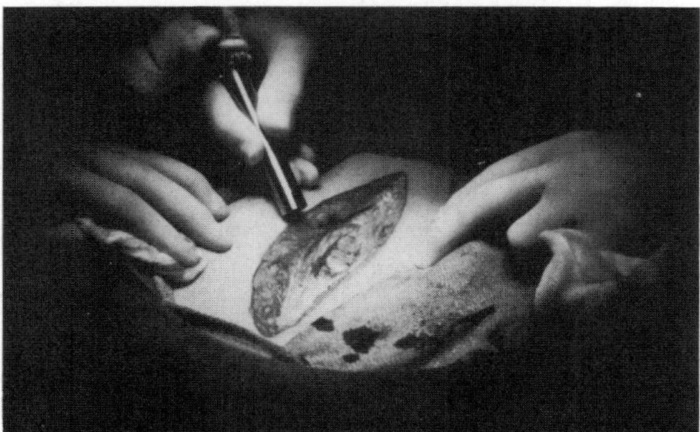

Figure 21-21 The incision above has been extended through the subcutaneous tissue. The laser beam begins to incise the rectus sheath.

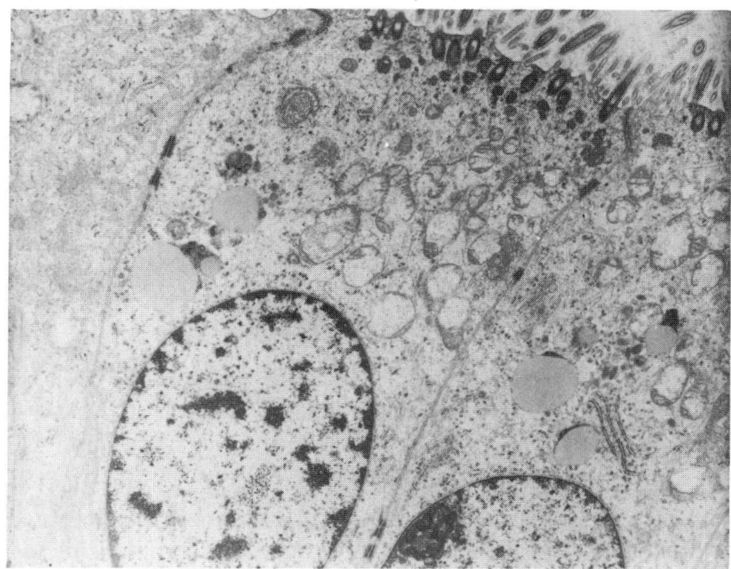

Figure 21-22 Transmission electron microscope (TEM) section of human oviduct at 500 μ GK 36 from impact. Swelling of mitochondria and electron transparency is shown. There are sparse cytoplasmic elements (27,800 ×).

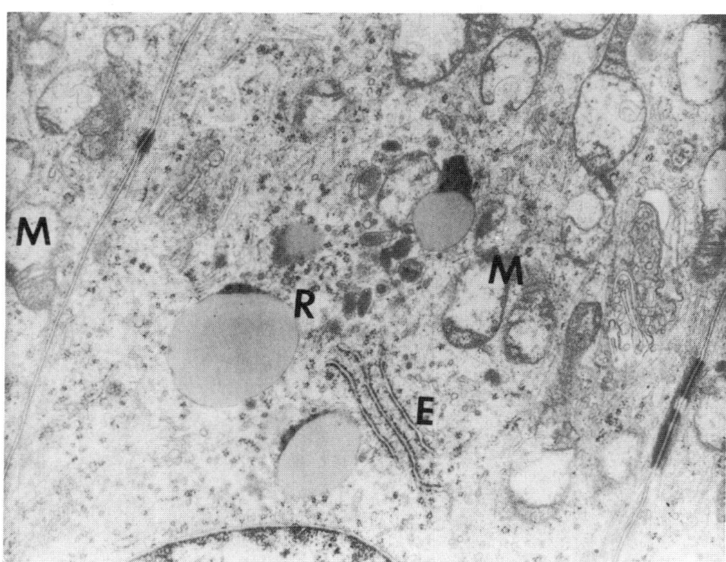

Figure 21-23 Transmission electron microscopic (TEM) section of human oviduct at 500 μ GK 36 from impact. Damage is indicated, ie, swollen mitochondria (M), with lack of cristae. Ribosomes (R) and endoplasmic reticulum (E) appear normal (27,800 ×).

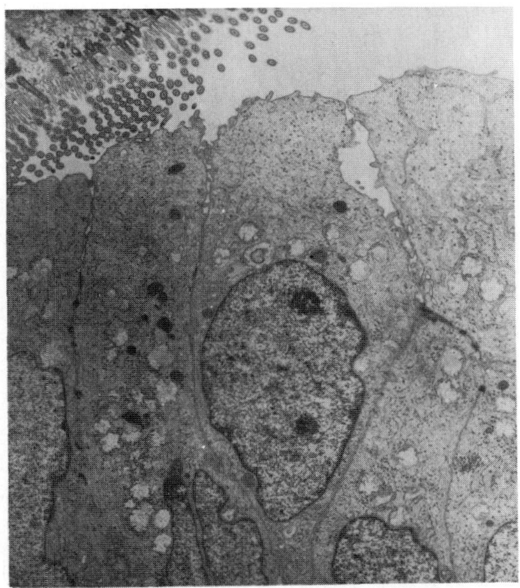

Figure 21-24 Transmission electron microscopic (TEM) section of human oviduct at 1000 μ GK 36 from impact. Normal appearance (9500 ×).

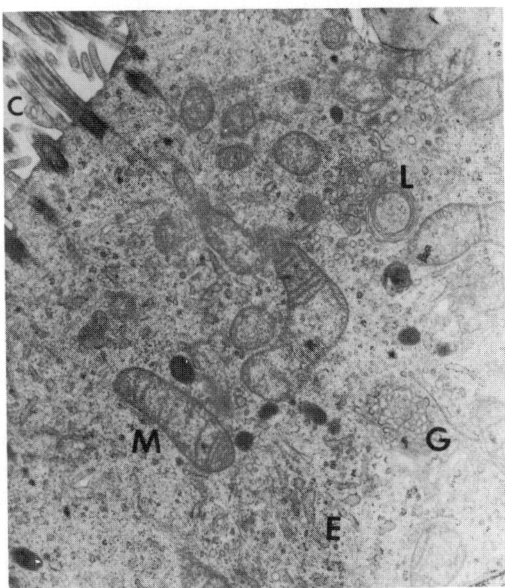

Figure 21-25 Transmission electron microscopic (TEM) section of human oviduct at 1000 μ GK 36 from impact. Normal mitochondria are shown. Endoplasmic reticulum (E), Golgi apparatus (G), and lamellar body (L). The cilia are seen on the upper left (C) (27,800 ×).

DISCUSSION

The intra-abdominal use of the laser in gynecology must, in the light of present knowledge, be considered in a developmental phase, since the current number of valid investigative studies are limited. Obviously, the only sound results for comparison are those which are worthy of publication in recognized gynecologic journals. Currently in the United States, only five or six surgeons have sufficient experience to apply the CO_2 laser for specialized intra-abdominal procedures. Therefore, sufficient patient material, together with appropriate follow-up data, will be accumulated slowly. To assess the value of laser techniques, a wide spectrum of pathological material must be evaluated; eg, in relation to tuboplastic surgery, experience must be generated with reconstruction after tubal ligation, electrocautery, Silastic band and clip sterilization. Similarly, obstruction at various anatomic sites in the tube secondary to infection, with or without IUD use, must be repaired with adjunctive laser surgery and compared to conventional techniques. Follow-up data will be meaningful only if some standardization of postoperative care is attained. Empiric regimens popularly reported are: 1) prophylactic antibiotics, 2) intra-abdominal dextran 70, 3) transcervical hydrotubation, and 4) parenteral adrenocorticosteroids. The "acid test" of success is apparent when the patient achieves intrauterine pregnancy.

The current requirements for articulated arms and for bulky draping apparatuses may be discouraging, but will be simplified as laser technology improves.

From the data presented here, one may deduce that the CO_2 laser is a useful adjunct to intra-abdominal surgery. Precision for delivering an incision to the exact site where it is wanted is a function of the microscopic power and the sensitivity of that delivery system. The sensitivity of the laser beam focused to a spot less than 1 mm, for cleaving cell layers (as a function of time and power) exceeds what can be accomplished with a steel knife regardless of the steadiness of the operating hand. In the final analysis, the combination of a skilled surgeon and advanced laser technology will produce the most favorable operative results.

Clearly, a bloodless operative field is advantageous to both the patient and the operating surgeon. When bleeding is controlled, tissue planes are easy to separate, and cleavage points between normal and diseased structures are reasonably identified. The opposite is of course true when hemorrhage obstructs the surgeon's view. The laser beam coagulates small vessels (ie, < 1 mm), but will not staunch the flow of blood from larger vessels. Dilute pitressin solution, injected into the tissue by means of a fine needle, will cause larger vessels to constrict and allow them to be sealed by the laser beam. Closing the abdomen without absolute hemostasis will invariably be followed by adhesion formation.

Laser-assisted microsurgery results in less adhesion formation and less scar tissue. Cicatrix occurs after tissue trauma. Devitalization, whether produced by infectious microorganisms or iatrogenic operative trauma, stimulates fibroblastic activity. The interaction between laser light energy and the target cells produces a net loss of tissue, which disappears as smoke or vapor. The impact zone, together with surrounding and underlying tissue, undergoes cell death or necrosis. On the basis of light and electron microscopic studies, cell injury may extend as far as 1 mm distal to the impact zone. Therefore, sutures must be placed at the 1 mm point to insure they will not pull through the tissue. The transitional injury zone of 500 μ may allow a projected estimate of approximately 1 mm of scar formation when the two opposing ends of the oviduct are joined together. This injured zone could be diminished by utilizing a smaller spot (ie, 0.5 mm) and perhaps pulsing a large surge of laser light to instantaneously cut away the diseased segments of tube. The preceding would result in less thermal conduction to surrounding tissue.

Endometriosis is exceptionally sensitive to the effects of CO_2 laser vaporization. Even the smallest visible implants may be treated expeditiously. At the same time, the patient's fertility is not jeopardized by trauma to surrounding structures. Current investigation channels the laser beam through the laparoscope, which may allow endoscopic treatment of ectopic endometrium. With the future development of a glass fiber to transmit low levels of laser power, the CO_2 laser may be directed into the uterine cavity to excise and vaporize lesions viewed through contact or conventional hysteroscopes.

Perhaps the most promising expectation for intra-abdominal laser application relates to the treatment of intraperitoneal implants of ovarian carcinoma. This cancer is the most lethal of the genital tract tumors in women. The patient's chances for survival are directly related to the degree of debulking that can be accomplished in cases of widespread tumor. The laser may prove especially invaluable to reach tumors located in the recesses of the peritoneal cavity. Bloodless vaporization may similarly allow more tumor to be destroyed than current operative methods technically can accomplish.

Finally, as more indications for intra-abdominal laser use become apparent, more surgeons will wish to use this modality. Of all the sites in which laser surgery is performed, this location is associated with the greatest risks for laser injury. Only the most experienced and facile surgeons should attempt to perform laser surgery within the peritoneal cavity until the techniques and complications have been established.

REFERENCES

1. Baggish MS: High power density carbon dioxide laser therapy for early cervical neoplasia. *Am J Obstet Gynecol* 136:117–125, 1980.

2. Baggish MS: Carbon dioxide laser treatment for condylomata acuminata venereal infections. *Obstet Gynecol* 55:711–715, 1980.

3. Baggish MS, Dorsey JH: CO_2 laser for the treatment of vulvar carcinoma in situ. *Obstet Gynecol* (in press).

4. Grosspietzsch R: Microtubular reanastomosis in animal model and early human results, in Bellina JH (ed): *Gynecological Laser Surgery.* New York, The Plenum Press (in press).

5. Intraphuvasak J: Improvement of microsurgical techniques in tubular microsurgery, in Bellina JH (ed): *Gynecological Laser Surgery.* New York, The Plenum Press (in press).

6. Klink F, Grosspietzsch R, Klitzing L, et al: Animal in vivo studies and in vitro experiments at human tubes for end to end anastomotic operation by CO_2 laser technique. *Fertil Steril* 30:100–102, 1978.

7. Fry TL, Gerbe RW, Botros SB, et al: Effects of laser, scalpel, and electrosurgical excision on wound contracture and graft *Take. Plast Reconstr Surg* 65:729–731, 1980.

8. Baggish MS, Chong A: Carbon dioxide laser microsurgery of the uterine tube. *Obstet Gynecol* (in press).

PART IV
Other Applications of the CO_2 Lasers in Surgery

22 Dermatology

Leon Goldman, MD
Elizabeth I. McBurney, MD

Carbon dioxide (CO_2) lasers with handheld focusing systems generally have been used in dermatology. More recently, CO_2 lasers attached to surgical microscopes have been employed. With the microscope attachment, small areas of pigment from a tattoo can be removed by aiming the laser beam with a micromanipulator. Alternatively, the microscope can be used to identify the target area and to follow the results of tissue exposures obtained with the hand piece. In view of the limited experience with the CO_2 laser in dermatology, the clinical experience of the operator is paramount and demands critical comparison with the scalpel, high frequency electrosurgery, cryosurgery, and other methods. The same rule applies to dermatology as applies to surgery with lasers: if you do not need the laser, do not use it. In contrast to the CO_2 laser, the neodymium-YAG laser has been used mostly for vascular lesions.[1]

From the early days of the development of the CO_2 laser, investigative studies were done both in animals and man (see Chapters 1, 5 and 6).

The parameters of healing of animal skin incisions regarding energy output and cutting velocities were evaluated.

Hishimoto and Rockwell[2] derived the formula given below to relate cutting speed *v*, with the depth *x*, of the cut:

$$v = Wd/Kx$$

(W is the power density in watts/cm^2, d the diameter of the beam, and K the energy required to transform a unit volume of tissue at 36.5° C into steam at 100° C.)

For a 0.4 mm spot diameter, this formula is given:

$$V = 1.3 \times 10^{-5}\ W/x$$

(V is the velocity of beam movement in cm/sec, W the power density in watts/cm^2, and x is the depth of the cut in cm.)

Graft replacement studies on animal skin were also done by Fidler in the Laser Laboratory of the Medical Center of the University of Cincinnati.[3] From all these experiments on animals, experience was gained for the use of the CO_2 laser for excision and for extensive thermal coagulation necrosis of tissue.[4] The CO_2 laser has been used to excise and perform graft replacement of melanomas. It may be utilized as an instrument for palliative oncological surgery.

The first primary tumors of the skin to be excised with the CO_2 laser were basal cell carcinomas, especially those in solar-damaged skin with secondary poikiloderma and excessive bleeding.[5,6] In these areas, comparable scalpel excisions were done to evaluate amount of bleeding and healing in this highly vascularized, atrophic, telangiectatic skin. As with the use of lasers in excision of the scars in burn surgery and immediate graft replacement, the bleeding was less but the healing was slower. In solar-damaged skin, the scar was not as acceptable cosmetically as it was with the cold knife. The CO_2 laser has been used as a cauterizing agent by Adams and Price.[6] Excellent scars were found with other types of CO_2 laser excisions as, for example, those connected with burns, angiomas, and angiosarcoma.

The next clinical experiment in dermatology was excision of an angiosarcoma of the finger. An effort was made, even with this single primary tumor, to attempt comparisons with other modalities. The first biopsy was taken with the scalpel excision. The bleeding was marked and the tissue was satisfactory for histopathology. The next biopsy of a portion of the same lesion was taken with high frequency electrosurgery. This tissue was completely charred and unsatisfactory for tissue examination. The hemorrhage was less than with the cold knife. The final third portion was removed by the CO_2 laser. This showed excellent healing with good cosmetic results. The biopsy from the CO_2 laser showed only a minimal peripheral rim of thermocoagulation necrosis and excellent tissue structure. After eight years of observation, there has been no recurrence of the angiosarcoma.[7]

CO_2 LASER FOR VASCULAR LESIONS

Excisional CO_2 laser therapy has been performed on vascular lesions, including granuloma pyogenicum (Figure 22-1), acquired angiomas, angiomas found in disseminated blue rubber bleb nevus syndrome, superficial varicosities of the lower legs, telangectasias of the face, and lymphangioma.[8,9] The CO_2 laser use was indicated by previous animal skin and liver studies demonstrating a marked reduction in capillary oozing after CO_2 laser surgery[5] and collateral studies of CO_2 laser excision and graft replacement of burns, which showed a definite decrease in hemorrhage over scalpel excision.[6]

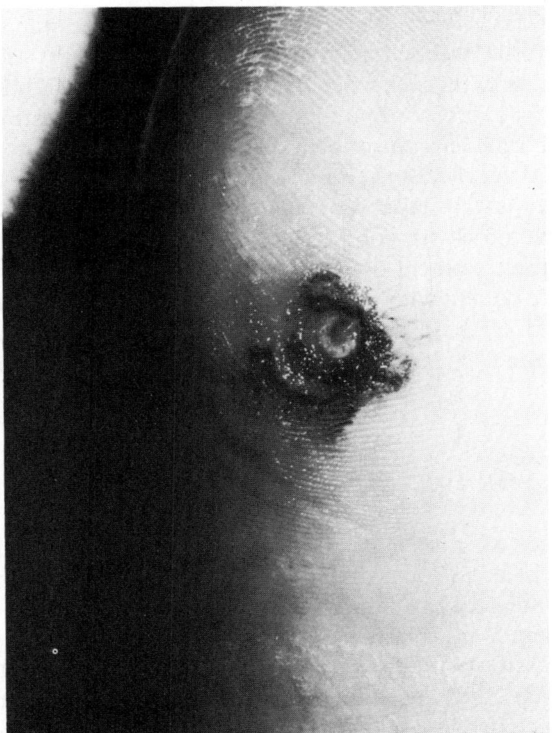

Figure 22-1 Postoperative CO_2 laser treatment of large granuloma pyogenicum of left heel.

In the patient with the blue rubber bleb nevus syndrome, the lesions frequently recurred after scalpel surgery and high frequency electrosurgery. Persistent healing without local recurrences of the angiomatous lesions was demonstrated in initial studies using different types of lasers (pulsed ruby, neodymium, CO_2). Fidler[10] performed extensive CO_2 laser surgical excisions and suturing with minimal blood loss and primary healing of many of the lesions without recurrences. CO_2 laser excision of the angiomatous lesions was done on the face, including the eyelids, and the palms and soles with excellent cosmetic results. The patient developed a resistant anemia, however, and died from hemorrhages of the visceral lesions.

Plastic surgeons in Japan have excised, with minimal bleeding, massive progressive cavernous angiomas of the skin in children, including those with Kasabach-Merrit syndrome.[11]

With such operations, the concern has been more with disturbances of cardiovascular dynamics after extensive removal of vascular tissue rather than with massive hemorrhage. The argon laser is preferred to the CO_2 laser for portwine marks.[12-14]

The CO_2 laser was not effective, from a cosmetic standpoint, in the treatment of the webbed telangiectasia of the thigh and superficial varicosities of women, even when this was done with the CO_2 laser attached to an operating microscope. With this instrument, the treatment spots are small and sharply circumscribed. Frequently, deep white linear scars resulted. However, McBurney and Ratz (personal communications) have recently tried the CO_2 laser for such telangiectasia and for telangiectasia of the face and nose with good results. Oshiro has also obtained excellent results with the treatment of telangiectasia of the nose.[15]

One male patient with extensive recurrent lymphangioma, which had been removed surgically with scalpel on four previous occasions, was treated with the CO_2 laser. The lesion has not recurred after 24 months' follow-up.[8]

CO_2 LASER FOR TATTOO REMOVAL

A number of investigators have tried two techniques for the CO_2 laser treatment of tattoos: direct volatilization with thermocoagulation necrosis and surgical excision.[12]

Since there is no selective color absorption in tattoos with the CO_2 laser, as is possible with lasers in the visible range, the direct destruction of the tattoos by thermocoagulation necrosis of the CO_2 laser may often lead to deep, extensive scarring. Bailin (personal communication) has used microscopic control with the CO_2 laser in an effort to minimize the post-treatment scarring. He has used 15-20 W with 0.05 to 0.1 sec exposure and a diameter of 2 mm. He believes that, with the bloodless field following CO_2 laser surgery, the pigment masses can be seen more easily and therefore, selective localized volatilization of these small masses can be done with minimal scarring. Examination under moderate magnification with a skin stereomicroscope helps to show these residual pigment masses. Bailin believes that with this technique, the postoperative scarring is less than that with the argon laser. He indicates also that these CO_2 laser vaporization studies are preliminary.

Similar results have been found by McBurney using the microscopic CO_2 laser vaporization technique for removal of professional and amateur tattoos and debris tattoos secondary to industrial explosions[14] (Figure 22-2A,B).

The argon laser and the pulsed ruby laser have been used to remove tattoos.[2,4,13] Controversy exists as to which type of laser used for tattoo removal yields the best cosmetic results. Adequate control experiments have not been done.

CO_2 LASER FOR VERRUCAE VULGARIS AND CONDYLOMATA ACUMINATA

In recent years at the Laser Laboratory of the Medical Center of the University of Cincinnati, the CO_2 laser has been used in dermatology most extensively for the treatment of verrucae (digital, plantar, and periungual types) and condylomata acuminata, including the giant con-

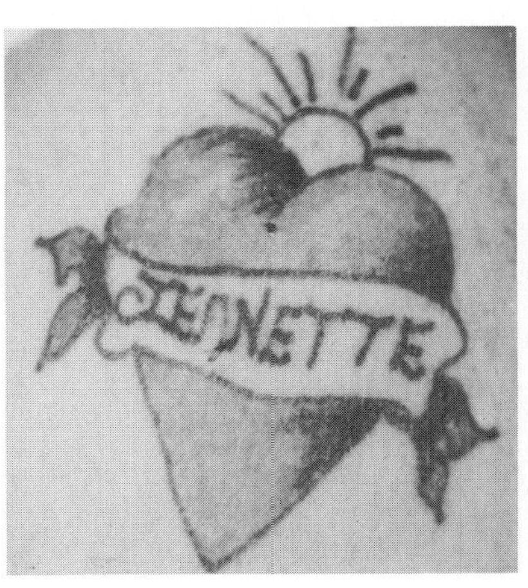

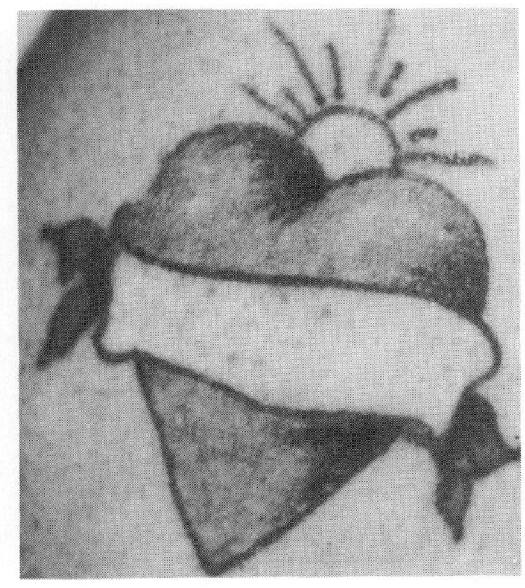

A **B**

Figure 22-2 **A** Tattoo on left upper arm. Patient requested removal of tattooed name only. **B** Five months after treatment with CO_2 laser.

dylomata acuminata of Buschke-Lowenstein.[2,4] Similar results for condylomata acuminata have been observed by Shellhas et al,[16] and by Fuselier et al.[17]

The CO_2 laser has been used as an adjunct therapy in the treatment program of warts, along with liquid nitrogen, cryosurgery, podophyllin, Euphorbia, and other cytotoxic agents.

McBurney (unpublished data) has used the CO_2 laser attached to the operating microscope to remove warts by direct volatilization in 45 patients. The patient population consisted of patients with recalcitrant and/or recurrent warts and immunosuppressed patients with extensive warts. The CO_2 laser was not used initially, but rather employed after the failure of the usual therapeutic modalities. Of the 45 patients treated, there was a 75% cure rate with a 6 to 36 month follow-up. The periungual areas showed some residual scarring after CO_2 laser removal of warts. One advantage of treating verrucae with a CO_2 laser with an attached operating microscope is that the wart tissue can be easily delineated from normal tissue (Figure 22-3A,B).

No immunological studies have been done to compare the immunological aspects of the different techniques of thermocoagulation necrosis with the laser or the high frequency electrical unit. Such necrosis in warts is supposed to induce antibody response. With the increasing number of studies in the immunobiology of warts, however, it would be of interest to determine the influence of the various techniques of thermocoagulation necrosis of warts.

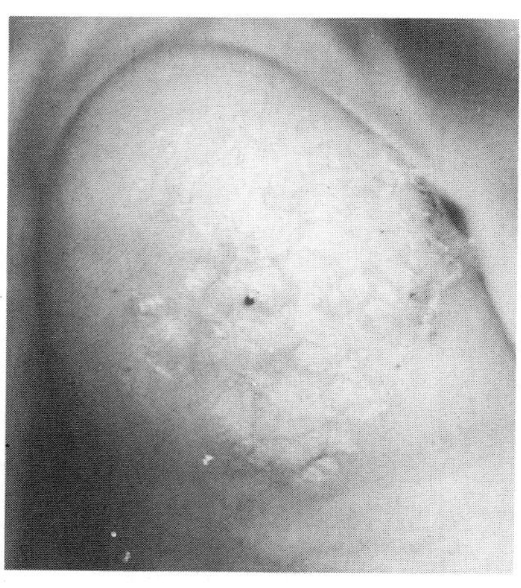

A

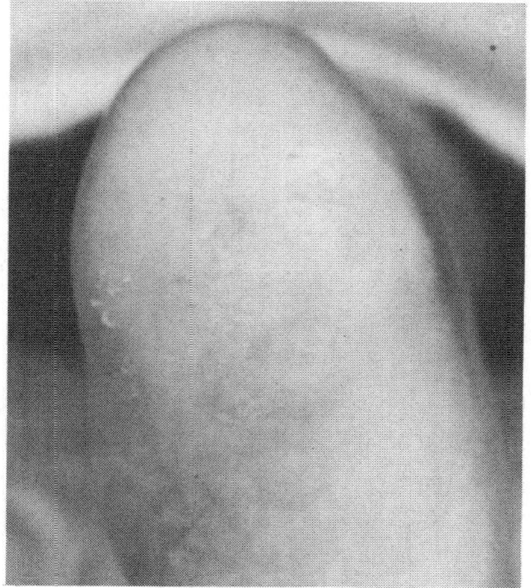

B

Figure 22-3A Extensive verrucae vulgaris, plantar surface of foot. **B** Six months after treatment with CO_2 laser. No recurrence.

At the Laser Laboratory of the Medical Center of the University of Cincinnati, high frequency electrocoagulation was used as the control to evaluate CO_2 laser removal of condylomata acuminata.[16] For example, for condylomata acuminata of the vulva, one side would be done with the laser; the other side would be done with the high frequency electrosurgical unit. Bleeding was less with the CO_2 laser, especially in the pregnant woman. The cosmetic appearance was also superior with the use of the CO_2 laser. Lesions in the vaginal vault, as well as lesions in men, were also treated with the CO_2 laser. The CO_2 laser colposcope often was used to detect small warts near larger areas of warts in both women and men. The colposcope also was used in the follow-up examinations, since new lesions might continue to develop rapidly in condylomata acuminata.[2,4,16]

In a series of ten patients with condylomata acuminata removed with the CO_2 laser, there was no recurrence of the warts after a 10 to 34 month follow-up. There was little or no residual scarring.[17]

CO_2 LASER FOR CUTANEOUS MALIGNANCIES

As discussed previously a basal cell carcinoma was the first primary skin tumor excised with the CO_2 laser. As excellent results presently are being obtained with the usual therapeutic modality of curettage and desiccation, CO_2 laser removal of basal cell carcinoma should be considered as an investigative procedure[18,19] (Figure 22-4).

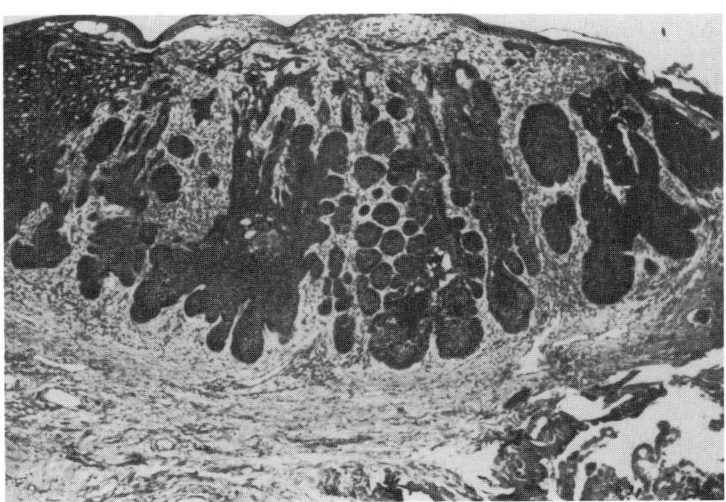

Figure 22-4 CO_2 laser biopsy of basal cell carcinoma of the neck, showing minimal peripheral thermocoagulation necrosis (hematoxylin-eosin 60 ×).

Recurrence rate following laser removal of basal cell carcinoma varies from 5%[8] to 50%,[6] which is inferior to those of current therapies.

SUMMARY

In the future, there will be increasing interest in clinical use of the CO_2 laser in dermatologic surgery, both for vaporization and excision. The laser will be used in investigative and clinical studies in cancer of the skin[19] and for vascular lesions of the skin. With increasing developments of CO_2 laser instrumentation flexibility, fiberoptic transmission, and more precise operating probes, the cosmetic results of the CO_2 laser in surgery and dermatology will be vastly improved. Increasing development of fiberoptics capable of transmitting high output CO_2 laser systems will increase the applications for the use of the CO_2 laser in dermatology for precision therapy and for CO_2 laser surgery for oral lesions (Albo, personal communication). As in other areas, smaller-sized flexible micro-attachments for microsurgery are all indicated.

As it is now in China, where laser surgery recently was developed more extensively,[11] CO_2 and argon lasers should be an integral part of current dermatology centers with a division of laser dermatology. There also should be ongoing critical evaluation of the laser surgery performed. Adequate programs for teaching laser surgery, which include safety guidelines, should be available to qualified practitioners.

ACKNOWLEDGMENTS

We would like to thank Dr. Deborah Rosen for reviewing this manuscript and Mrs. Gloria Abney for secretarial assistance in preparation of this chapter.

REFERENCES

1. Goldman L, Fraden D, Bloembergen N, et al: Studies in laser safety of new high-output systems 2. TEA CO_2 laser impacts. *Optics and Laser Technology,* April 1973, p 58.

2. Goldman L, Rockwell RJ: *Lasers in Medicine.* New York, Gordon & Breach, Science Publishers, 1971.

3. Fidler JP, Law EJ, MacMillan BG, et al: Comparison of carbon dioxide laser excision of burns with other thermal knives. *Ann NY Acad Sci* 267:254–263, 1976.

4. Goldman L: *Applications of the Laser.* Cleveland, CRC Press, 1970.

5. Goldman L, Rockwell RJ, Naprstek Z, et al: Some parameters of high-output CO_2 laser experimental surgery. *Nature* 228, 5278, 1334, 1971.

6. Adams EL, Price NM: Treatment of basal cell carcinomas with a carbon dioxide laser. *J Dermatol Surg Oncol* 5:803–806, 1979.

7. Goldman L, Johnston J: Laser surgery of a digital angiosarcoma. *Cancer* 39:1738–1742, 1977.

8. Goldman L: Laser dermatologic surgery, research clinical applications, in Goldschmidt H (ed): *Physical Modalities in Dermatologic Therapy.* New York, Springer Verlag, 1978, pp 245–256.

9. Kaplan I, Peled I: The carbon dioxide laser in the treatment of superficial telangiectasias. *Br J Plast Surg* 28:214–215, 1975.

10. Fidler JP, Hoefer RW, Polanyi TG, et al: Laser surgery in exsanquinating liver injury. *Am Surg* 181:74–80, 1975.

11. Goldman L: Laser dermatology in China. *Arch Dermatol,* to be published.

12. Goldman L: *Introduction to Modern Phototherapy.* Springfield, Charles C Thomas, 1978.

13. Apfelberg DB, Maser MD, Lash H: Extended clinical use of the argon laser for cutaneous lesions. *Arch Dermatol* 115:719–721, 1979.

14. McBurney EI: Carbon dioxide laser treatment of dermatologic lesions. *South Med J* 71:795–797, 1978.

15. Oshiro T: *Laser Treatment for Nevi.* Tokyo, Medical Laser Research Co. (MEL), 1980, p 68.

16. Shellhas HF, Fidler JP, Rockwell RJ Jr, et al: Resecting vulvar lesions with the CO_2 laser. *Contemp Obstet Gynecol* 6:35–38, 1975.

17. Fuselier HA, McBurney EI, Brannan W, et al: Treatment of condylomata acuminata with carbon dioxide laser. *Urology* 15:265–266, 1980.

18. Goldman L, Dreffer R, Rockwell RJ Jr: CO_2 laser surgery for cancer of man. *Laser Journal* 1:1–3, Jan–Feb, 1971.

19. Goldman L: The laser in skin cancer. *Int Adv Surg Oncol* 1:217–226, 1978.

23 Neurosurgery

Peter W. Ascher, MD

Neurosurgery is one of the most recent disciplines in modern medicine. In spite of having existed for such a short time, it has already achieved a very high level of perfection. In 1928 Bovie[1] and Cushing[2] presented the electrosurgical apparatus and its use in neurosurgery.

For a long time increased surgical skill was the only contribution of neurosurgeons to the development of neurosurgery. The main achievements of this discipline depended on those of other fields of medicine such as diagnostic innovations, improvement of anesthesia, and pre- and postoperative therapy.

From 1960 to 1965 a new method, namely, microsurgery was introduced to neurosurgery, which had been used since 1921 in other surgical disciplines. This accomplishment offered neurosurgeons new and unexpected possibilities. Numerous investigators[2-9] developed the new method and the instruments. However, instruments such as the microscope and the bipolar forceps can be used only within certain limits set by the sensitivity of the central brain tissue.

These apparently natural limitations to operability were exceeded in Graz, when Heppner and Ascher[10,11] introduced the CO_2 laser in June 1976. This method has also been applied in other disciplines of surgery for quite a few years. It would only seem logical that the introduction of an immaterial knife, meant that a true "non-touch" technique should have its focus on neurosurgery. But, surprisingly enough, this was not the case. Early attempts by Rosomoff[12] using a pulsed ruby laser in neurosurgery were unsuccessful. Stellar et al,[11] using the CO_2 laser without the microsurgical mode, obtained unsatisfactory results although he did recognize the potential of this new modality of surgery.

It is quite obvious today that surgical and gynecological instruments must be adapted in order to be used in neurosurgery. This is also true for the use of the CO_2 laser and was the reason why we specified some important modifications in the construction of the CO_2 laser.

The laser, of course, is simply a surgical tool on a more sophisticated level. We expected little more than a clean-cutting instrument for the "non-touch" technique. Before a pioneer for a new surgical technique can introduce his new method convincingly, he must produce evidence for its absolute indications and that it will be superior to previously used techniques. In addition to this specific use of the laser, we found many relative indications which were of advantage either for the patient or the surgeon.

DEVELOPMENT OF THE NEUROSURGICAL LASER AND TECHNICAL DATA

We modified the CO_2 laser (Sharplan 791) in two principal ways.[9] The first was the replacement of mechanical devices by a pilot laser (helium laser). This made a "contact-free" technique, as had been originally envisaged, available for the first time. The other modification was the coupling of the laser to the operating microscope in order to accommodate the increasing proportion of microsurgical procedures in neurosurgery.[14-16] Practical considerations have since been amply confirmed by experience and have led to the development of an electromechanical guiding device for the beam under the microscope (Figure 23-1).

Technical Data

We use the Sharplan 791 CO_2 laser with following specifications:

Output

Laser	Flowing gas, 50 W CO_2 laser.

Output power	45 W at the system focus, continuous or pulsed.
Wavelength	10.6 μ.
Mode structure	TEM_{00}.
Spot size	0.12 mm with 50-mm focal length focusing head. 0.30 mm with 125-mm focal length focusing head.

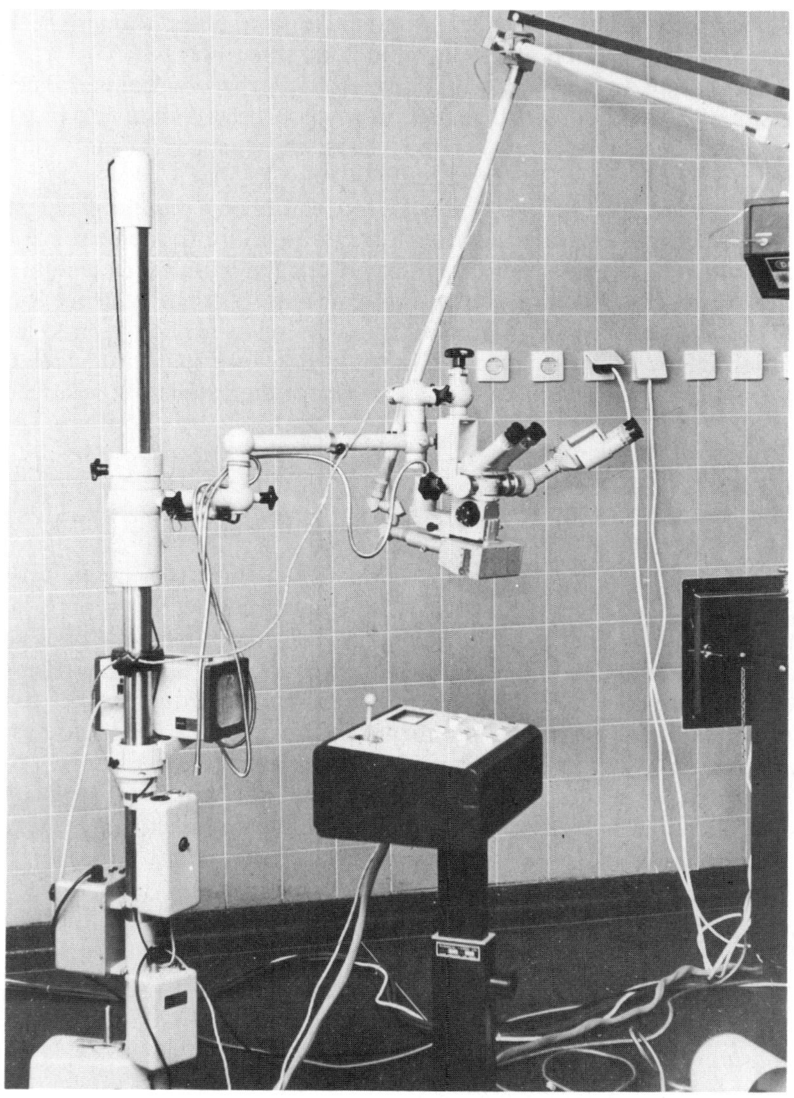

Figure 23-1 Sharplan 791 with Microslad 733 Zeiss OPMI 1 and optic adapter.

Operation

Maneuverability	The light, pen-like focusing head held by the surgeon has 6° of freedom and can be moved on a 2.2-m radius around the main cabinet.
System activation	Turn-on sequence: key switch circuit breaker mode-selector switch Output control: one or two foot switches
System modes	a. Standby b. Manual: continuous operation c. Timed: 0.1 sec, 0.05 sec, 0.01 sec pulse, preselected.
Laser operating data	Tube pressure: 25 to 35 mm Hg Current: up to 90 mA.

Input

Electrical power	115 volts AC, 25 amp 50/60 Hz single phase
Laser medium	Gas mixture: 4.5% ± 0.5% CO_2 13.5% ± 1.0% N_2 Balance He Container: ICC rating 3AA2265 cylinder with CGA 350 valve fitting. Regulated working pressure: 30 psi (2 atm) Minimum cylinder pressure: 100 psi (7 atm) Working hours per cylinder: approximately 100 hours.
Inert gas	Dry nitrogen Container: ICC rating 3AA2265 cylinder with CGA 350 valve fitting Regulated working pressure: 3 to 6 psi Minimum cylinder pressure: 100 psi (7 atm)
Cooling system	Open loop water flow Minimum water flow rate: 4 liters/min. Minimum water pressure: 20 psi difference (1.5 atm difference) Maximum inlet water temperature: 70°F(21°C)

Physical characteristics

Main cabinet & laser	Floor space: 80 cm × 100 cm Overall height: 270 cm adjustable Working radius from telescopic beam: approximately 220 cm
Overall weight	270 kg

For microsurgical use we combined the Sharplin 791 He laser with the Microslad 722 (microsurgery laser adapter). The Microslad 722 system enables the surgeon to operate with the Sharplan 791 CO_2 surgical laser while observing and controlling the laser via a standard operating microscope. The control of the laser is done by using the Microslad control unit. Two red aiming beams enable the user to aim the laser to the desired area, showing exactly the point of the laser focus. Laser beam movements are controlled by the "joystick" on the control unit panel which governs the *optical* unit attached to the microscope. The aiming beam system is incorporated into the new type 791/He and 733 laser head. Recently, we designed the 4th generation of the optical attachment (Figures 23-2, 23-3).

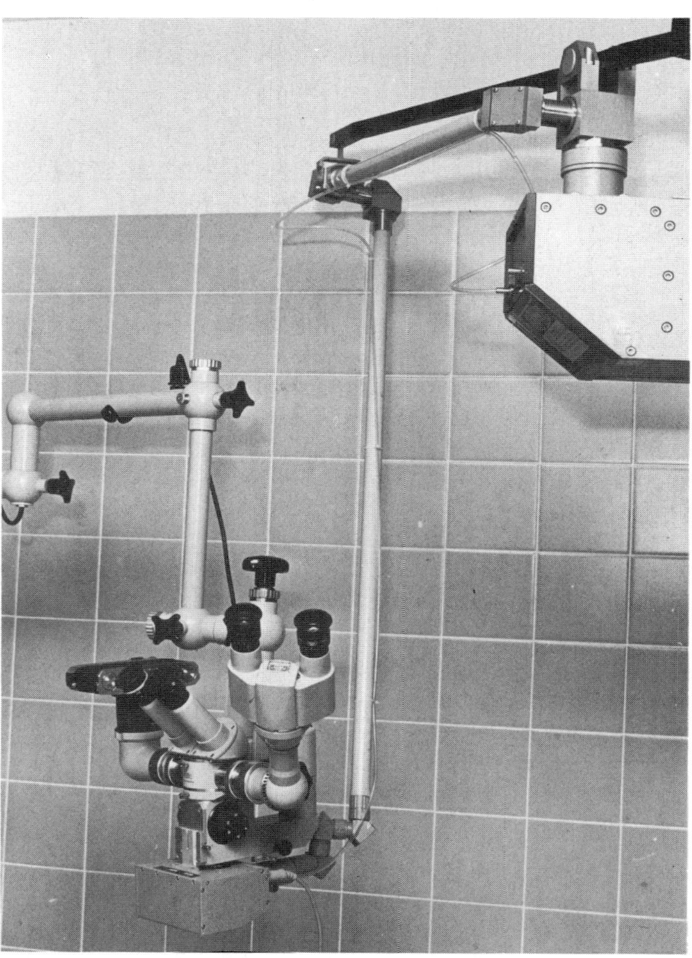

Figure 23-2 Microadapter attached with Zeiss operating microscope OPMI 1, second generation.

INTERACTION OF THE LASER BEAM WITH NERVOUS TISSUE[15-17]

When introducing a new method, the first and most important thing is to show that there are no specific risks to the patient. Therefore, we conducted a large series of experiments starting in 1975. As reported earlier, we were able to prove that cutting with the laser caused less trauma of the surrounding tissue than the cold or electric knife. We found three typical zones of tissue damage with the laser:

1. Zone of 10–15 μ of lased tissue.
2. Zone of 150 μ of coagulated tissue.
3. Outer zone of edema varying between 100 μ and 200 μ.

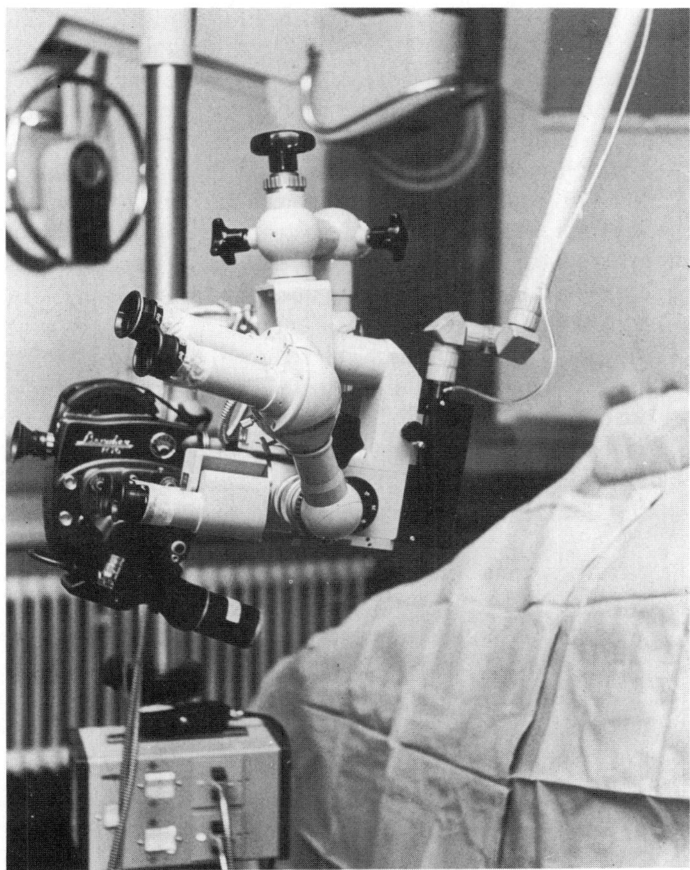

Figure 23-3 Microadapter attached with Zeiss operating microscope OPMI 1, third generation.

In a comparative study we demonstrated that the cold and the electric knife damages the brain tissue about one-third more than the laser. Besides this decreased morphological damage with the CO_2 laser we can avoid any electrical or mechanical alterations beyond the thermal damage caused by the use of the laser.

LASER-SPECIFIC SURGICAL TECHNIQUES

We used the CO_2 laser in three different ways.[19,20]

1. Freehand use of the laser is similar to the use of the scalpel except power and speed of movement rather than pressure control the depth of cut.[14]
2. Freehand laser surgery with observation through the operating microscope is useful in microvascular procedures utilizing special handpieces.
3. The electromechanical use of the micromanipulator opened up unexplored territory. Almost every operation seemed to extend the boundaries of established operability. The new prototype of microadapter is attached to the objective lens of the operating microscope (Zeiss OPMI 1–6) connected to the laser arm and surgically draped. The mirror in the microadapter is moved electromechanically by the manipulating table with the left hand to aim the beam in any direction. It is possible to operate up to 5 mm over and under the focal level of the laser without losing a significant amount of energy.

For coagulation it is necessary to reduce the energy intensity. This can be done by changing the lens, shortening the radiation time, or by reducing the output energy. Similarly, the laser power can be preselected in three stages. A rough estimate of the depths of the penetration is thereby achieved. Delicate membranes are not cut continuously, but with interrupted single "shots" in series. This is made possible by the design of the latest models.

Apart from cutting and coagulation, a third possibility under the microscope is in the form of vaporization of the diseased tissue. This technique has been found to be the least traumatic when applied to tumors of limited size (3 to 5 cm^3). Larger tumors would require more powerful lasers but their depth of penetration and destructiveness would be too dangerous for use in sensitive areas of the brain.

CASE REPORTS

On July 28, 1976 one member of our team (Heppner) performed the first successful neurosurgical laser operation in Graz. Since then we have carried out 395 neurosurgical operations with this instrument. Most of the cases were only relative indications for the use of the laser. Approximately 10% of the cases were absolute indications. As examples, we shall present four cases. Two deal with diseases of the spinal cord and two with diseases of the brain.

Case 1: Extirpation of an intramedullary ependymoma from C2 to C5 by laser vaporization.

S.F. was a 40-year-old male with a 1½-year history of sensory disturbances on the right side of the body and frequent headaches. The patient related his symptoms to a previous fall from a truck. Prior to admission, the sensory disturbances increased, his right upper arm became progressively weak, and he experienced severe constipation. Physical and neurological examinations were within normal limits.

Roentgenograms of the cervical spine revealed spondylosis at C5–C6 with degenerative changes in the joints from C2 to C4. Electromyograms were normal. Descending myelography demonstrated an intramedullary enlargement from C2 to C6. Computed tomography also revealed an expanding lesion at the same level (Figure 23-4).

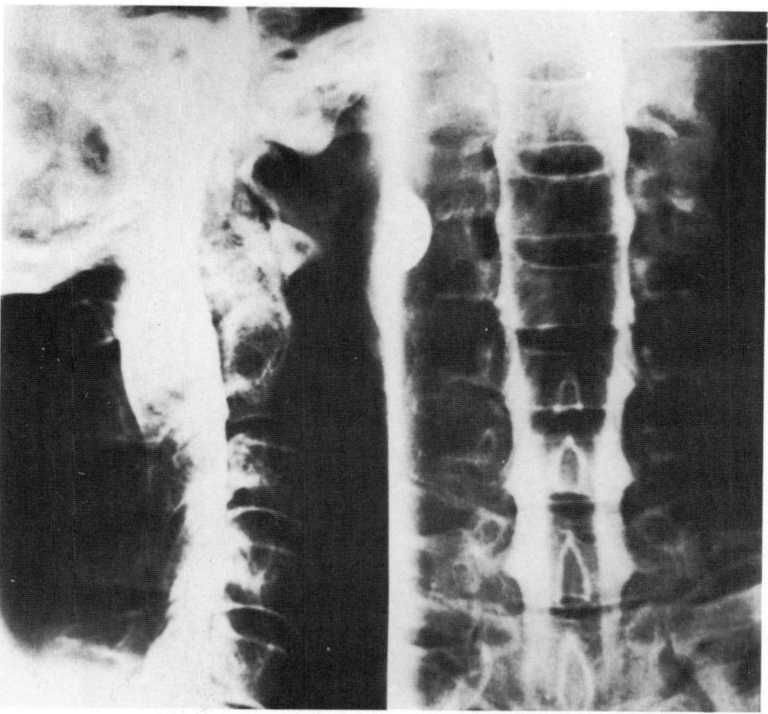

Figure 23-4 Myelotomy, showing the intramedullary tumor C2 to C5.

The enlarged spinal canal was completely filled with a soft tissue mass of homogeneous density, demarcated by a less dense area compatible with edema. Differentiation between the normal neural tissue and the tumor was made possible only by the zone of edema. All other auxiliary examinations were normal (Figure 23-5).

After detailed discussion, the patient agreed to an operation and an attempt at extirpation of the tumor. The operation was performed in April 1978. The patient was given a general anesthetic plus local anesthesia, and placed in a sitting position. A skin incision from C1 to C7 was made and the dorsal aspect of the spinal column exposed in the usual fashion. A laminectomy from C2 to C5 was then carried out. The laminae

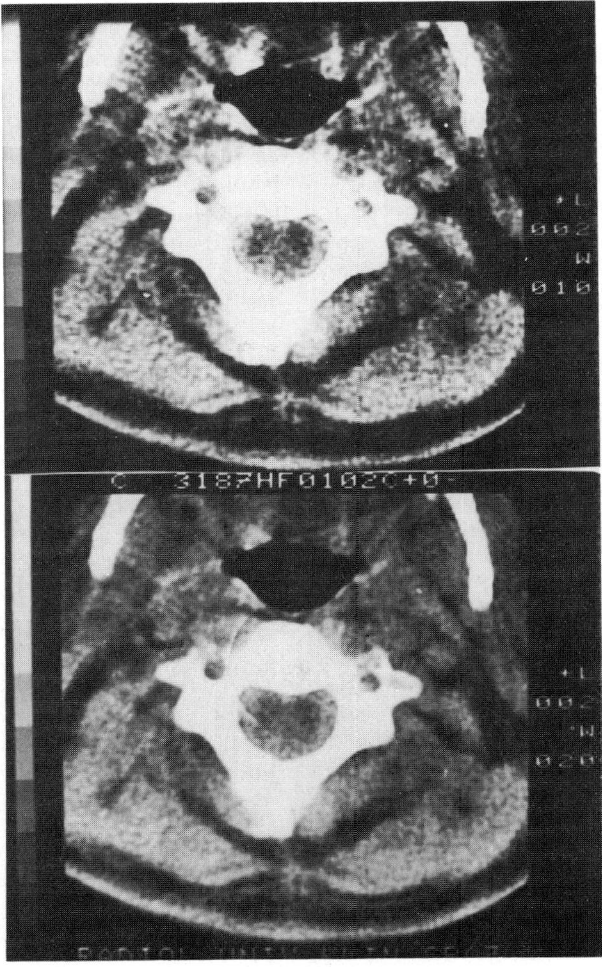

Figure 23-5 Computer tomography of the tumor.

were found to be paper-thin. In the area of laminectomy, the dural sac was widened in a biconvex shape. Its greatest enlargement was at the level of C4. The dura was opened and sutured to the adjacent muscles. The underlying cord was swollen and completely filled the dural sac.

The operating microscope with the laser adapter was brought into the field. Using magnification of 6 and 12 power, we found foreign tissue in the midline, 3.5 cm in length and 0.5 cm in width. The surface of the tumor was clearly demarcated.

The tumor was dissected with the pulsed laser (15 W, pulsed mode, 1/20 sec, in focus, 250-mm lens) on the surface, first on the left side and then on the right. At a depth of 2 mm the tumor margins became indistinct. At that point, the tumor mass was vaporized step by step with 20 W, slightly out of focus. The laser absorption was clearly more intense in the tumor tissue. Thus, it was easy to differentiate tumor from intact cord. With two microscope adaptations, the entire length of the tumor was vaporized layer by layer to the depth of 1.5 cm, at which point the anterior commissure was reached. There was no bleeding during the procedure.

The entire operation, from opening to closure of the dura, was performed without mechanical contact or contamination of the operating field. Using an "immaterial" knife, literally a light beam, we followed the principle of not touching the spinal cord in order to keep the postoperative complications to an absolute minimum. For decompressive reasons, the dura was closed with a plastic patch implant. The bone defect was covered with a gelatin sponge and the soft tissue sutured.

The patient was awake immediately after the operation and could move all his extremities. Within 24 hours a tetraplegia developed, predominantly in the right upper extremity. On the third day the neurological deficit receded rapidly. On the seventh postoperative day the patient was able to leave his bed with assistance. Along with the motor disturbances we found hyperesthesia of all four extremities, most marked at the tips of the toes and fingers. On the seventh day only a strong burning sensation of the fingers of the right hand remained. Micturition and defecation were never impaired. At discharge on the 19th postoperative day, there was only minimal spinal ataxia with slight paresis of the right hand. For further treatment the patient was transferred to a rehabilitation center. In July he was discharged from that institution, having regained full neurological function.

Case 2: Extirpation of an intradural arterial venous malformation T12 to L1 by laser coagulation.

D.M. was a 64-year-old female with a history of a slowly increasing paraparesis over a seven-month period. At the time of admission to the University Clinic for Neurosurgery in Graz, she had a paraplegia with sensory impairment from L3, as well as loss of bladder and bowel control.

Descending myelography revealed a narrow spinal canal from T11 to T12. Tomography of T11–T12 showed an old compression fracture of T12. Electromyograms showed signs of peripheral nerve damage in the L2 to L4 roots on the left side. Ascending myelography showed signs of arachnoid adhesions. All other auxiliary examinations were within normal limits.

The operation was carried out under general anesthesia with the patient in a lateral decubitus position. The skin incision was made from T11 to L2, and a T11–L2 laminectomy was performed. Opening of the dura was accomplished in the usual fashion. The operating microscope, in combination with the microadapter, was brought into the field. Using magnification of 6 and 12 power, we discovered an unexpected finding: an arterial venous malformation on the left side, extending from the level of T12 to L1. The diseased veins were draining mainly into the dorsal vein. The vessels were sealed step by step with the CO_2 laser (5 to 10 W, 0.01 sec to 0.05 sec, pulsed in focus, 250 mm lens). Complete coagulation and resection by vaporization (10 W, continuous wave, in focus, 250-mm lens) of the malformation was carried out. Free passage cephalad and caudal to the lesion was confirmed. Closure of the dura was accomplished with continuous sutures. The operation was completed in the routine manner.

Postoperatively, neurological function as well as bladder and bowel function returned very slowly, and the patient was transferred to a rehabilitation center.

Case 3: Resection of a large para- and endosellar malignant meningioma by laser vaporization.

F.G. was a 29-year-old male with a one-year history of hormonal dysfunction. At examination, a visual defect led to an ophthalmological consultation. He was sent to our hospital with a diagnosis of tumor of the hypophysis. Neurologically, we found nothing abnormal except bitemporal hemianopsia. Tomograms of the sella, computertomograms of the brain and the sella, angiography of both carotid arteries, and hormonal status confirmed the diagnosis of an endosellar tumor. All other auxiliary examinations were normal (Figures 23-6, 23-7).

The operation was performed in June 1979. The patient was given a general anesthesia and placed in the supine position. A coronal skin incision was made on the forehead. The skull was opened bifrontally with the electric drill and Hall instruments. The dura was opened bifrontally by making two curved incisions and severing the falx. Between the two optic nerves, the meningioma-like tumor appeared. The operating microscope with the laser adapter was brought into the field.

Using magnification of 6 and 12 power, we incised the tumor capsule with the laser (15 W, continuous wave, in focus, 250-mm lens). Using the

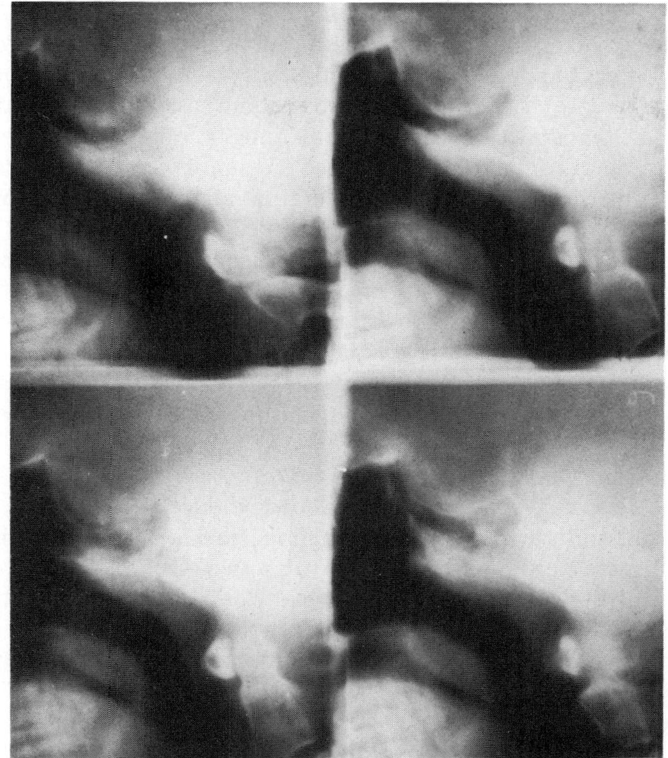

Figure 23-6 Tomogram of the sella.

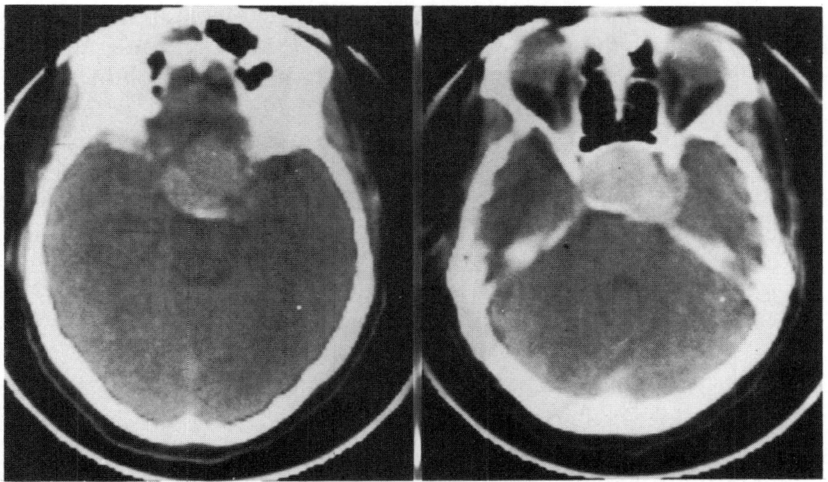

Figure 23-7 Computer tomograms of the tumor.

laser we could extend this incision to the optic nerves on both sides. The capsule was then split in a rectangular fashion. In the following procedure the tumor was vaporized (25 W, continuous wave, 150-mm out of focus, 250-mm lens). It was possible to remove about two-thirds of the diseased tissue. The remainder of the tumor had a slight connection to the wall of the sinus. Since complete extirpation of the tumor would have meant risking sinus bleeding, we ended the operation at this stage as a resection. Closure of the skull and skin was performed in the usual way.

Histologically, we found an angioblastic meningioma with malignant, degenerative cells. The patient was placed into the intensive care unit for 24 hours. He was allowed to get out of bed on the seventh postoperative day. His visual defects improved almost to the point of complete recovery. In the following month the patient was given radiation treatment (5000 R). In May 1980 he finished his studies as a lawyer.

Case 4: Giant lipoma of the corpus callosum.

G.P. was a 20-year-old, right-handed woman, who suffered for two years from minor epileptic seizures and increasing headaches. Disturbed consciousness was noted repeatedly over a two-week period and was accompanied by transitory sickness, uncontrolled speech, and motor automatism followed by rigidity lasting a few seconds. Two months prior to admission, anticonvulsive therapy was terminated by the patient as no improvement was noticed.

Neurologically, findings were normal, except for slight nystagmus. Skull x-rays showed calcification in the corpus callosum. Pneumoencephalography showed a space-occupying lesion compressing the roof of the 3rd ventricle. Bilateral carotid angiography revealed a midline expansion of both pericallosal arteries. Computer tomography verified a calcified tumor in the corpus callosum. In the electroencephalogram, subcortical irritation without epileptic potential was found. Ophthalmological examination showed edema of the disc; the blind spot was enlarged but vision was normal. All laboratory values were normal (Figures 23-8, 23-9, 23-10).

We operated through a left frontoparietal craniotomy extending over the superior sagittal sinus. The tumor was found at a depth of 3–4 cm in the interhemispheric fissure. It was embedded in a network of arteries which originated from both left and right pericallosal arteries. It extended from the genu corporis callosi to the splenium. The falx cerebri was narrowed, causing a median sagittal groove in the tumor.

The arteries surrounding the tumor were dissected free and partly coagulated, sparing both pericallosal arteries and all vessels entering the brain substance. Tough parts of the tumor were divided by the laser knife, simultaneously cutting the tumor into pieces (35 W, continuous wave, in focus, 125-mm lens). Employing microsurgical techniques, the right

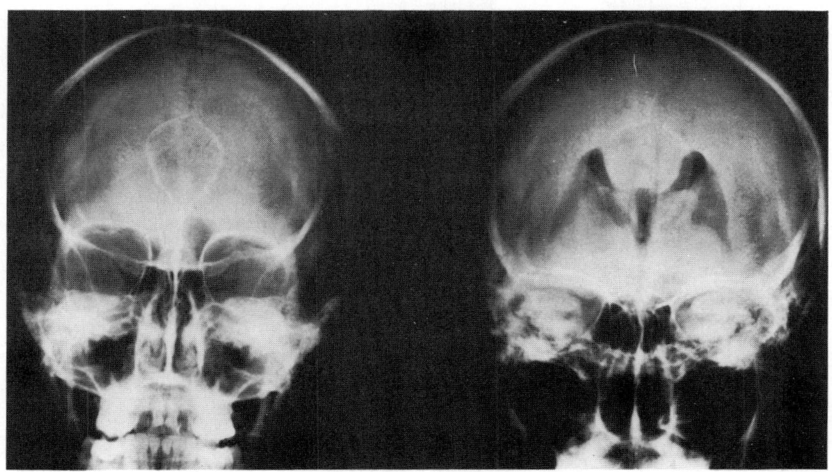

Figure 23-8 Plain x-ray of the skull and pneumoencephalogram in antero-posterior view with the lipoma.

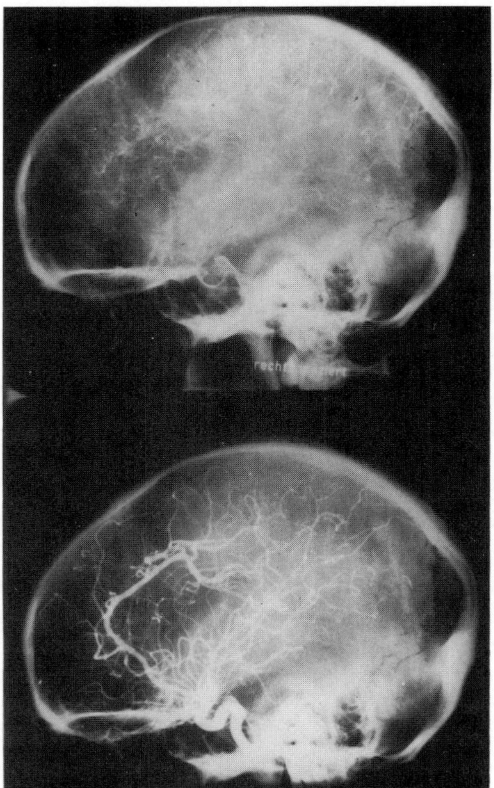

Figure 23-9 Carotid angiogram lateral view of the lipoma.

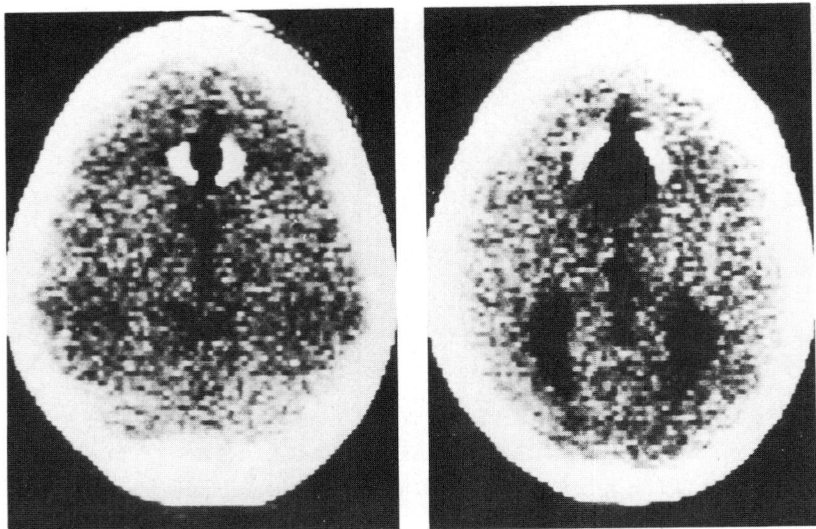

Figure 23-10 Computer tomograms of the corpus callosum lipoma.

pericallosal artery and the great vein were also freed from the tumor.

Immediately after operation the patient was alert but aphasic, showing a marked paresis of the right side which improved rapidly after the second postoperative day. On the 15th postoperative day the patient regained her speech, and one week later she was able to get out of bed. Recovery was complicated only by occasional hyperthermia (39.5°C), tachycardia (200/min), and transient drowsiness. Four years after the operation she was still working as a travel agent.[21]

SUMMARY

After more than four years of clinical experience we believe that the CO_2 laser has extended the limits of operability. With increasing experience we are finding new indications and new advantages of this technique. It should be strongly emphasized that this method requires a new concept of neurosurgery and also requires a new approach to surgical training. In order to benefit from the achievements in the field of neurosurgery, surgeons will have to undergo at least two years of special training to master this new method.

We want to stress that the CO_2 laser is only an additional tool with new indications in neurosurgery, but not a replacement for successful traditional techniques.

ACKNOWLEDGMENTS

Appreciation is expressed to Dr Susanne Neubauer for her translation, and to Miss Gertraud Machinger for her secretarial assistance.

REFERENCES

1. Bovie WT: New electro-surgical unit. *Surg Gynecol Obstet* 47:751–752, December 1928.

2. Cushing H: Electrosurgery as an aid to the removal of intracranial tumors. *Surg Gynecol Obstet* 47:751–784, December 1928.

3. Kurze T, Doyle JB Jr: Extradural intracranial approach to the internal auditory canal. *J Neurosurg* 19:1033–1037, 1962.

4. Jacobson JM II, Suarez EL: Microsurgery in anastomoses of small vessels. *Surg Forum* 22:243–245, 1960.

5. House WF: Transtemporal bone microsurgical removal of acoustic neuromas (monography). *Arch Otolaryngol* 80:599–756, 1964.

6. Rand WR (ed): *Microsurgery*. St Louis, CV Mosby, 1966.

7. Donaghy RMP: Patch and bypass in microsurgery, in Donaghy RMP, Yasargil MG (eds): *Microvascular Surgery*. Stuttgart, Thieme Verlag, 1967, pp 75–86.

8. Yasargil MG, Donaghy RMP: *Microvascular Surgery*. Stuttgart, Thieme Verlag, 1967.

9. Malis LI: Petrous ridge compression and its surgical correction. *J Neurosurg* 26 (suppl):163–167, 1967.

10. Heppner F, Ascher PW: Über den Einsatz des Laserskalpells in der Neurochirurgie. *Akt Med Techn* 24:424–426, 1976.

11. Ascher PW: *Der CO_2-Laser in der Neurochirurgie*. Wein-Zürich, Molden-Verlag, 1977, pp 16–17.

12. Rosomoff ML: Effect of ruby laser on brain and neoplasms. Presented at 1st Annual Biomedical Laser Conference, Boston, 1965.

13. Stellar S, Polanyi TG, Bredemeier NC: Laser surgery, in Wolbarsht ML (ed): *Laser Application in Medicine and Biology,* vol 2. New York, Plenum Press, 1974, pp 241–293.

14. Ascher PW, Oberbauer R, Holzer P, et al: Vorteile und Möglichkeiten des CO_2-Lasers in der Neurochirurgie. *Wien Med Wschr* 127:260–262, 1977.

15. Ascher PW: The use of the CO_2-Laser in neurosurgery, in Kaplan I (ed): *Laser Surgery II*. Jerusalem, Jerusalem Academic Press, 1978, pp 28–30.

16. Ascher PW, Oberbauer R, Clarici G: Laserstrahl, ein modernes neurochirurgisches Instrument, in Argyropoulos G, Lanner G (eds): *Neurochirurgie von Heute*. Wien Kwizda, 1977, pp 53–57.

17. Ascher PW: The effect of CO_2-laser beam on neutral tissue: Light and electromicroscopic findings. *Acta Neurochir* (in press).

18. Ascher PW, Ingolitsch E, Walter G, et al: Ultrastructural findings in CNS tissue, with CO_2-laser, in Kaplan I (ed): *Laser Surgery II*. Jerusalem, Jerusalem Academic Press, 1978, pp 81–90.

19. Ascher PW, Ingolitsch E, Walter G: Neuere histologische Untersuchungsergebnisse nach Gebrauch des CO_2-Lasers am Zentralnervensystem. *Kongreßbericht 19. Tag.d.Österr.Ges.f.Chir.*, Wien, Egermann-Verlag, 1979, pp 479–482.

20. Ascher PW: Neurosurgical laser technique, in Goldman L (ed): *Laser Biomedical Engineering,* in press.

21. Clarici G, Heppner F: The operative approach of lipoma of the corpus callosum. *Neurochirurgia* 22:77–81, 1979.

24 Polyps and Tumors of the Rectum and Sigmoid Colon

R.C.J. Verschueren, MD
J. Oldhoff, MD

Electrosurgery on polyps and superficially growing malignancies of the rectum, performed through rigid rectoscopes, is a widely accepted technique.[1-3] In order to be eligible for curative electrosurgical treatment the rectal cancer should meet certain criteria:

1. The tumor should be a well differentiated adenocarcinoma.
2. The tumor should not cover more than one-third of the circumference of the rectum.
3. The growth pattern must be exophytic.
4. Digital examination must rule out infiltration into the rectal wall.
5. The tumor should be localized in the extraperitoneal part of the rectum.

The use of electrosurgery has some drawbacks. We use the electrosurgical unit to slowly vaporize the tumor. This may be time-consuming and, in order to be locally radical, we must take the risk of full-thickness, thermal devitalization of the rectal wall. This is why cancers located above the peritoneal reflection (more than 9 cm away from the anus) are not suitable for this type of therapy. After electrosurgery a thick layer of thermally devitalized tissue is left behind. Premature release of this necrotic area can cause serious hemorrhage. A predominant drawback of electrosurgery is the lack of visual control over the depth of thermal damage, hence lack of control of radicality.

The availability of a CO_2 laser in our hospital prompted us to consider this new modality as an alternative to electrosurgery in this field. The introduction of the CO_2 laser as a surgical tool provided us with an instrument allowing step-by-step vaporization of a malignant tumor in a confined space.

The mechanism of such tissue vaporization has been described elsewhere.[4,5] The thermal damage in the wall of the crater after vaporization is very limited. The penetration of the heat destruction after using the CO_2 laser to vaporize tissues has been investigated in our laboratory by enzyme-histochemical methods, and proved to be determined by the time a particular part of the tissue is exposed to the laser beam. For exposure times varying between one and six seconds, the thickness of this layer of thermal damage varied between 200 μ and 800 μ.[6] During preliminary laboratory experiments, it became obvious that the mucosa could be vaporized, leaving a small amount of necrotic tissue behind, and the defects healed promptly.

Before attempting the use of the CO_2 laser on rectal cancers, this instrument was used on lesser tumors of the rectosigmoid colon.

INSTRUMENTATION

1. The CO_2 laser used for this clinical work was the Sharplan 791 (Kaplan, 1974).
2. The micromanipulator was designed and manufactured by the American Optical Corporation.[7]
3. The microscope was an OPMI 1 from Zeiss, on which a 400-mm lens was fixed. The magnification (16:1) proved to be the most convenient.
4. The rectoscopes.

Two laser rectoscopes were designed for this purpose: one for the lower rectum and one for microsurgery above the peritoneal reflection. Both were manufactured from copper and subsequently chromium-plated. Their internal and external diameters were, respectively, 34 mm and 38 mm for the former, and 28 mm and 32 mm for the latter (Figure 24-1). Their length was 25 cm. A handle, perpendicular to the axis of the tube, facilitated manipulation inside the rectum and subsequent fixation of the rectoscope to the operating table (Figure 24-2). A suction tube inside the wall of the rectoscope provided the possibility of evacuating smoke during laser surgery. An external light source linked to a fiber cable allowed visualization of the rectum while positioning the rectoscope. A movable suction device inside the rectoscope enabled us to "grasp" and move pedunculated polyps in order to stretch the stalk and make it visible.

PREPARATION OF THE PATIENT

Initially, all patients had a three-day preparation of the bowel with a low-residue diet and an enema the evening before operation. Later in this series, the patients with polyps in the distal part of the rectum received only enemas the evening before and the morning of the operation.

Most operations were carried out under general anesthesia. However, a single-dose caudal block proved to be adequate for the operation in those patients who were at risk for general anesthesia.

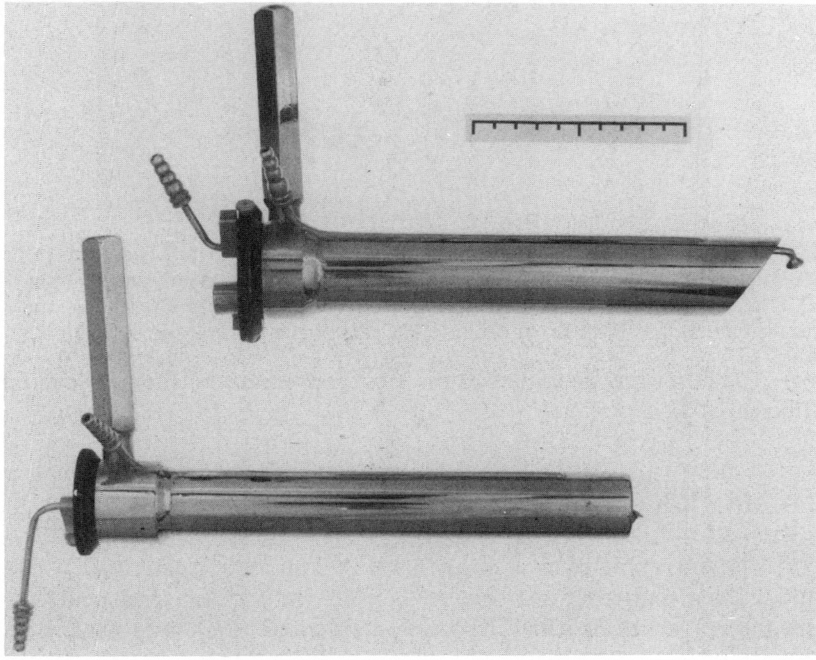

Figure 24-1 The two laser rectoscopes. The thick one at the top is for the lower rectum.

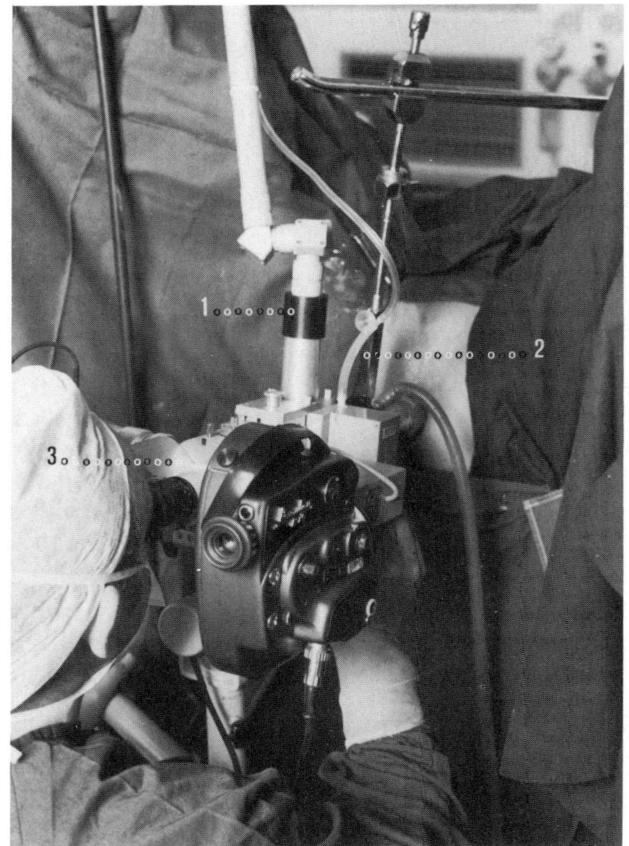

Figure 24-2 Technical arrangement for laser microsurgery in the rectum: 1) The beam manipulator of the Sharplan 791 mounted on top of the micromanipulator. 2) The rectoscope suspended on a gimbal. 3) The Zeiss operating microscope. A movie camera has been fitted on the right side of the microscope body.

The lithotomy position was the most convenient for these procedures (Figure 24-2).

TECHNIQUE

The micromanipulator, when used in conjunction with a CO_2 laser and a Zeiss operating microscope, delivers the focused laser beam at a distance of about 35 cm. This micromanipulator has been used in the surgery of the upper aerodigestive tract by Strong and Jako.[8] The working mechanism of this delicate instrument has been elaborately described in the publications of these authors.

While looking at the operating field through the microscope, the surgeon sees a green marker spot on the target tissue. This marker spot informs the surgeon as to the exact position of the laser beam focus. A "joystick" linked to the mirror system of the micromanipulator makes it possible to move the marker spot and thus the position of the laser beam over the operating field, while providing accurate control of these movements by simultaneous viewing through the binocular microscope.

After anal dilatation, the rectoscope is introduced. In order to facilitate the introduction of the thick rectoscope above the peritoneal reflection, the optical system of a diagnostic rectoscope is fixed at its proximal end, thus providing illumination and allowing insufflation of the bowel with air. When the rectoscope has been centered around the polyp or tumor, its handle is firmly attached to a gimbal mounted on the operating table (Figure 24-2).

Excision of Pedunculated Polyps

A thin, metal suction tube is introduced into the lumen of the rectoscope. The end of this suction tube is angulated and has the form of a "sucker." The surface of the polyp is aspirated into the "sucker" by applying suction to the tube and the tube is then fixed onto a rotating ring mounted at the proximal end of the rectoscope. The stalk of the polyp can now be stretched by adjusting the depth of the tube and rotating the ring in a convenient position (Figures 24-3, 24-4). The external light source is

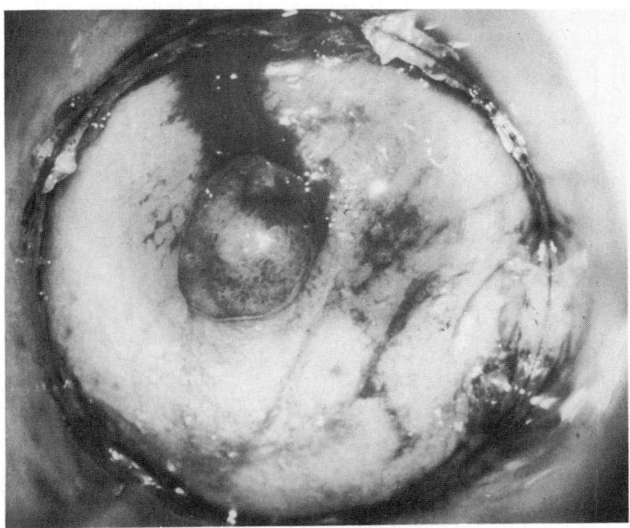

Figure 24-3 View of a pedunculated polyp.

removed from the rectoscope, and the microscope with the micromanipulator and the beam manipulator of the Sharplan are positioned in front of the rectoscope. The stalk of the polyp is then transected at its base. In most cases some hemorrhage occurs. Hemostasis is achieved by moving the laser spot over the bleeding zone with swift movements, thus coagulating the tissue (Figure 24-5). The entire polyp is removed from the rectoscope and examined histologically. In case of malignancy the histologic examination indicates whether or not the resection was sufficiently radical.

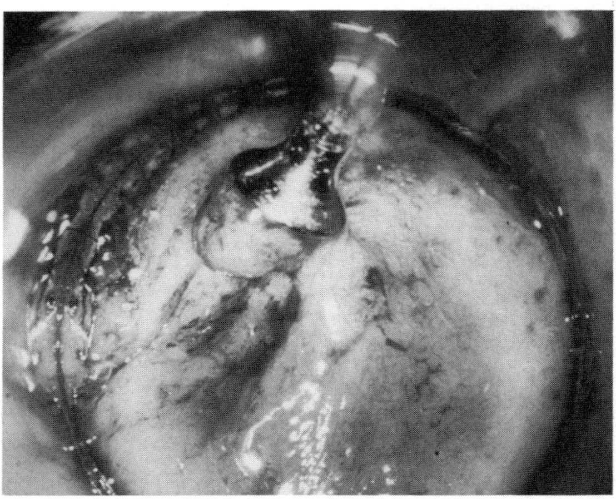

Figure 24-4 The stalk can be stretched when the polyp has been grasped with the suction device.

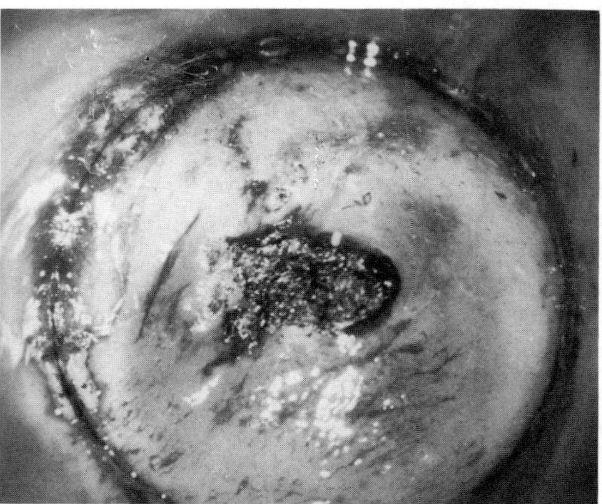

Figure 24-5 After transection of the stalk, the cut surface has been coagulated for hemostatic purposes.

Destruction of Sessile Polyps and Broad-Based Tumors

The decision to carry out laser destruction of these tumors was taken only when several biopsies proved that the growth was benign. These tumors are not excised but are destroyed in situ by laser evaporation (Figures 24-6, 24-7). This is achieved by continuously moving the beam over the tumor surface and thus gradually vaporizing the pathologic tissue. Visual control through the microscope is so accurate that the change of color from pink to gray warns the surgeon when the vaporiza-

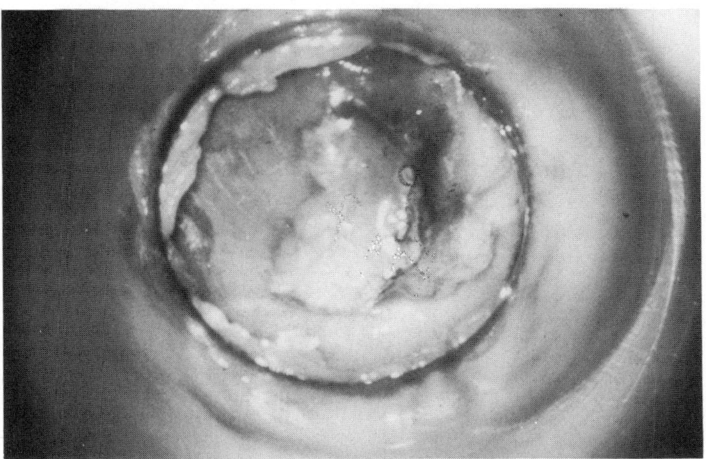

Figure 24-6 Sessile polyp in the rectal wall.

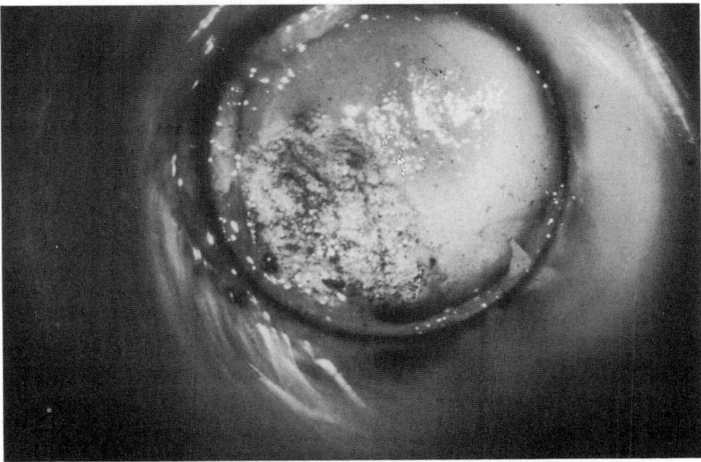

Figure 24-7 View of the rectal wall after vaporization of the sessile polyp.

tion reaches the connective tissue underlying the mucosa. The depth of vaporization can easily be influenced by changing the output of the laser or the speed of movement of the laser spot. This technique proved to be very reliable since perforations never occurred, notwithstanding the fact that a number of these tumors were located above the peritoneal reflection.

In some patients with a sessile adenoma close to the anus, the tumor mass can be vaporized by means of one of the handpieces. After dilatation of the anus, the introduction of a speculum provides enough space for safe surgery with one of the slender handpieces of the Sharplan (Figures 24-8, 24-9).

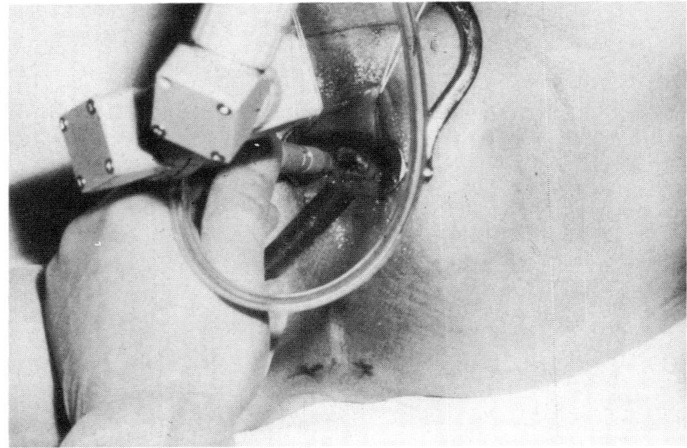

Figure 24-8 Laser vaporization of a sessile polyp located close to the rectoanal junction.

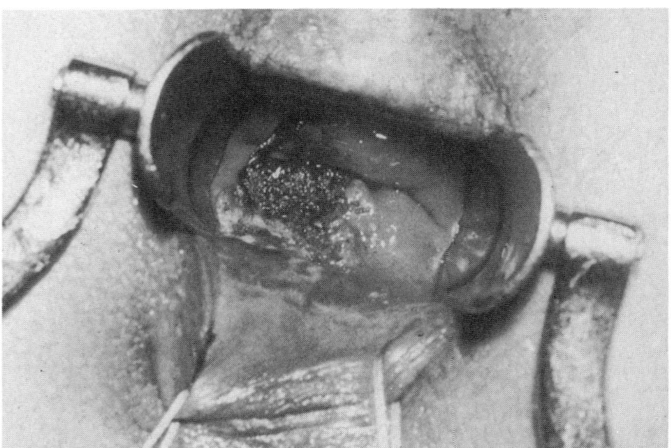

Figure 24-9 Close-up of the defect remaining after vaporization of polyp shown in Figure 24-8.

RESULTS

Between February 1975 and June 1976, 44 operations were carried out on 28 patients. Some required two or three procedures because of the large tumor volume which had to be vaporized or the great surface covered by the adenomatous growth. Three patients had had subtotal colectomy for familial polyposis prior to laser surgery for the multiple polyps in the remaining rectal stump. No scarring could be seen after vaporization of these small polyps. Notwithstanding the fact that some patients had very large tumors, there were no problems with hemostasis, and we saw a mild late hemorrhage in a patient using anticoagulant drugs on only one occasion.

In seven patients a sessile tumor located above the peritoneal reflection was vaporized without causing a perforation.

DISCUSSION

Our experience is too small and the follow-up too short to make definite statements about the specific indications and limitations of the use of the CO_2 laser in the rectosigmoid colon.

Several advantages of the use of the CO_2 laser became obvious:

1. The micromanipulator allows precise positioning and movement of the laser beam; the microscope provides good vision.

2. The minimal amount of thermal damage to remaining tissues is evidenced by prompt healing and the absence of recognizable scar tissue upon rectoscopy six weeks postoperatively. Electrosurgery in the rectum usually causes heavy scarring due to slow healing.

3. The hospital stay is shorter than for electrosurgery. Electrocoagulation boils the pathologic tissue, transforming it into a thick necrotic slough. In order to decrease the risk of later hemorrhage due to premature release of this necrotic tissue, bowel preparation is required and the patient must be hospitalized for three or four days postoperatively. There is no need for these precautions when laser surgery is performed, since no appreciable slough is left behind. The laser operation can be carried out the day following admission and the patient can be discharged the next day.

4. Laser evaporation by this procedure can be safely carried out up to 25 cm from the anus, while electrocoagulation above the 10-cm level is debatable because of the risk of perforation.

During treatment of this series of patients, one shortcoming of the instrumentation, the insufficient power output, became evident. The 35 watts delivered by the Sharplan yields a rather low-power density in the focal spot when using a 400-mm lens and, consequently, a small volume of vaporized tissue per unit time. A laser device delivering two or three times more power might enable us to operate more rapidly when dealing with large tumors for which vaporization is required. In the very near future we shall start using the American Optical 100 W CO_2 laser[9] for the eradication of small rectal cancers.

SUMMARY

The CO_2 laser is a superior substitute for electrosurgery in the treatment of polyps and small cancers in the rectosigmoid colon. More experience is needed before establishing the exact criteria for its use.

REFERENCES

1. Klok PAA: The treatment of some forms of rectal cancer by electrocoagulation. *Arch Chir Neerl* 16:173–183, 1964.
2. Swerlow DB, Salvati EP: Electrocoagulation of cancer of the rectum. *Dis Colon Rectum* 15:228–232, 1972.
3. Crile G Jr, Turnbull RB: The role of electrocoagulation in the treatment of carcinoma of the rectum. *Surg Gynecol Obstet* 135:391–396, 1972.
4. Hall RR, Hill DW, Beach AD: A carbon dioxide surgical laser. *Ann Roy Coll Surg* 48:181–188, 1971.
5. Mihashi S, Jako GJ, Incze J, et al: Laser surgery in otolaryngology: Interaction of CO_2 laser and soft tissue. *Ann NY Acad Sci* 267:263–294, 1976.
6. Verschueren R: *The CO_2 Laser in Tumor Surgery.* Amsterdam, Van Gorcum & Comp. B.V., 1976.
7. Stellar S, Polanyi TG, Bredemeier HC: Lasers in surgery, in Wolbarsht ML (ed): *Laser Applications in Medicine and Biology,* vol II. New York, Plenum Press, 1974, pp 241–290.
8. Strong MS, Jako GJ: Laser surgery in the larynx: Early clinical experience with a continuous wave CO_2 laser. *Ann Otol Rhinol Laryngol* 81:791–798, 1972.
9. Polanyi TG, Bredemeier HC, Davis TW Jr: A CO_2 laser for surgical research. *Med Biol Eng* 8:541–548, 1970.

25 Genitourinary Surgery

R.R. Hall, MS, FRCS

The role of the CO_2 laser has become well defined in some surgical specialities but in urology this is not yet the case. This is not for want of clinical interest or lack of experimentation, although technical difficulties and the absence of a flexible fiberoptic instrument to conduct the laser beam adequately have limited the development of CO_2 laser cystoscopy.

ENDOSCOPIC SURGERY

The most important advance in modern urology has been the development of endoscopic surgery. The technical innovations of fiberoptic lighting, solid-rod telescopes, continuous irrigation, and solid-state diathermy sources have made the urological resectoscope the most versatile of all endoscopes. However, there is still room for improvement and it seems logical that the unique thermal optical properties of lasers could be used to advantage in endoscopic urology. The rigidity of the resectoscope makes access difficult to certain parts of the bladder, particularly high on the posterior wall and on the anterior wall. The speed of tissue removal is relatively slow compared with open surgery so that most urologists still favor suprapubic enucleation for very large prostates, despite the disadvantages of open surgery, because it is faster than endoscopic resection. Even with the careful use of the electrocautery, hemostasis can be time-consuming and hemorrhage may be considerable during endoscopic resection of bladder tumors or the prostate. Solid-state electrocauterization apparatus provides an improved current for cutting tissue, but postoperative scarring can still reduce the capacity of the bladder following extensive and repeated resections, and limits its usefulness in the urethra. In view of these limitations a variety of workers have investigated the possibility of improving upon diathermy transurethral resection by the use of lasers.

Access Within the Bladder

Staehler and associates[1,2] have attacked the problem of access within the bladder by passing the Nd-YAG laser along a flexible quartz fiber introduced through the cystoscope. By this means small tumors anywhere within the bladder have been reached with ease for fulguration. Many patients have been treated successfully for tumors as large as a hazelnut, the lesions being coagulated in situ by repeated pulses of 1.06 μ energy. The system has also been used to irradiate the tumor bed following conventional transurethral resection of invasive bladder tumors in the hope of reducing the incidence of local tumor recurrence.[3,4] These investigators selected the Nd-YAG laser in preference to the CO_2 and argon lasers on the basis of preliminary animal experiments which suggested that the CO_2 laser was insufficiently hemostatic and the argon laser carried too great a risk of bladder perforation.[5,6] Long-term results of this treatment are not yet available nor has a controlled comparison with diathermy fulguration or transurethral resection been reported. Rothauge[7] has used an argon laser cystoscope for a similar purpose in 38 patients, reporting satisfactory preliminary results and noting that pulsed laser treatment in the bladder could be performed without anesthesia.

Wilscher et al[8] have constructed and tested a CO_2 laser cystoscope and have demonstrated the feasibility of treating lesions anywhere within the bladder by reflecting the laser beam in the gas-distended bladder cavity from the end of a rigid cystoscope.

Bülow and Levene[9] in a preliminary report describe a hand-held 20 watt CO_2 laser small enough to allow direct connection to a cystoscope. The focused laser beam was coaxial with the instrument and thus could be used for incision of the urethra or base of the bladder, but could not be directed within the bladder cavity.

Certainly, from these preliminary developments, the ability to reach small lesions anywhere within the lower urinary tract by means of a reflected laser beam or flexible fiber is a practical proposition which is worthy of further investigation.

Time for Tissue Removal

To date, the Nd-YAG laser does not present any advantage in time that is immediately apparent for ablation of lesions in the lower urinary tract. Diathermy fulguration is as rapid as the Nd-YAG laser and neither can compare with resection, which is preferred by most urologists and which removes tissue in bulk rather than coagulating it in situ and waiting for separation of the necrosed tissue days or weeks later. It should be noted, however, that heating of the bladder wall was found to be more homogeneous with Nd-YAG energy than with coagulation diathermy,[10] which could provide theoretical, if not practical, advantage for those who prefer this to resection. Bladder perforation has not been observed with this laser, and adjacent organs are safe if the applied power is no greater than 40 watts with a 2-mm spot size and pulse duration of two seconds.[11]

The time taken by Bülow[12] to divide a urethral stricture with a 40-watt focused Nd-YAG laser (20 minutes for a 1 cm stricture) was also considerably slower than conventional practice when a "cold knife" optical urethrotome is used. Bülow and Levene[9] made no comment on the speed of incision with their 20-watt CW CO_2 laser cystoscope. Using a prototype CO_2 laser cystoscope producing approximately 12 watts focused to a 2-mm spot within the bladder, Hall (unpublished data) vaporized part of a human papillary tumor and found the time for vaporization to be very slow (Figure 25-1). Based on the results of an experiment which vaporized resected human prostatic tissue we calculated that at least 80 watts of available, focused CO_2 laser power would be required to perform laser prostatectomy at a speed comparable with conventional instruments, assuming there was no bleeding during vaporization with the laser.[13] In view of this it is suggested that the instrument developed by Bülow and Levene[9] may prove useful for urethral strictures, but it is unlikely to be of practical value within the bladder or for prostatic resection.

Hemostasis

One of the main features emphasized in the promotion of the CO_2 laser for surgery has been the "bloodless" nature of its incision and vaporization of tissue. Were this true in the lower urinary tract, it would certainly be a major advantage.

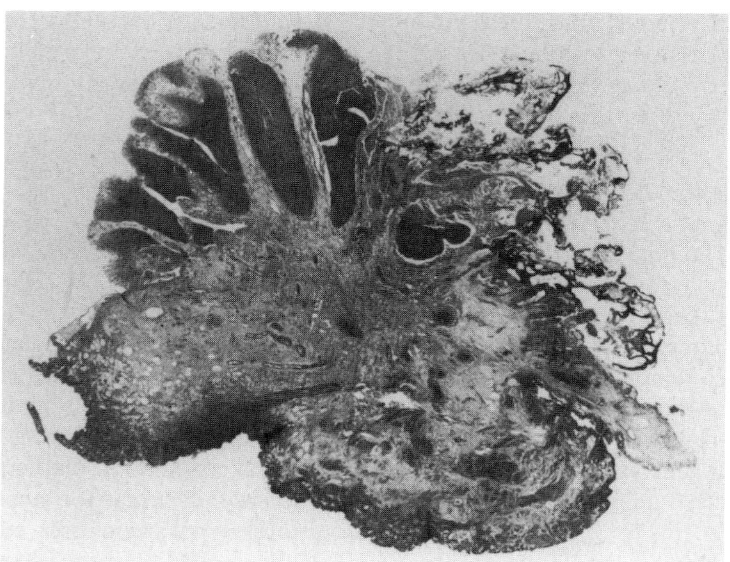

Figure 25-1 Section of a 5-mm human papillary transitional cell carcinoma of bladder partly vaporized by a CO_2 laser. Half of tumor vaporized, remaining tumor viable. Minimal thermal damage in underlying bladder wall. Instrument used: prototype CO_2 laser cystoscope by Karl Storz Ltd and Laser Industries.

There are no published reports concerning the control of bleeding with CO_2 laser cystoscopes; only the inference that experience gained in otolaryngology will apply in urology, namely, that bleeding is minimal if vessels encountered are less than 0.5 mm in diameter.[8,14] Clinical experience shows that this will apply in the urethra, but unfortunately many of the arteries and veins in the human bladder wall and prostate are considerably larger than 0.5 mm.

To clarify this point the author has used the Sharplan CO_2 laser to open the human bladder and vaporize bladder mucosa, bladder wall muscle, and benign prostatic tissue during conventional transvesical prostatectomy. Using power levels from 10 to 40 watts with spot sizes varying from 1.5 mm to 5 mm in diameter, it was found that bleeding occurred which obscured the site of laser impact, thus preventing the removal of any significant amount of bladder mucosa, muscle, or prostate. In two patients with multiple superficial tumors of the bladder undergoing open resection, papillary tumors less than 5 mm to 6 mm in diameter could be destroyed satisfactorily, albeit slowly, but attempts to vaporize or excise larger sessile tumors failed because of hemorrhage.

In experiments on chemically induced bladder tumors in animals,[15] hemostasis was satisfactory with the CO_2 laser, but the size of vessels encountered in rabbits and even dogs, does not compare with the human bladder and prostate. Pariente and d'Ovidio[16] found that in one patient with bladder papillomatosis bleeding was "much reduced" and "nothing compared to the hematic coloring (of the urine) which we are used to seeing in conventional urologic surgery." Despite this, with increased experience and larger tumors, it is unlikely that the CO_2 laser will prove sufficiently hemostatic for urological endoscopy if used alone. Several workers[13] have suggested the combination of CO_2 lasers with argon or Nd-YAG lasers to provide both hemostasis and rapid vaporization, but this has not been achieved in clinical trials to date.

Scarring

Many investigators have reported that CO_2 laser incisions heal with very little scarring, particularly in mucous membranes. Wilscher et al,[8] Hughes and Scott[17] and Troitsky et al[18] have confirmed this for CW CO_2 laser incisions of the urinary epithelium, and Rattner[19] noted similar findings for superpulsed CO_2 laser lesions in the rabbit bladder. This should be an important advantage for the treatment of multiple, frequently recurring bladder tumors if it can be exploited endoscopically. Similarly, on theoretical grounds it could improve the management of urethral strictures as previously suggested,[9] but this has yet to be demonstrated.

Bülow et al[12,20] have reported the successful excision of urethral strictures in five patients with a 40-watt Nd-YAG laser focused to a 1.5 mm spot. This is rather surprising, as the relatively deep penetration of this laser would be expected to produce further periurethral fibrosis and recurrent stenosis, so it may be significant that these patients have only been followed for a short period. It is possible that the precise excision of all the fibrous tissue of the strictures by laser vaporization is so much more effective than the simple incision achieved with conventional urethrotomes that a small amount of late periurethral fibrosis is not significant. More recently, after considering Nd-YAG, argon, and CO_2 laser radiation, Bülow[21] has suggested that the latter would be the most appropriate for the excision of strictures.

NONENDOSCOPIC UROLOGY

The particular feature of laser action on tissue that appealed to pioneers of this type of surgery was the rapid, intense, localized heating that could seal blood vessels and lymphatics during primary incision, sterilize the wound, facilitate incision of infected tissues, and vaporize small lesions in situ with great precision or larger volumes without extensive dissection or operative manipulation. All these factors are relevant in urological surgery where it is well known that the kidney, bladder, prostate, and genitalia are particularly vascular and frequently the site of primary or secondary infection. It was thus with good reason that a number of surgeons have put the potential advantages of the laser to the test in nonendoscopic urological surgery.

Animal Studies

Mulvaney and Beck[22] first reported an attempt at wedge resection of the dog kidney with a 50-watt CW CO_2 laser, but found the incision to be slow and hemostasis unsatisfactory. Hughes and Scott[17] used a similar laser in dogs for vasectomy, partial nephrectomy, ablation of the bladder mucosa, and prostatic surgery. They found that the vas deferens could be transected easily with one pulse from the laser, but recanalization of the vas occurred in one-third of cases by six weeks, and it was concluded that the laser would be unsuitable for human vasectomy because recanalization would occur too frequently. Partial nephrectomy was successful with the laser if performed with synchronous renal ischemia, although large segmental renal arteries required suture ligature in the conventional manner. Destruction of 80% of the bladder's epithelial surface was performed with the unfocused laser beam; the bladder healed without undue scarring and reepithelialization proceeded normally. Attempts at wedge biopsy of the dog prostate failed because of bleeding from the prostate which obscured further laser action. It was considered that the laser would have no advantage for prostatic surgery because of its poor hemostasis in this anatomical location.

Breitwieser et al,[23] following similar studies of partial nephrectomy, did not report any advantage from the laser, particularly because conventional ligatures were required for hemostasis. Meiraz et al[24] undertook partial nephrectomies in cats with a CO_2 laser and found it to be a safe and effective procedure, free of complications. Barzilay[25] confirmed this observation when performing lower-pole, partial nephrectomy in dogs, but noted that although incision with this laser prevented capillary and venous bleeding, for the parenchymal branches of the renal artery, ligation was required in the usual way. Serial histological examination confirmed normal healing of the kidney and pelvicalyceal system and no evidence of secondary hemorrhage.

Clinical Experience

Mulvaney and Beck[22] were among the first to treat urological lesions with a laser. They destroyed a metastatic adenocarcinoma in the urethra with a pulsed ruby laser, but the tumor recurred two months later. Vainberg[26] successfully treated 50 patients with urethral polyps and condyloma acuminatum of the penis by means of a CO_2 laser. Laser vaporization was simple, effective, and uncomplicated, and was recommended for possible use in outpatient practice. Barzilay[25] has performed lower-pole, partial nephrectomy and an extensive nephrolithotomy in a small number of patients with satisfactory results, although the CO_2 laser incision was found to be slow. Pariente and d'Ovidio[16] performed laser nephrotomy for renal calculi in an unspecified number of patients. They reported that "incision of the renal parenchyma was always bloodless though we never practiced the clamping of the renal pedicle." This is a rather surprising observation, particularly in the absence of renal ischemia, and is contrary to the findings of previous observers.

Hall[13,27] has used the CO_2 laser for a wide variety of nonendoscopic urological operations in routine clinical practice and, at the conclusion of each operation, recorded the opinions of the operating surgeon, surgical assistants, the anesthetist, and visiting surgeons concerning the advantage of the laser compared with conventional techniques. The operations performed or attempted with the laser included nephrectomy, upper- and lower-pole partial nephrectomy, nephrostomy, nephrolithotomy, pyelolithotomy, ureterolithotomy, transvesical prostatectomy, open excision of multiple bladder tumors, simple and radical cystectomy, scrotal flap urethroplasty, anterior urethroplasty, excision of squamous cell carcinoma of the glans penis, total penectomy, radical block dissection of the inguinal and iliac lymph nodes, excision of suprapubic, scrotal, and perineal fistulae and abscesses, and vaporization of condyloma acuminatum.

Hemostasis was generally disappointing with the exception of the renal parenchyma where incision was slow and renal ischemia time prolonged. Incision of dense fibrous tissue was good and the use of the laser in a case of xanthogranulomatous pyelonephritis was particularly impressive. Laser incision of infected tissues and vaporization of abscess cavities was simple, but none of these wounds healed by primary intention despite the supposed sterilizing effect of the laser. Postoperative lymphatic drainage in several patients undergoing pelvic or superficial inguinal lymphadenectomy was not noticeably reduced. The inability of this laser to perform significant bladder and prostatic resection has been described above.

SUMMARY

It is quite possible to perform almost any open urological operation with the CO_2 laser. Animal experiments have indicated that it could prove particularly advantageous in renal surgery and for superficial lesions of the lower urinary tract. In clinical practice these advantages have been less apparent, mainly because the blood vessels encountered are significantly larger than those in animal models. In renal calculus surgery the laser adds nothing to established techniques employing hypothermia and, with a few unusual exceptions, does not present any significant advantages for nonendoscopic urology in general.

It should be recognized that modern urologists spend an increasing proportion of their operating time using a resectoscope. As in other specialities, it is the endoscopic application of lasers that has been the most promising to date. It is clear that, for reasons of poor hemostasis, the CO_2 laser will be of limited value in urological endoscopy if used alone, but its combination with the Nd-YAG laser may become a practical possibility[28] which may prove more fruitful. Alternatively, the growing possibility of flexible cystoscopy may make the Nd-YAG laser a more attractive proposition for outpatient treatment of the lower urinary tract without anesthesia. Thus it is possible that lasers may yet lead to the next major technical advance in urology.

REFERENCES

1. Staehler G, Gorisch W, Hofstetter A: Ein Laser-Zystoskop. *Akt Urol* 7:363–366, 1976.
2. Staehler G, Hofstetter A, Schmiedt E, et al: Endoskopische Laser-Bestrahlung von Blasentumoren des Menschen. *Fortschr Med* 95:1–5, 1977.
3. Staehler G, McCord RC, Hofstetter A, et al: Nd:YAG laser irradiation of the normal and tumorous bladder wall, in Kaplan I (ed): *Proceedings of the 2nd International Symposium on Laser Surgery.* Jerusalem, Jerusalem Academic Press, 1978, pp 180–184.
4. Staehler G, Hofstetter A: Transurethral laser irradiation of urinary bladder tumors. *Eur Urol* 5:64–69, 1979.
5. Staehler G, Hofstetter A, Gorisch W, et al: Endoscopy in experimental urology using an argon-laser beam. *Endoscopy* 8:1–4, 1976.
6. Staehler G: Personal communication, 1977.
7. Rothauge CF: Transurethrale Behandlung von Blasentumoren mit Laser. *Helv Chir Acta* 45:233–236, 1978.
8. Wilscher MK, Filoso AM, Jako GJ, et al: Development of carbon dioxide laser cystoscope. *J Urol* 119:202–207, 1978.
9. Bülow H, Levene S: Development of a carbon dioxide laser endoscope without a mobile arm system. *Urol Res* 7:31, 1979.
10. Hofstetter A: *Proceedings of the 3rd International Symposium on Laser Surgery.* Jerusalem, Jerusalem Academic Press, 1979.
11. Staehler G, Halldorsson T, Langerholc J, et al: Dosimetry of neodymium: YAG laser applications in urology. *Lasers in Surgery and Medicine* 1:191–197, 1980.
12. Bülow H, Bülow U, Frohmüller HGW: Transurethral laser urethrotomy in man: Preliminary report. *J Urol* 121:286–287, 1979.

13. Hall RR: Urological laser cystoscope. *Proceedings of the 3rd International Symposium on Laser Surgery.* Jerusalem, Jerusalem Academic Press, 1979.

14. Strong, MS, Jako GJ, Polanyi TG, et al: Laser surgery in the aerodigestive tract. *Am J Surg* 26:529, 1975.

15. Rattner W, Rosemberg S, Fuller T, et al: Carbon dioxide laser in bladder surgery, in Kaplan I (ed): *Proceedings of the 2nd International Symposium on Laser Surgery.* Jerusalem, Jerusalem Academic Press, 1978, pp 185–188.

16. Pariente R, d'Ovidio M: First experiences in the use of CO_2 laser in urological surgery, in Kaplan I (ed): *Proceedings of the 2nd International Symposium on Laser Surgery.* Jerusalem, Jerusalem Academic Press, 1978, pp 169–179.

17. Hughes BF, Scott WW: Preliminary report on the use of a CO_2 laser surgical unit in animals. *Invest Urol* 9:353–357, 1972.

18. Troitsky RA, Vishnevsky AA, Polonsky AK, et al: Healing of the wound of the urinary bladder inflicted by the laser under experimental conditions. *Urol Nefrol* 40:35–37, 1975.

19. Rattner WH, Rosemberg SK, Fuller T: Difference between continuous wave and superpulse carbon dioxide laser in bladder surgery. *Urology* 13:264–266, 1979.

20. Bülow H, Bülow U, Frohmüller GW: Laser investigations of the strictured dog urethra. *Invest Urol* 16:403–407, 1979.

21. Bülow H: Present status of endoscopic laser techniques in urology. *Endoscopy* 4:240–243, 1979.

22. Mulvaney WP, Beck CW: The laser beam in urology. *J Urol* 99:112–115, 1968.

23. Breitwieser P, Herbrich H, Nöske H-D, et al: CO_2 laser als Operationsinstrument in der experimentellen Urologie. *Biomed Tech* 18:6, 1973.

24. Meiraz D, Peled I, Gassner S, et al: The use of the CO_2 laser for partial nephrectomy: An experimental study. *Invest Urol* 15:262–264, 1977.

25. Barzilay B, Perlberg S, Caine M: The use of CO_2 laser beam for kidney surgery: Experimental and clinical experience preliminary report, in Kaplan I (ed): *Proceedings of the 2nd International Symposium on Laser Surgery.* Jerusalem, Jerusalem Academic Press, 1978, pp 164–168.

26. Vainberg ZS, Vishnevsky AA, Likhter MS: Use of laser for surgical treatment of the urethral polyps and condylomata of the penis. *Urol Nefrol* 42:44–47, 1977.

27. Hall RR: The carbon dioxide laser in non-endoscopic urological surgery, in Kaplan I (ed): *Proceedings of the 2nd International Symposium on Laser Surgery.* Jerusalem, Jerusalem Academic Press, 1978, pp 197–201.

28. Pinnow DA, Gentile AL, Standlee AG, et al: Polycrystalline fiber optical waveguides for infrared transmission. *J Quantum Electronics* 13:91D, 1977.

26 Orthopedic Surgery

H. Horoszowski, MD
I. Farine, MD
M. Heim, MD

The laser beam has been utilized in medicine since the early 1960s. In orthopedics a first attempt was made in 1972 by Moore.[1] In June 1975 we introduced the Sharplan CO_2 laser scalpel in orthopedic surgery and defined the criteria for its use. The CO_2 laser scalpel seemed to be convenient in orthopedic surgery because its biological properties are related to the wavelength. Israel Industries have developed the Sharplan CO_2 laser scalpel, the wavelength of which is 10.6 μ. Biologically, the cutting power is good, the hemostatic properties sufficient, the paraincisional necrotic zone only 0.6 mm, and the water penetration is low (0.1%).

MATERIAL AND RESULTS

In order to establish our criteria, more than 300 patients were operated on using the laser, specifically patients with fractures, joint problems, hand problems, bleeding diathesis, tumors, and infections. We were then able to establish the best indications for the laser.

Hemophiliac Patients

This group of patients enabled us to study the hemostatic properties of the laser scalpel.[2] The most homogeneous series of operations consisted of five synovectomies of the knee in which we eliminated one of the normal precautions taken for surgery of such patients. The first patient, 10 years old, previously operated on his left knee, underwent a right knee synovectomy in 1976 with the laser scalpel. He suffered from chronic synovitis which failed to respond to conservative therapy.

For this first operation with the laser, a standard preoperative preparation was performed. The day prior to surgery, cryoprecipitate was infused. On the operating table, Factor VIII was administered up to a 100% circulating rate, a tourniquet cuff was inflated on the operated limb, and postoperative replacement was conducted classically. The postoperative hospitalization period was shortened by one half in comparison with the previous surgery. The range of movements and muscle power in the right leg were better in a shorter time than in the left one. After four years follow-up, no subsequent significant hemarthrosis has occurred and a full range of movements exists.

Four identical cases of knee synovitis were operated upon. We eliminated the tourniquet (cases 2 to 5), the peroperative infusion of Factor VIII (case 3) (operating at a 14% circulating rate of Factor VIII), the preoperative and operative infusion of Factor VIII (cases 4 to 5), operating without a tourniquet, at 1% of Factor VIII. In case 5, even the postoperative rate of Factor VIII was lowered to 30%.

Other operations were successfully performed on severe hemophiliacs with this technique, including hip release, knee release, and patellectomy. This demonstrates not only the hemostatic properties of the CO_2 laser, but also the diminution of postoperative oozing.

Thus the CO_2 laser scalpel is a further step in the operative treatment of hemophiliacs with antibodies to Factor VIII.

Surgery of Tumors

The CO_2 laser scalpel was used advantageously for removing benign and malignant tumors.

Benign tumors The group of benign tumors includes osteoid osteomas and aneurysmal bone cysts. Osteoid osteoma, characterized clinically by night pains, causes extensive sclerosis of the long bones; the tumor itself is not more than 2 mm to 5 mm in diameter. By using the CO_2 laser scalpel, it is possible to cut the sclerotic bone very close to the nidus, avoiding further weakness or iatrogenic fractures. Postoperative and functional results are better, especially in femur neck localization, or when the tumor is close to ligaments or the growth plate. In our last case, we exposed the tumor through the cortex without bone resection, allowing immediate function. In bone cysts, especially aneurysmal bone cysts, the CO_2 laser allows virtually bloodless operations.

Malignant tumors The group of malignant tumors includes Ewing's sarcoma, osteosarcoma, and rhabdomyosarcoma. The CO_2 laser scalpel can be used for biopsies or for resection of the tumor. Biopsies of malignant tumors, such as Ewing's sarcoma, are easy and bloodless. We presume that there is much less diffusion of malignant cells than with conventional biopsies. Therefore, we extended the application of the CO_2 laser to resection biopsies, where the tumor is removed en bloc, such as in osteosarcoma, chondrosarcoma, and rhabdomyosarcoma.

Joint Replacement Surgery

We used the CO_2 laser scalpel in 20 total hip replacements and three knee replacements. We were able to perform the knee replacements without a tourniquet cuff. It resulted in better quadriceps power and no thrombophlebitis. In such procedures, performed in elderly people, often fat and always suffering from varicose veins, the lack of a tourniquet cuff was a great advantage.

Total hip replacements were performed with the CO_2 laser scalpel in patients suffering from rheumatoid arthritis and familial Mediterranean fever (FMF). These systemic diseases destroy the joints and alter the capsule, ligaments, and muscles. Operations performed by classical techniques are often complicated by hemorrhage, infections are more frequent, and the range of movements of the replaced joint is always poor. In six rheumatoid and FMF patients operated on bilaterally, one hip classically and the second with the laser scalpel, the results of the laser-operated hip were significantly better. Operative bleeding and postoperative oozing were reduced by one-third. The mean range of flexion two weeks after the surgery was 120° instead of 80°. All patients noted less pain than after the previous operation and an easier rehabilitation.

DISCUSSION

The coagulative properties of the CO_2 laser were best demonstrated in surgery on severe hemophiliac patients,[2] and on cases of bilateral joint replacement. The blood loss was reduced by one-third, the postoperative oozing by 40%. Our studies have shown that the sealing properties are optimal on a surface equivalent to two-thirds of the Gaussian distribution of the energy of the focal point, ie, a good seal is possible on vessels up to 1 mm in diameter. Larger vessels (up to 1.5 mm) may be sealed when emptied of blood between two hemostats. The CO_2 laser in our opinion is responsible for more hemorrhage when cutting large vessels. When the wall of a dilated vein is partially cut, bleeding occurs which absorbs the energy of the laser scalpel. The cutting properties diminish almost completely and there is no coagulative or cutting effect. Therefore, large vessels have to be individualized and ligated or cauterized.

Hospitalization time is markedly reduced following laser surgery. Less oozing and postoperative edema reduce the number of complications. The possibility of operating without a tourniquet reduces thromboembolic phenomena. Decreased pain attributable to these factors, and possibly to the sealing of the cut nerves, facilitate an easier rehabilitation. The reduction of hospitalization time is from 30% to 50%.

Tumor surgery is, for us, an absolute indication for laser surgery.[3–5] Three problems must be discussed: the depth of the cut of the bone, bone consolidation, and metastatic diffusion of malignant tumors.

The depth of the cut of the bone and its breadth were studied on fresh animal bone, cut in such a way that the laser was fixed, the bone moving at a predetermined speed; the only variable was the output. We determined that the depth of the cut at high voltage is related to the time during which the beam remains on the bone. When augmenting the voltage by 80% (hyperpulsed beam), the cut is not deeper but is narrower by up to 50%. The laser beam alters the organic substance of the bone and melts the inorganic ones which deposit like a char in the depth of the cut. If one activates the laser scalpel a second time on the same cut, the energy of the beam is partially absorbed by the char. The laser scalpel loses its cutting properties, so only the thermal effect remains. This results in a broad destroyed area surrounded by more devitalized bone. A cut of bone has to be done at one passby leaving the beam enough time to penetrate into the medullary canal. If the cut is not deep enough, the char has to be removed with a thin osteotome prior to the second pass of the laser scalpel on the same cut.

Bone consolidation was studied experimentally.[6] We found no significant difference with respect to the consolidation time or percentage of pseudarthrosis, although the histological studies have shown devitalized osteocytes on both sides of the cut. The thermal devitalization zone extends 2 mm from the cut edge of the bone.

In studies performed in Basel (personal communication), it was shown that the first phase of callus formation is slower following laser osteotomy; the callus then hardens massively and the final time of ossification is similar to classical osteotomy. We presume that the hydroxyhepatite crystals liberated and crystallized by the thermal effect of the laser beam could be a catalyst of osteogenesis. Nevertheless, we always use a dynamic compression system for osteosynthesis following laser surgery and, if possible, external fixation, which enhances further compression even days after the operation.

Diminution of the rate of metastasis following tumor surgery on muscles or bones cannot be demonstrated. Kaplan, in a prospective study on melanoma, showed a significant decrease of metastasis following laser knife excision of such tumors. It is logical to presume that in orthopedic surgery we face the same phenomenon. This is due to the possibility that broad excision at a distance from the tumor, by a nontouch technique and without chiseling the bone reduces the metastasis rate.

The sealing of lymphatic vessels and veins is another element for the prevention of malignant dissemination. Cellular destruction by sublimation in places where radical excision is technically impossible is a technique which can be used in tumor surgery. Cultures of cells that were exposed to the laser beam have proved they were totally destroyed. For this reason we think that the CO_2 laser scalpel is an absolute indication in tumor surgery as one step of a comprehensive treatment.

Fine-structure surgery in orthopedics by the laser scalpel was of no advantage in our hands. Furthermore, a high complication rate makes us believe that the existing device is dangerous. The proximity of the nerves, vessels, and tendons in the hand, for instance, obliged us to use protective techniques for those elements. It is best to use the absorbing power of water for the beam. In the region of the knee or elbow, it is easy to infiltrate 100 ml of saline solution, but in fine structure surgery only a few milliliters can be injected. This small quantity of fluid is immediately vaporized by the beam, and the thermal diffusion creates damage incompatible with a good functional result. Only further developments (very fine focal zone), by diminishing the cutting surface and the paraincisional necrotic zone, and without loss of cutting power, will enhance proper utilization of the laser scalpel in fine-structure surgery.

Surgery on infective tissues with the laser scalpel is acceptable to plastic surgeons. We found the same advantages in orthopedic surgery, and the CO_2 laser scalpel was used for excision of infected postoperative wounds, especially for the treatment of infected total hip joints. The advantages of the laser scalpel are due to the possibility of broad excision with thermal effects at a distance from infected tissues, and without touching the infected zones.

The best use of the CO_2 laser beam is for removal of an artificial joint. It is always difficult to remove the bone cement. The laser beam sublimates the bone cement, which disappears. There is an emission of irritative smoke which has to be aspirated.[5] Toxicologic studies have shown that there is no toxic product in the smoke. The ease of destruction of the cement facilitates previously difficult operations.

However, there are some disadvantages with the use of the CO_2 laser scalpel. Smoke and unpleasant odor are due to the lased cells. The richer the tissue in water, the more smoke and steam will be produced. Therefore, it is mandatory to use a powerful vacuuming device.

The CO_2 laser cuts slower than the knife. Considering only the cutting time, the operating time is prolonged by one-third; on the contrary, the hemostasis time is nearly nonexistent, the laser scalpel sealing the vessels up to 1 mm in diameter. In fact, there is nearly no difference in total operating time. In patients with blood dyscrasias, the total operating time is shortened even more.

The final inconvenience is in operative technique. The laser is a beam of light which destroys the tissues. There is no contact between the cutting device and the tissues. Therefore, tactile sensations must be replaced by visual ones. This necessitates special training before clinical use of the laser.

SUMMARY

The CO_2 laser is of definite surgical importance. Its properties are different from the electrocautery and from the scalpel and, therefore, its indications must be carefully considered. In our opinion, coagulopathies and malignant tumors are an absolute indication for surgery with the CO_2 laser scalpel. Joint surgery in inflammatory diseases is a relative indication. There are some advantages to the laser scalpel in surgery of infections. The CO_2 laser is still contraindicated for fine-structure surgery in orthopedics.

REFERENCES

1. Moore YH: Laser energy in orthopedic surgery. *Proceedings of International Congress of Orthopaedic Surgeons.* Amsterdam, Excerpta Medica, 1973, p 1077.
2. Horoszowski H, Seligshon U, Heim M, et al: Laser in hemophilia in Seligshon U, Rimon A, Horoszowski H (eds): *Haemophilia,* London, Castle House Publication, 1981, pp 189–193.
3. Horoszowski H, Farine I, Engel J: The laser in orthopaedic surgery, in Kaplan I (ed): *Proceedings of the 1st International Symposium of Laser Surgery.* Jerusalem, Jerusalem Academic Press, 1976, pp 139–144.
4. Farine I, Horoszowski H: The use of laser scalpel in orthopaedic surgery, in Kaplan I (ed): *Proceedings of the 2nd International Symposium on Laser Surgery.* Jerusalem, Jerusalem Academic Press, 1978, pp 351–353.
5. Ganel A, Farine I, Horoszowski H, et al: Bone cement melting by a laser beam, gaz analysis. *Lasers and Electro-optics* 1:12–13, 1981.
6. Tauber C, Farine I, Horoszowski H, et al: Fracture healing in rabbits after osteotomy using the CO_2 laser. *Acta Orthop Scand* 50:385–390, 1979.

27 Ophthalmology

Hugh Beckman, MD
Terry A. Fuller, PhD

HISTORY

For centuries man has known that staring into the sun during an eclipse might cause damage to the eye. After the invention of the ophthalmoscope, many ophthalmologists described the appearance of solar retinopathy, which represented retinal photocoagulation by rays of sunlight focused onto the retina by the cornea and lens. In the late 1800s and early 1900s many investigators reported on their ability to create lesions in the retina using focused sunlight or light emitted by a carbon arc. Meyer-Schwickerath[1,2] first reported on his clinical experiences with photocoagulation of the retina in the early 1950s. At that time he utilized sunlight or a Beck arc. He later replaced these energy sources with the xenon lamp and created the xenon photocoagulator manufactured and commercially distributed by Zeiss. In 1956 Meyer-Schwickerath[3] described the use of the xenon arc photocoagulator to produce holes in the iris for the treatment of pupil block glaucoma. This may be the first recorded use of light energy as a means of vaporizing tissue. Since the xenon arc photocoagulator is a relatively low-powered source of energy, exposure times were long, and a great deal of heat was conducted from the target site into surrounding areas, thus creating excessive tissue damage surrounding the treatment sites.

In the early 1960s the ruby laser was developed. The use of its high-powered monochromatic energy for tissue coagulation and vaporization placed ophthalmology in the forefront of medical laser investigation. Ruby lasers have been used[4–7] in the treatment of such retinal diseases as macular degeneration and diabetic retinopathy. Beckman[8] and Perkins[9] in 1971 described the formation of iridectomies with ruby lasers in human eyes. The treatment of intractable glaucomas by transscleral, transconjunctival irradiation of the ciliary body was described by Beckman in 1972,[10] and in 1973 Krasnov[11] described ruby laseropuncture of the anterior chamber angle in the treatment of some glaucomas.

In 1968 L'Esperance[12] described the design of an ophthalmic argon laser photocoagulation system, and in 1969 he reported on its use in the treatment of retinal vascular diseases.[13] This exciting new energy source created a major breakthrough in ophthalmic therapy. It replaced the ruby laser and supplemented the xenon arc photocoagulator, and became the prime energy source for the treatment of retinal diseases. The argon laser's ability to traverse the optically transparent media of the eye, and cut or coagulate the rest of the inner pigmented structures, resulted in investigators developing techniques for argon laser iridectomy[14] and laser trabeculotomy.[15]

CO_2 LASER

Until recently, all the applications of lasers in ophthalmology were dependent upon the transmission of the laser beam through the transparent outer ocular coats with absorption of the energy by the pigmented inner layers. The CO_2 laser with its emission at 10.6 μ is unlike those other wavelengths previously used in that all layers of the eye, including the cornea and sclera, almost totally absorb the energy.

The earliest observations on the effects of CO_2 laser energy on the eye related to the great amount of damage it caused. Fine[16,17] used 10 watts of CW CO_2 energy for one second and created corneal ulcers. With 20 watts, scleral perforations were made and vitreous poured out of the wound. Retinal tears were formed. Campbell[18] in 1968 reported similar findings. Indeed, the continuous wave CO_2 laser at large spot sizes and moderate powers seemed a poor choice for ocular surgery as the microtechniques required precluded charring and shrinkage of tissue. Thus, these two factors had to be eliminated before the laser became competitive with conventional ophthalmic microsurgery.

In 1971 we reported on the development of a laser especially designed for ophthalmic use[19] (Figure 27-1). It is a combined CW and rapid superpulse (RSP) Hill laser.[20] The rapid superpulse portion of this laser has a peak output of 10,000 watts with a maximum average output of 20 watts (CW rating). The average power is a function of its pulse rate which is variable from 75 to 200 pulses per second. The pulse width is 5200 microseconds. It is controlled by a digital control panel with which the laser is capable of firing in timed bursts or a series of bursts both in CW and RSP modes. The laser operates in the TEM_{00} mode (Figure 27-2). A helium-neon tracer light focuses coaxially with the beam through a Zeiss operating microscope OPMI 6. With the microscope, the surgeon views the impact site and can direct the beam by means of a "joystick." With the prototype of this instrument, we performed experimental glaucoma surgery on rabbits and evaluated its performance in corneal surgery. In the ensuing years, the possibilities of the use of the CO_2 laser emission in ophthalmic surgery attracted other investigators into the field.

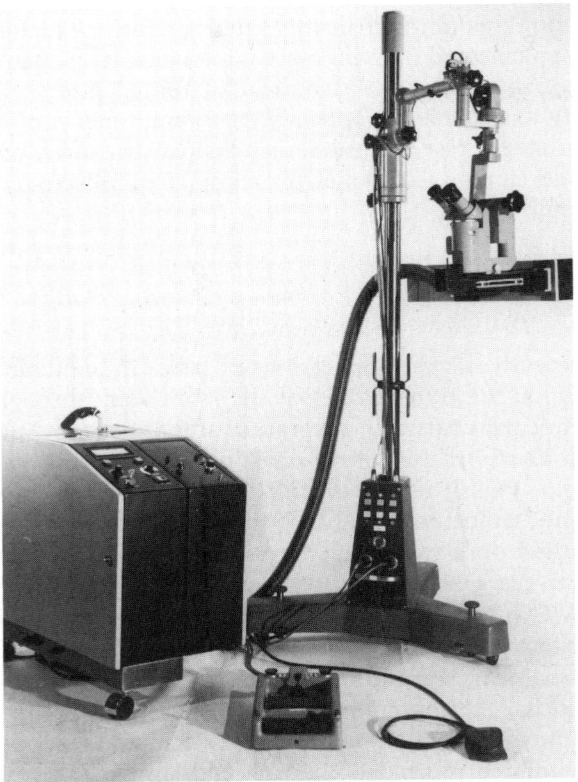

Figure 27-1 Combined rapid superpulse and continuous wave CO_2 laser delivered through operating microscope under "joystick" control.

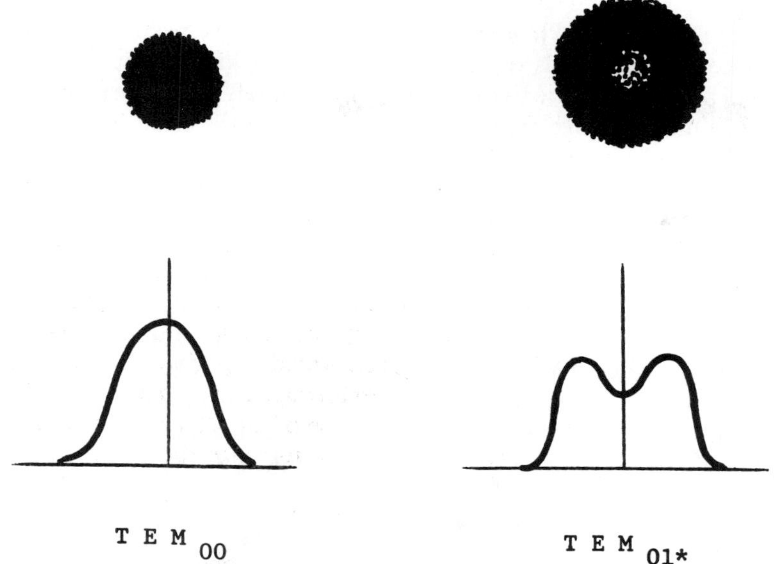

Figure 27-2 Distribution of energy TEM_{00} and TEM_{01*} modes.

Glaucoma Surgery

In 1978 Ticho et al[21] and Beckman and Fuller described techniques utilizing the CO_2 laser to perform filtering procedures in the treatment of glaucoma. Ticho used a hand-held probe to deliver a 1-mm spot onto the corneal-scleral junction. He used 3.8 watts of CW CO_2 laser energy for 0.8 seconds. In all his cases, a 1-mm hole was formed into the anterior chamber. These limbal holes were created under a conjunctival flap. No iridectomy was performed. All patients had neovascular glaucoma. Four of his eight cases were successful, with lasting filtering blebs and intraocular pressures below 20 mm Hg. In the four cases that failed, there were twigs of peripheral iris adherent to the inner surface of the opening, and Ticho felt that, had he created iridectomies, he might have prevented this complication and increased his success rate.

We utilized the etching properties of the relatively cold-cutting rapid superpulse emission to create a two-layer filtering procedure, which might best be termed a subscleral CO_2 laser sclerostomy. In this procedure, a conjunctival-Tenon's flap is dissected in the usual surgical fashion. Utilizing the laser beam, a one-third depth incision is etched 5 mm × 5 mm based at the superior limbus (Figure 27-3A). This incision is 0.5 mm wide. The flap is then undermined conventionally with a lamellar dissector until the blue-white limbal interface is visualized (Figure 27-3B). Originally, we just created a 1.5-mm laser sclerostomy into the anterior chamber at this interface (Figure 27-3C). Recently, however, we have been etching furrows into the two-thirds thickness scleral base, which radiate from the eventual sclerostomy site to the edges of the wound. Our hope is that this creates 1) more surface area within the flap for absorption of aqueous, and 2) directs fluid from the sclerostomy to the external filtering edges of the flap. The iris prolapses through the sclerostomy and a surgical iridectomy is performed in all cases. The flap is then closed with #8-0 collagen sutures. Tenon's capsule and the conjunctiva are closed separately with interrupted collagen sutures.

Utilizing this procedure, we have had the following results. There were 20 eyes treated. Of the 11 eyes with open-angle glaucoma, all have had successful lowering of pressure below 20 mm Hg with only one eye requiring topical medication. Of the nine secondary glaucomas, there was failure in two of the four cases of neovascular glaucoma and in one eye with traumatic glaucoma. Two cases were controlled below 20 mm Hg, and two below 25 mm Hg.

The possible advantages of the laser filtering procedure over a conventional filtering procedure might be:

Safety Since no sharp instrument penetrates into the anterior chamber, damage to the lens or penetration into the vitreous is impossible. The rate of infection would be kept to a minimum.

Technical ease The microdissection is performed under direct observation through the microscope. No blade obscures the base of the wound. Precise depth can be regulated. Softness of the eye is not a factor as scleral resistance is not necessary to facilitate cutting. Hemostasis is obtained with the laser beam (CW being slightly more hemostatic than RSP). Less blood in the field lends itself to better surgical technique.

Adjunct to filtration It has been noted that thermal injury may inhibit the healing of the wound margins due to coagulation of tissue. This may not be the case but, certainly, further studies in this area should be performed to determine whether inhibition of scleral healing occurs. Creating the scleral flap by outlining it with the laser beam, thus creating a 0.5-mm wide incision, is not thought to yield predictably flat uniform blebs. Since instituting the grooved "well-and-tree" in the scleral bed, we have had consistently good results. Unfortunately, this extensive equipment is not uniformly available to ophthalmic surgeons at this time.

Vitreous

Both Karlin[23] and Miller[24] have investigated the use of CO_2 laser energy in the vitreous. Karlin's work was performed with a conventional air-tissue interface in which the beam is directed into the vitreous. Miller's

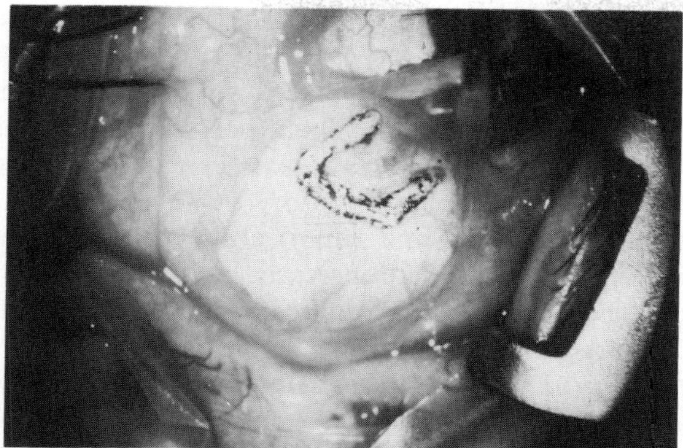

Figure 27-3A One-third scleral thickness groove etched with rapid superpulsed laser.

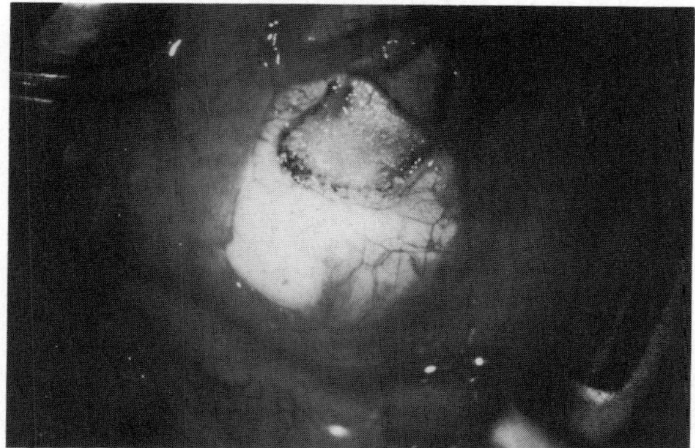

Figure 27-3B Flap of sclera dissected up, revealing scleral base.

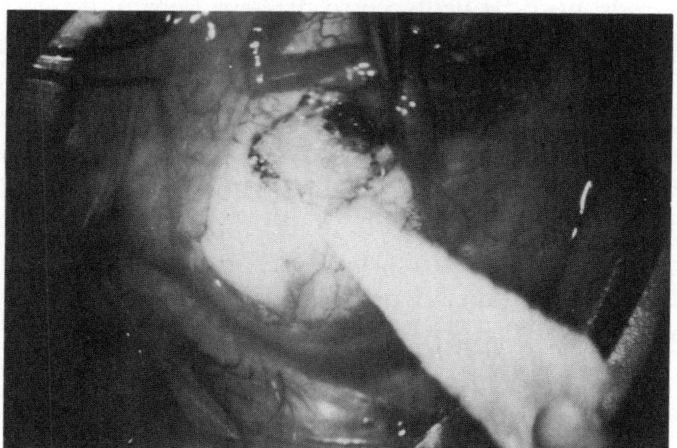

Figure 27-3C Rapid superpulse CO_2 laser sclerostomy into anterior chamber showing iris prolapse through hole.

work was done with an ingenious 1.5-mm probe with an infrared output window. This window allows the delivery of the energy onto a surface within a fluid medium. It can be placed directly in apposition to the vitreous without an air interface. The absorption of CO_2 emission by vitreous is exceptionally high; thus the laser's greatest effect is at the first point of contact with it. In our laboratory we noted that in CW mode at low energy levels, a boiling and vaporization of the vitreous occurred while, as the energy levels were increased, a tunneling of the vitreous began. With rapid superpulse even at high repetition rates, little effect was noted on the vitreous.

All investigators have noted that fibrous bands can be severed with the CO_2 emission. As of now, exact techniques for this have not been satisfactorily worked out for clinical use, but the ability to transect bands within the vitreous without mechanically pulling on the retina during the transection holds great promise for clinical application. Miller has also used his windowed probe to photocauterize blood vessels off the surface of the optic disc, and this may hold promise in the care of patients with proliferative diabetic retinopathy. Photocoagulation of the retina can be performed transvitreally with this probe.

Lens

Photovaporization of the crystalline lens has been reported by Karlin, Miller, and us.[25] Vaporization of the anterior and posterior capsule can be performed with ease. Tunneling of lens material is also performed quite easily. Around the tunnel, the coagulated lens material takes on what we described as a hardened consistency. Miller called it a rubbery consistency. This charring effect was less evident when RSP energy was used than with CW. Since the laser beam has no mass, an infinite number of tunnels would need be drilled into the lens before complete vaporization would take place. For this reason, our feeling is that the laser will eventually have to be wedded to some type of mechanical *chewing* or oscillating probe to effect complete dissolution of the cataractous lens on a practical basis. Anterior capsulotomy could be performed with an actual vaporization of the anterior lens capsule to any configuration desired. Another possible important use might be the performance of posterior capsulotomies and division of secondary membranes without damaging the vitreous face. A new CO_2 carrying fiberoptic might make these ocular techniques more feasible.

Sclera

Scleral dissection has been described by Karlin, Miller and us. Hemostatic bloodless dissection of the sclera is quite possible with the laser. In

CW mode there is more hemostasis, particularly when the beam impinges on the choroidal surface beneath the sclera. The combined experience would seem to indicate that high-powered CW lasers used in extremely small spot sizes would be the most efficient method of through-and-through scleral dissection. The rapid superpulse laser beam seems preferable when partial penetration with minimal charring and shrinkage of tissue is desired, such as in filtering procedures for glaucoma. A histopathologic comparison between RSP, CW, and electrocautery can be seen in Figures 27-4A, 27-4B, and 27-4C. The RSP laser yields the most parallel walled cut with least tissue necrosis, with CW next best, and electrocautery yielding the most tissue damage.

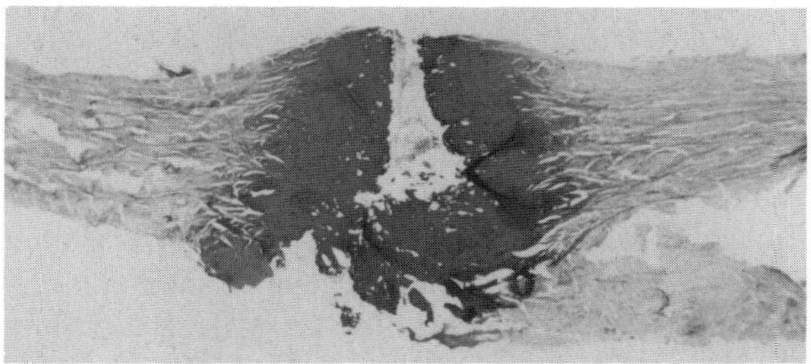

Figure 27-4A Rapid superpulse scleral incision showing parallel walls and relatively little coagulation necrosis (4×).

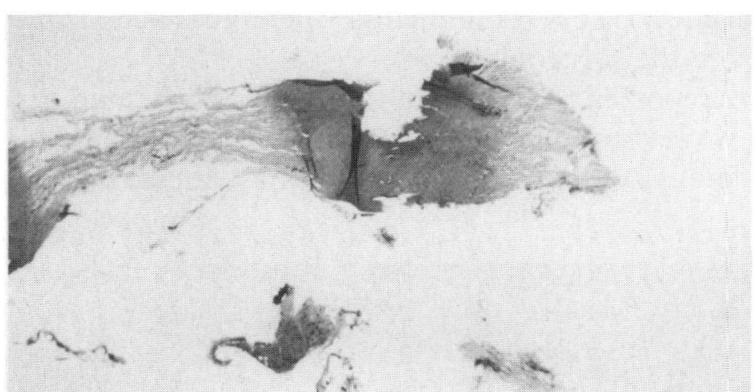

Figure 27-4B Continuous wave scleral incision showing less parallel cut and wider area of coagulation necrosis (4×).

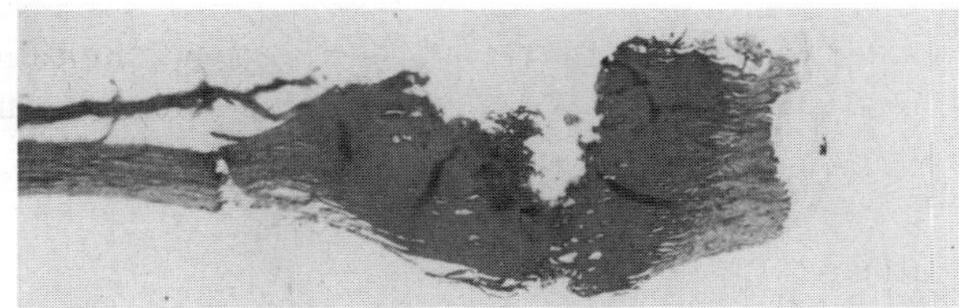

Figure 27-4C Electrodiathermy incision showing least parallel cut and widest area of coagulation necrosis (4×).

Cornea

Peyman[26] and we have reported on the use of CW CO_2 laser energy in an attempt to change the refractive power of rabbit corneas. Although immediate high changes in refractive power can be induced, due probably to shrinkage of corneal collagen, the memory of the cornea causes a resumption of the original refractive power within a month in almost all cases. It might be that, as finer spot sizes are available, a computerized CO_2 laser keratotomy would be a possible method of changing refractive error but, at the present time, this remains a program with many problems to be solved.

Treatment of Lesions of the Lid and the Paraocular Skin

One should generally think of using the laser to improve on those techniques in which one might consider using electrocautery or cryotherapy. Since the laser beam is convergent, a smaller necrotic zone is created than is created by the spreading type of tissue injury caused by either the electrocautery or cryotherapy. One can, therefore, create a hemostatic incision or ablation with the extent of the lesion easily visualized and, therefore, easily regulated. The tissue being treated is under direct observation through the microscope, and no instrument obscures the tissue from the surgeon's view.

We have reported on the use of the laser in both rapid superpulse and continuous wave modes in the treatment of such lesions as papillomas, verrucae, hemangiomas, basal cell carcinomas, and basal cell papillomas.

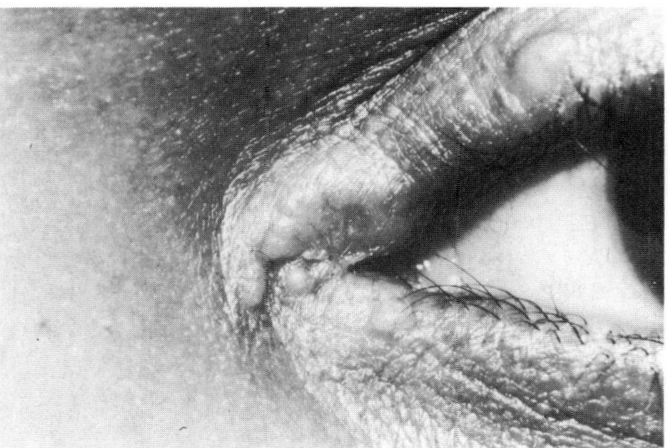

Figure 27-5A Papillomata involving lids and medial canthus.

We found that CW energy resulted in a faster removal of tissue, but that charring and puckering was increased as compared with the rapid superpulsed laser with which a finer, more controlled cutting could be performed. Figures 27-5A, 27-5B, and 27-5C show the laser's ability to ablate papillomata microsurgically at the inner canthus, while sparing important structures such as the lacrimal puncta, which are in close contact with the lesions. Healing was excellent and, interestingly enough, patients did not report as much local pain postoperatively as would be reported with either scalpel surgery or the electrocautery. A Ziegler-type procedure for minimal ectropion was successfully performed under topical anesthesia. This utilized the tissue-puckering effect of continuous wave CO_2 laser emission to shrink the inner conjunctival surface of the lower lid, thus pulling the lid closer to the globe.

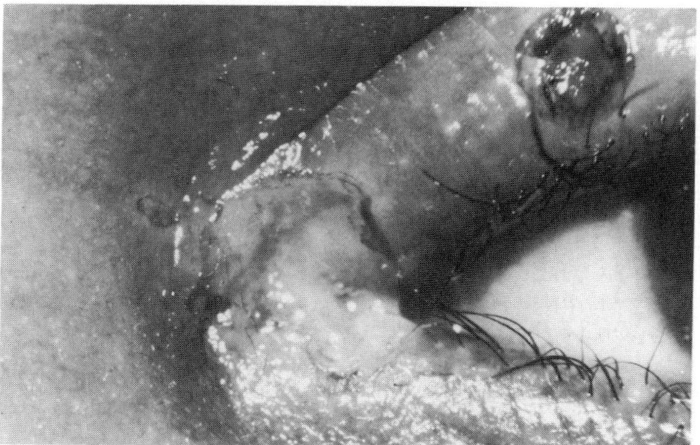

Figure 27-5B Immediately postoperative RSP CO_2 laser ablation of papillomata.

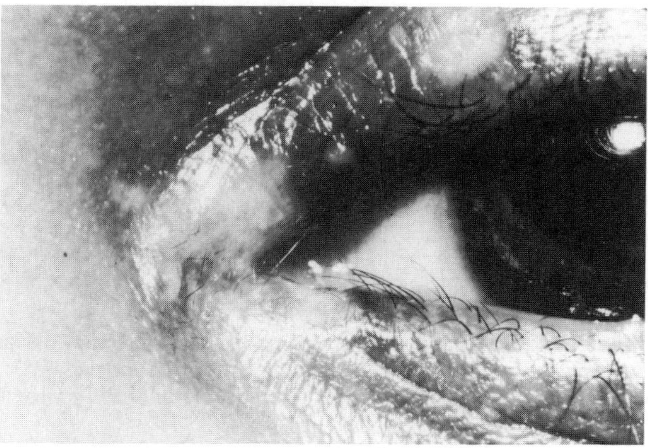

Figure 27-5C One week postoperatively, showing healing of lesions. Vitiliginous appearance in deeply pigmented skin disappeared in one month.

SUMMARY

Although the use of lasers in photocoagulation has been commonplace in ophthalmology for many years, techniques involving the use of lasers as an extraocular and intraocular surgical tool are just beginning to gain clinical favor. Experience with the CO_2 laser has lagged far behind, primarily because the high-powered, large-spot-sized lasers developed for such specialties as gynecology and otolaryngology were not suitable for ophthalmic microsurgery. As newer instrumentation becomes available, it is believed this technology will yield many applications for ophthalmic surgery.

REFERENCES

1. Meyer-Schwickerath G: Lichtkoagulation: eine Methode zur Behandlung und Verhutung der Netzhautablosung. *Albrecht v. Graefe Arch Ophthalmol* 156:2, 1954.

2. Meyer-Schwickerath G: *Lichtkoagulation.* Stuttgardt, Enke-Verlag, 1959.

3. Meyer-Schwickerath G: Erfahrungen mit der Lichtkoagulation der Metzhaut und der Iris. *Doc Ophthalmol* 10:91, 1956.

4. Zweng HC, Flock M, Kapany NS, et al: Experimental laser photocoagulation. *Am J Ophthalmol* 58:353, 1964.

5. Zweng HC, Paris GL, Vassiliadis A, et al: Laser photocoagulation of the iris. *Arch Ophthalmol* 84:193–199, 1970.

6. Beetham WP, Aiello LM, Balodimus MC, et al: Ruby laser photocoagulation of early diabetic neovascular retinopathy: Preliminary report of long term controlled study. *Trans Am Ophthalmol Soc* 67:39–67, 1969.

7. Campbell CJ, Rittler MC, Koester CJ: Laser photocoagulation of the retina. *Trans Am Acad Ophthalmol Otolaryngol* 70:939–943, 1966.

8. Beckman H, Barraco R, Sugar HS, et al: Laser iridectomies. *Am J Ophthalmol* 72:393–402, 1971.

9. Perkins ES: Laser iridotomy for secondary glaucoma. *Trans Ophthalmol Soc UK* 91:777–779, 1971.

10. Beckman H: Transscleral ruby laser irradiation of the ciliary body in the treatment of intractable glaucoma. *Trans Am Acad Ophthalmol Otolaryngol* 76:423–437, 1972.

11. Krasnov MM: Laseropuncture of anterior chamber angle in glaucoma. *Am J Ophthalmol* 75:674–678, 1973.

12. L'Esperance FA: An ophthalmic argon laser photocoagulation system: Design, construction, and laboratory investigations. *Trans Am Ophthalmol Soc* 6:870, 1968.

13. L'Esperance FA: The treatment of ophthalmic vascular disease by argon laser photocoagulation. *Trans Am Acad Ophthalmol Otolaryngol* 73:1077, 1969.

14. Abraham RK, Miller GL: Letter to editor. *Ann Ophthalmol* May 1973, p 613.

15. Worthen DM: Argon laser trabeculotomy. *Trans Am Acad Ophthalmol Otolaryngol* 78:371, 1974.

16. Fine BS, Peacock GR, Geeraets WJ, et al: Preliminary observations on ocular effects of high power continuous CO_2 laser irradiation. *Am J Ophthalmol* 64:209, 1967.

17. Fine BS, Fine FL, MacKeen D: Corneal injury threshold to carbon dioxide laser irradiation. *Am J Ophthalmol* 66:1, 1968.

18. Campbell CJ, Rittler MC, Bredemeier H, et al: Ocular effects produced by experimental lasers: II. Carbon dioxide laser. *Am J Ophthalmol* 66:604, 1968.

19. Beckman H, Rota A, Barraco R, et al: Limbectomies, keratectomies, and keratostomies performed with a rapid-pulsed carbon dioxide laser. *Am J Ophthalmol* 71:1277–1283, 1971.

20. Hill AE: Multijoule pulses from CO_2 lasers. *Applied Physics Letter* 12:9, 1968.

21. Ticho U, Monselize M, Levene S, et al: Carbon dioxide laser filtering surgery in hemorrhagic glaucoma. *Glaucoma* 1:114, 1979.

22. Beckman H, Fuller TA: Carbon dioxide laser scleral dissection and filtering procedure for glaucoma. *Am J Ophthalmol* 88:73–77, 1979.

23. Karlin DB, Patel CKN, Wood OR, et al: CO_2 laser in vitreoretinal surgery. *Ophthalmology* 290:86, 1979.

24. Miller JB, Smith M, Pinkus F, et al: Transvitreal carbon dioxide laser photocautery and vitrectomy. *Ophthalmology* 85:1195–1200, 1978.

25. Beckman H, Fuller TA, Boyman R, et al: Carbon dioxide laser surgery of eye and adnexa. *Ophthalmology* (in press).

26. Peyman GA, Larson B, Raichand M, et al: Modification of rabbit corneal curvature with use of carbon dioxide laser burns. *Ophthalmic Surg* 11:325–329, 1980.

28 General Surgery

R.C.J. Verschueren, MD
J. Oldhoff, MD

The CO_2 laser has been at the disposal of surgeons for more than ten years[1] and has been widely used in the past decade. For some indications the use of this laser has proved to be of no benefit. After the pioneering work of Goodale[2] the CO_2 laser was no longer used for the hemostasis of bleeding gastric ulcers. It was soon replaced by the argon and neodymium-YAG laser. Initially, it was thought the CO_2 laser might be the ideal hemostatic instrument for hepatic surgery, and the early reports about experimental work were promising.[3-5] Subsequent reports of major liver resections in patients are scarce and less enthusiastic.[6]

Early reports about the use of the CO_2 laser for the excision of burns suggested the superiority of this new modality,[7,8] but when the electrosurgical unit and the CO_2 laser were compared, the benefits of the latter were much less convincing.[9] Fidler[10] stated "there is a marked variation of results with adult patients with inconsistent advantages of the CO_2 laser over the electrosurgical thermal knife."

During the past decade, use of the CO_2 laser has been expanding greatly. CO_2 lasers are now being used as a substitute for the scalpel in a variety of procedures in the field of general surgery. A comprehensive review of all these applications can be found in the proceedings of the meetings of the International Society for Laser Surgery.[11,12] This chapter will critically review the benefits of the CO_2 laser in those procedures that were carried out in a satisfactory and safe way with conventional instruments before the advent of the laser. Up-to-date knowledge was obtained during the last meeting of the International Society for Laser Surgery (Graz, Austria, 1979) and by means of a questionnaire sent to surgeons using the CO_2 laser in general surgery. Before discussing the potential advantages and drawbacks of the CO_2 laser, a short review of the interaction between the CO_2 laser beam and the tissues is necessary.

EFFECT OF THE CO_2 LASER BEAM ON TISSUES

When the focused beam of the CO_2 laser impinges on the tissue surface, vaporization in the focal point creates a crater. Moving the focal spot in a linear fashion creates an incision. The depth of the incision is inversely proportional to the speed of this movement, and increases when a higher energy output is used. As soon as the integrity of the tissue surface has been interrupted, the elasticity of the tissue pulls the edges apart and thus creates an incision. During tissue vaporization the thermostatic effect of boiling water keeps the temperature at the edges at about 100° C.[13] The heating of the edges of the incision has a hemostatic effect, but also creates thermal necrosis of the tissues. This thermal tissue damage has been studied in detail in our laboratory by means of enzyme-histochemical methods.[14] The penetration of the thermal damage into the edges of the incision was found to be determined by the time the fraction of the incision had been exposed to the vaporizing beam.

While incising tissues, the focused CO_2 laser beam seals minor blood vessels in its path. The larger vessels are not thermally sealed by the tissue-vaporizing, focused beam and must be coagulated separately. For this purpose, the distance between the focusing lens and the tissue is increased, thus defocusing the beam. The energy density in the spot of the defocused beam is not strong enough for tissue vaporization to take place, and the exposed tissues slowly become dehydrated and even carbonized. The shrinking effect of this dehydration closes the vessel to be coagulated. Exposing the tissue surrounding a bleeding vessel to the defocused laser beam causes considerable thermal damage since the thermostatic effect of boiling water stops being effective as soon as the tissue has been dehydrated. The temperature can rise as high as 300° C, the point required for tissue combustion and carbonization to take place. The high temperature at the surface is responsible for deep penetration of the conducted heat and, hence, a thicker layer of necrotic tissue. The presence of this necrotic tissue after laser surgery is known to be responsible for slower healing[15] and to increase the hazard of postoperative infection.[16]

ADVANTAGES OF THE CO_2 LASER IN GENERAL SURGERY

The early prototypes manufactured by the American Optical Corporation were reliable machines, but had a very bulky manipulator arm which made them less suitable as surgical instruments. With the advent of Sharplan in 1973,[17] general surgeons had a surgical CO_2 laser with a maneuverability that made it acceptable as a surgical instrument. Soon, the CO_2 laser was used all over the world for a variety of surgical procedures, and manufacturers developed various models. The advocates of this new instrument claimed a variety of advantages.

A critical review of this is necessary to determine to what extent these claims justify the use of these expensive instruments and if they outweigh the drawbacks that are not always cited.

Bacteriostatic Action

It has been claimed repeatedly that the heat generated by the laser beam sterilizes the wound edges and thus allows surgery to be carried out in heavily contaminated tissues such as decubitus ulcers.[18] This claim is no more than an oversimplification of the pathophysiology of infections and the factors determining the healing of wounds. The surgical treatment of decubitus ulcers consists of the removal of all necrotic and infected tissues, and covering the resulting defect with a rotation flap or a free skin graft. Healing is not determined by the instrument used for the excision of the necrotic area, but by factors such as the extent of the excision, viability of the resulting defect, vascular supply of the skin flap and, most importantly, the metabolic condition of the patient. We are convinced that the results published by Stellar[18] can be duplicated by using the electrocautery or the scalpel. The use of the CO_2 laser may offer a slight benefit in that it vaporizes fragments of necrotic bone and ligaments in the depth of the ulcers. Using the CO_2 laser for debridement of the necrotic bone has the disadvantage that the extent of the procedure is difficult to control. Using a chisel or bone forceps to carry out this debridement, the appearance of healthy viable bone can be visually assessed. When using the laser to vaporize this necrotic material, the edges of the defect are more or less carbonized and, as a result, the viability of the tissue may be difficult to assess.

Hemostatic Action

The incision made by the CO_2 laser is indeed relatively bloodless and, therefore, thoughts were initially entertained that the laser would be the hemostatic light knife of the future. However, the hemostatic effect of the cutting beam of the CO_2 laser is rather limited. Once a vessel with an internal diameter exceeding about 1 mm is transected, hemorrhage will result, and the defocused beam is required to stop bleeding. Several years ago, the CO_2 laser was used in our institution to carry out translobar resection of the liver in mongrel dogs. As soon as the liver surface was incised, blood started oozing from the parenchyma and completely absorbed the laser beam, thus reducing the cutting efficiency to zero. Once the liver was incised, blood started oozing from the incision, making further cutting impossible since the incident laser light was absorbed by the layer of blood. This blood soon started to boil and formed a coagulum, shielding the underlying tissue from the laser beam. Obtaining hemostasis by means of the defocused beam was difficult in this situation. The coagulum covered the oozing vessels and precluded any attempt to seal them by coagulation.[14] A surgical team in Australia used a CO_2 laser for wedge excision from the liver and for one partial hepatectomy. On these occasions, the laser was slow to cut and the authors were not convinced that there was any less bleeding from the liver.[6]

When performing orthopedic surgery in hemophiliacs, a group in Israel saw a distinct advantage in using the CO_2 laser for incision of the soft tissues. The diffuse oozing was drastically reduced and the amount of clotting factors required for the normalization of the coagulation was considerably less than during conventional surgery.[19] These results were recently confirmed by others.[20]

The CO_2 laser is a hemostatic instrument but there is no proof yet that it is any better than an electrosurgical unit as far as general surgery is concerned.

Limitation of Tumor Spread During Surgery

Sealing blood vessels and lymphatics on its pathway, the CO_2 laser is believed to decrease operative hematogenic and lymphatic tumor spread. Frishman[21] reported a reduction in the mortality and occurrence of pulmonary metastases after excising a subcutaneous fibrosarcoma with the CO_2 laser. Unfortunately, his results were biased by not randomizing the animals after tumor implantation.

The influence of the CO_2 laser on operative tumor spread was carefully investigated in our laboratory. The model was the Cloudman S_{91} melanoma in mice. Factors such as local recurrence rate, pulmonary metastases, and lymphatic spread were studied, but no oncological benefits could be credited to the CO_2 laser. Fortunately, no detrimental effects could be detected, and Oosterhuis[22,23] concluded that the use of this modality in cancer surgery is permissible, but indicated only when it offers technical advantages.

Belief in the oncological benefits of the CO_2 laser for the excision of malignant tumors is the personal responsibility of the individual surgeon. This belief, however, is dangerous when it leads to less extensive resection, assuming that the use of the CO_2 laser justifies smaller margins. Until now, no clinical series proving the oncological benefits of the CO_2 laser has been reported.

Decreased Postoperative Pain

Pain is a subjective interpretation of a somatic perception and, therefore, very difficult to quantify. Moreover, since pain is subjective, investigation into postoperative discomfort can easily be biased. Many surgeons are very enthusiastic about the lack of postoperative pain when the CO_2 laser is used for mastectomy, an abdominoperineal resection, or a partial glossectomy.[24]

For some surgeons the decreased pain is the main motivation for using the laser.[25] If there is less pain after surgery with the CO_2 laser, we consider this only important enough when it outweighs the drawbacks.

CO_2 Laser Microsurgery

Inspired by the pioneer work of Strong and Jako[26] we started using the CO_2 laser in conjunction with a micromanipulator and an operating microscope for surgery in the rectum. Several rectal cancers and sessile polyps were vaporized by means of the laser beam. Healing was prompt and no complications were seen.[14]

Recently, we started using the same technic for the eradication of leukoplacia of the oral mucosa. In the vast majority of the patients the surgery is done on an outpatient basis and under local anesthesia. Recurrences were not seen; healing was prompt without functional impairment. For the oral mucosa, the CO_2 laser enables us to obtain results that cannot be obtained with other modalities.

DISADVANTAGES OF THE CO_2 LASER IN GENERAL SURGERY

Thermal Damage in the Edges of a CO_2 Laser Incision

Because the CO_2 laser is a thermal instrument, a certain degree of devitalization of tissue in the edges of the incision must be expected. The factors determining the extent of this thermal damage were elaborately investigated in our laboratory.[14] This layer of necrotic tissue, although very thin, will delay healing and increase susceptibility to infection.

Madden[16] investigated the resistance to infection of surgical wounds produced by a scalpel, the electrosurgical unit, and the CO_2 laser. Incisions were made in the paravertebral area of the back of albino guinea pigs. These incisions were inoculated with a strain of *Staphylococcus aureus.* All wounds made with the CO_2 laser or the electrocautery developed purulent discharge, whereas only 30% of the wounds made with the scalpel exhibited gross infection. In other animals, incisions were made with the three instruments, but were not contaminated. In the wounds made with the scalpel, the advancing sheets of epithelium bridged the wound after 24 hours, and collagen fibers were evident on the sixth day. In the wounds made with the electrocautery, epithelial bridging was not even seen on the sixth day, and collagen formation was absent. Advocates of the use of the CO_2 laser disagree with these results because the CO_2 laser used by Madden, unlike newer machines, was a multimode laser.[27] In the single mode lasers, the spatial distribution of the energy at the focal spot is more efficient and might cause less thermal damage in the edges of the incision.

Hall, investigating the healing of skin and fascia incised with the CO_2 laser, found similar delays.[13] The delay in healing of wounds made by thermal instruments like the CO_2 laser was again confirmed three years later.[28]

The reports of clinical work with the CO_2 laser only briefly mention the consequences of the thermal damage, to the extent that one might believe that the CO_2 laser is the magic instrument of the future and that "the advantages in many procedures make it almost indispensable."[29] McCarthy[30] reported transient erythema surrounding laser incisions and "excessive amounts of tissue fluid secreted by laser excised areas."

Because of our concern about thermal damage and the lack of convincing benefits, we do not advocate the use of the CO_2 laser as a substitute for the scalpel.

Lack of Maneuverability and Technical Problems

In the design of recent CO_2 lasers, attention has been given to the required versatility of the instrument. The manipulator arms, nevertheless, still have a degree of awkwardness likely to prolong the operation. Because the articulated manipulator arm is suspended over the operating site, it is in constant competition with the overhead lights, making frequent light adjustments an almost invariable feature of the use of the laser.[5]

In addition, the surgeon is burdened by the need to preserve sterility by adequately draping the manipulator arm and to evacuate the smoke arising during the procedure.

Operating theaters are unfriendly environments for delicate instruments, and the slender manipulator arm is likely to be damaged in the hands of attendants who move the laser apparatus from one place to another. Loss of alignment of the mirrors and loss of coaxiality of the beam will be the consequence. A minor alignment problem may be enough to disturb the focus, and the confused surgeon will burn the tissues instead of incising them.

Lack of Mechanical Contact with the Tissues

When using the CO_2 laser as a light knife, the focus of the beam projects beyond the tip of the handpiece. The surgeon has good visual control of what the laser beam is actually doing but, being deprived of mechanical contact with the tissues, he cannot foresee what will happen the next second. This lack of tactile feedback makes it difficult to stay in the correct anatomical plane, and makes surgery with the CO_2 laser in the vicinity of major vessels and nerves hazardous. Some surgeons use the CO_2 laser as a cutting instrument in the vicinity of the vessels during axillary or groin dissection. Others use the CO_2 laser for amputation of the breast, but switch to conventional surgery for the dissection of the lymph nodes in the axilla.[31–33] White[31] carried out mastectomies with the laser and concluded that "clearing the axillary vein in a Patey or radical mastectomy was somewhat hazardous and slow." After using the CO_2 laser for a perineal dissection, White[31] saw no complications and healing was prompt, but there was no technical advantage in using the laser.

When using the CO_2 laser to dissect flaps, it may be difficult to stay in the correct anatomical plane. A report about an accidental laser incision of a skin flap during subcutaneous mastectomy has been published. Aronoff[29] also had problems with skin flaps: "On turning the skin flap, one must be careful not to make the flap too thin, for the effect of the laser spreads out slightly as one is undercutting skin and one can lose flaps." Sound reasons are needed to justify the exposure of patients to this increased hazard of the CO_2 laser.

SUMMARY

The CO_2 laser has been used in clinical surgery for about ten years. For some of the applications that were promising initially, such as excision of burns and hepatic surgery, enthusiasm is fading. For cancer operations and surgery of the soft tissues, enthusiasm is still present, and belief in the alleged benefits is strong. However, the advantages claimed for the use of the CO_2 laser in general surgery as a light knife have not been substantiated to date. Prospective randomized clinical trials will be needed to show if patients actually benefit from laser surgery.

Used in conjunction with an operating microscope and a micromanipulator, the CO_2 laser beam can be used in confined spaces and considerably increases the possibilities of local therapy.

REFERENCES

1. Polanyi TG, Bredemeier HC, Davis TW Jr: A CO_2 laser for surgical research. *Med Biol Eng* 8:541–548, 1970.
2. Goodale RL, Okada A, Gonzalez R, et al: Rapid endoscopic control of bleeding gastric erosions by laser radiation. *Arch Surg* 101:211–214, 1970.
3. Hall RR, Beach AD, Hill DW: Partial hepatectomy using a carbon dioxide laser. *Br J Surg* 60:141–144, 1973.
4. Fidler JP, Hoefer RW, Polanyi TG, et al: Laser surgery in exsanguinating liver injury. *Surg Forum* 23:350–352, 1972.
5. Fidler JP, Hoefer RW, Polanyi TG, et al: Laser surgery in exsanguinating liver injury. *Ann Surg* 181:74–80, 1975.
6. Stephens FO, Jones PH: Laser surgery. *Med J Aust* 2:589–590, 1970.
7. Stellar S, Levine M, Ger R, et al: Excision of acute third degree burns followed by immediate autograft replacement: An experimental study in the pig. *J Trauma* 13:45–53, 1973.
8. Levine M, Ger R, Stellar S, et al: Use of the carbon dioxide laser for the debridement of third degree burns. *Ann Surg* 179:246–252, 1974.
9. Levine MS, Salisbury RE, Peterson HD, et al: Clinical evaluation of the carbon dioxide laser for burn wound excisions: A comparison of the laser, scalpel and electrocautery. *J Trauma* 15:800–807, 1975.
10. Fidler JP, Law E, MacMillan BG: Comparison of carbon dioxide laser excision of burns with other thermal knives. *Ann NY Acad Sci* 267:254–262, 1976.
11. Kaplan I: *Proceedings of the 1st International Symposium on Laser Surgery*. Jerusalem, Jerusalem Academic Press, 1976.
12. Kaplan I: *Proceedings of the 2nd International Symposium on Laser Surgery*. Jerusalem, Jerusalem Academic Press, 1978.
13. Hall RR, Beach AD, Baker E, et al: Incision of tissue by carbon dioxide laser. *Nature* 232:131–132, 1971.
14. Verschueren RCJ: *The CO_2 Laser in Tumor Surgery*. Assen, Van Gorcum, 1976.
15. Hall RR: The healing of tissues incised by a carbon dioxide laser. *Br J Surg* 58:222–225, 1971.
16. Madden JE, Edlich RF, Custer JR, et al: Studies in the management of contaminated wound: IV. Resistance to infection of surgical wounds made by knife, electrosurgery, and laser. *Am J Surg* 119:222–224, 1970.
17. Kaplan I, Ger R, Sharon U: The carbon dioxide laser in plastic surgery. *Br J Plast Surg* 26:359–362, 1973.
18. Stellar S, Meijer R, Walia S, et al: Carbon dioxide laser debridement of decubitus ulcers: Followed by immediate rotation flap or skingraft closure. *Ann Surg* 179:230–237, 1974.

19. Horoszowski H, Farine I, Engel J: The laser in orthopaedic surgery, in Kaplan I (ed): *Proceedings of the 1st International Symposium on Laser Surgery.* Jerusalem, Jerusalem Academic Press, 1976, pp 139–144.

20. Morscher E, Rittmann WW, Marbet GA, et al: Die Anwendung von Laserstrahlen bei Operationen an Hämophilen. *Therapeut Umschau* 36:316–321, 1979.

21. Frishman A, Gassner S, Kaplan I, et al: Excision of subcutaneous fibrosarcoma in mice. *Isr J Med Sci* 10:637–641, 1974.

22. Oosterhuis JW, Verschueren RCJ, Oldhoff J: Experimental surgery on the Cloudman S91 melanoma with the carbon-dioxide laser. *Acta Chir Belg* 74:422–429, 1975.

23. Oosterhuis JW: *Tumor Surgery with the CO_2 Laser: Studies with the Cloudman S91 mouse melanoma.* PhD Thesis—State University, Groningen, The Netherlands, 1977.

24. Carruth JAS: Personal communication, 1979.

25. Kott I: Personal communication, 1980.

26. Strong MS, Jako GJ, Polanyi TG, et al: Laser surgery in the aerodigestive tract. *Am J Surg* 126:529–533, 1973.

27. Slutzki S, Shafiri R, Bornstein LA: Use of the carbon dioxide laser for large excision with minimal bloodloss. *Plast Reconstr Surg* 60:250–255, 1977.

28. Hishimoto K, Rockwell RJ Jr, Epstein RA, et al: Laser wound healing compared with other surgical modalities. *Burns* 1:13–22, 1974.

29. Aronoff BL: CO_2 laser in surgical oncology. *Int Adv Surg Oncol* 1:243–263, 1979.

30. McCarthy WH, Shaw HM, Jones PH: Laser surgery for malignant melanoma and superficial malignancies. *Aust NZ J Surg* 48:656–661, 1978.

31. White H: Personal communication, 1980.

32. Aronoff BL: Personal communication, 1979.

33. McCarthy WH: Personal communication, 1970.

INDEX